IMMEDIATE COLPOSCOPY

Vulvoscopy and Anoscopy

Giovanni Miniello

IMMEDIATE COLPOSCOPY
Vulvoscopy and Anoscopy

edra

Publishing Manager: Arianna Ribichesu

Paper, Print and Binding Manager: Michele Ribatti

Illustrations: Giovanni Miniello

ISBN 978-88-214-5512-4
eISBN 978-88-214-5513-1

Edra S.p.A.
Via G. Spadolini, 7
20141 Milano
Tel. 02 881841
www.edizioniedra.it

Printed in Italy in May 2021 by "Printer Trento S.r.l.", Trento

(*) Edra S.p.A. is part of LSWR GROUP

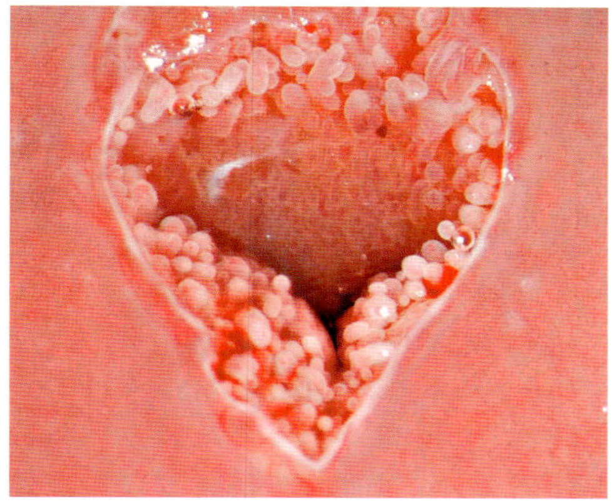

At the bottom of everything,
there is always a heart.
Just look for it.

g.m.

CONTENTS

INTRODUCTION

Colposcopy concerns the study of surface epithelium at the cervix, vagina and vulva along with the underlying stromal connective tissue and its vascular network, to help locate changed or abnormal cells.
This procedure is not only a useful diagnostic tool for evaluating women who have had abnormal PAP smears and delineating the location, size and extent of the lesion for targeted biopsies and directed treatment, but must be considered as an extension of the routine gynecological checkup which deserves widespread use.
In this monograph, we have decided to avoid details regarding description of the colposcope, colposcopic terminology, procedures for colposcopic examination, techniques for cervical biopsy, treatment modalities for cervical intraepithelial neoplasia (CIN), suggestions for preventing errors in the colposcopic assessment of the cervix, the merits and demerits of colposcopy and so on, masterfully treated in other books, in order to give space to some diagrams and the many pictures concerning physiology of the cervix, vulvar and perianal lesions, cervico-vaginal infections, metaplastic changes, dysplastic conditions, cancer and rare colposcopic findings.
This monograph contains a full set of more than 500 colpophotographs, some correlated wet mount microphotographs and diagrammatic representations, along with detailed captions, providing a useful, quick or in-depth consultation for postgraduates, gynecologists, health professionals, pathologists, biologists as well as, novices and advanced colposcopists.
We hope that this monograph will be beneficial in meeting these goals.

Giovanni Miniello
Gynecologist
Visiting Professor of Colposcopy and Uro-Gynecologic Microscopy
International Consultant of Colposcopy for the United Nations

IMMEDIATE COLPOSCOPY

The colposcope allows the epithelial surface to be examined at a relatively low-power magnification which usually ranges from 4x to 40x. More recent instruments provide greater magnification but most colposcopic examinations can be accomplished within the magnification range of 6x to 15x.

It is convenient to have colposcope fitted with a green (or blue) filter (Figure 1) which filters out the red light in order to highlight the vascular pattern, by making the vessels darker. It is advisable to use the green or blue filter after applying normal saline solution and before the application of acetic acid. In fact, this solution may cause tissue swelling and consequent opacity, potentially obscuring important details of the vascular pattern which are closely related to histologic changes.

It is worth noting that no single colposcopic finding is pathognomonic of any one lesion.

Most times, no vascular pattern is observable on the original squamous epithelium.

The surface of the original cervical squamous epithelium is completely smooth and displays a translucent pinkish or reddish tinge (Figure 2). The external orifice of the uterus known as external os, through which the endocervical canal communicates with vagina, appears as a somewhat circular aperture. The external os is bounded by two lips, an anterior and a posterior lip, of which the anterior is usually the shorter and thicker, although, on account of the slope of the cervix, it projects lower than the posterior.

Sometimes, the external orifice can appear particularly stenotic (Figure 3). There may be an association

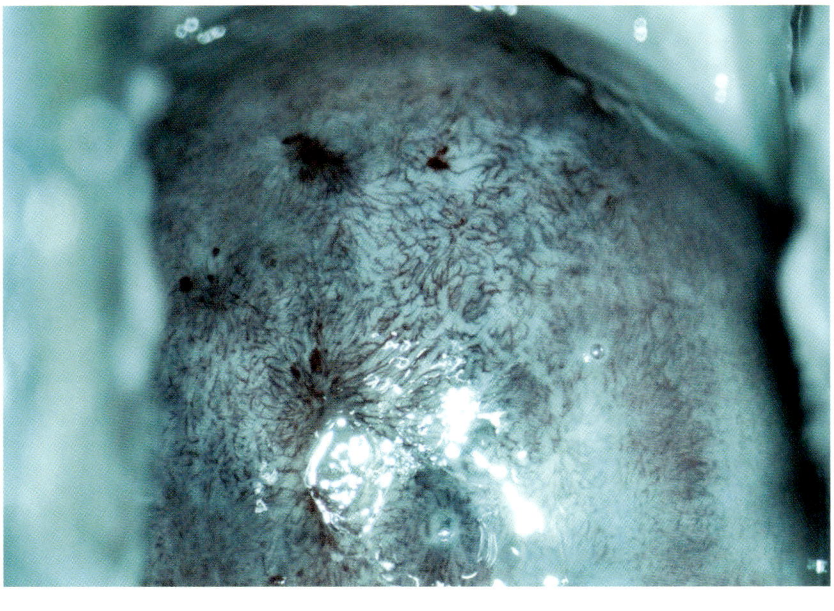

Figure 1 - Saline colposcopy view with the aid of a green filter. The green filter enhances visualization of blood vessels by making them appear darker in contrast to the surrounding epithelium.

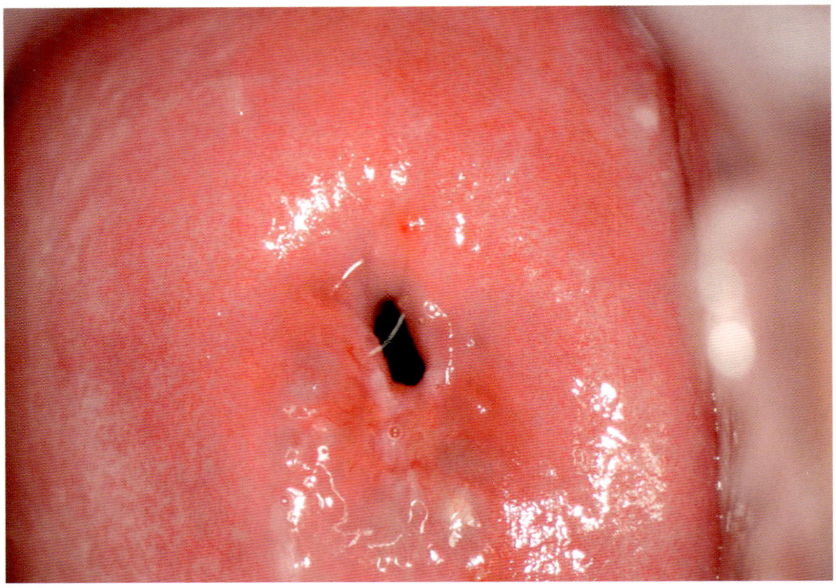

Figure 2 - A normal cervix displays a translucent pinkish or reddish tinge and a completely smooth epithelial lining.

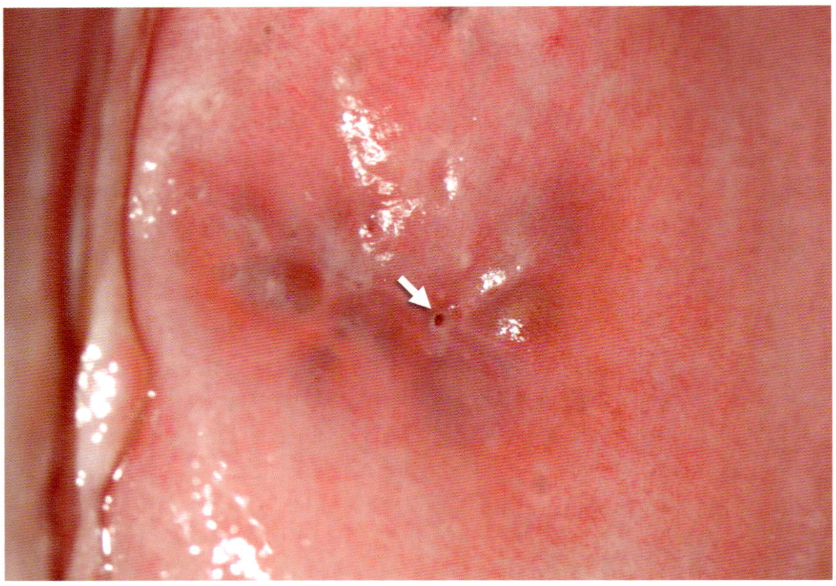

Figure 3 - Stenotic external os (arrow).

between external os cervical stenosis and endometriosis in women with pelvic pain. On the contrary, if the external os is particularly wide and the anterior lip is everted, the distal portion of the *arbor vitae* can be observed (Figure 4).

The mucous membrane of the endocervix is crossed by two longitudinal ridges, anterior and posterior, from which numerous secondary folds emerge out peripherally, creating a palm tree-like pattern, referred to as arbor vitae. The posterior longitudinal ridge of arbor vitae is less frequently observable (Figure 5). This arrangement increases the surface area of mucus secreting columnar cells. When the anterior longitudinal plica is hypertrophic (Figure 6), its distal portion visible at the external os may mimic an endocervical polyp. The broad anterior insertion to ectocervix can provide helpful diagnostic hints. There exist particular anatomical conditions that may limit the colposcopic inspection. In fact, a congenital stenosis of the proximal tract of vagina (Figure 7) or a stenosis due to fibrous bridles (Figure 8) limit the complete detection of the cervix. Furthermore, surgical outcomes following total hysterectomy, may hinder a complete investigation of the vaginal vault. In this case, the vaginal vault is frequently distorted with mucosal recesses at the 3 and 9 o'clock positions (Figure 9). These lateral indentations usually termed as "dog ears" must be inspected with Desjardin's or Kogan's forceps, and carefully scraped when PAP smear is carried out, because this can harbor granulation tissue (Figure 10) or even neoplasia (Figure 11).

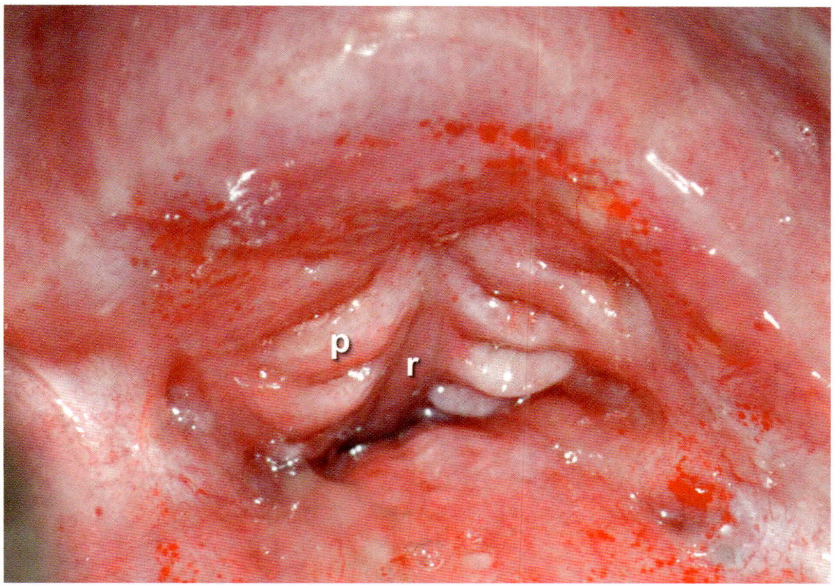

Figure 4 - Small oblique columns, the palmate folds (p), proceed from the anterior longitudinal ridge (r) of the endocervical canal. This structure gives the appearance of branches from the stem of a tree, called arbor vitae.

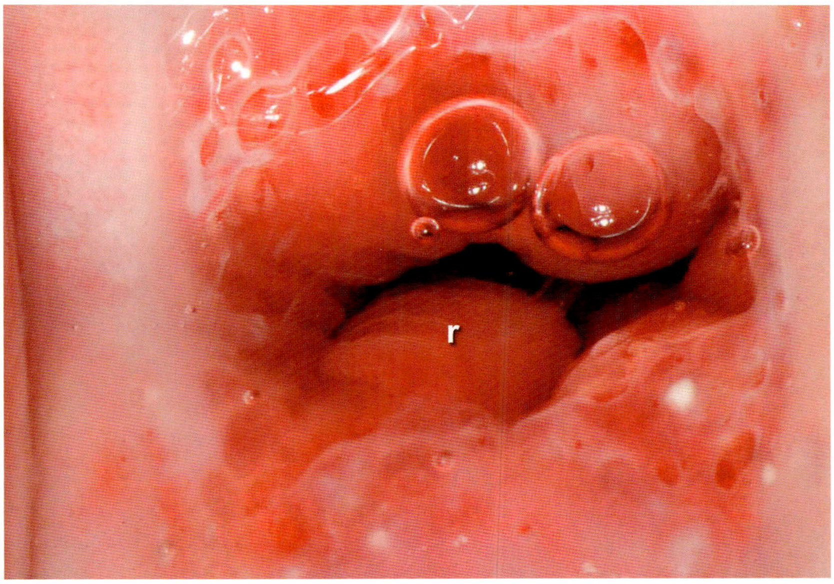

Figure 5 - Posterior ridge (r) of arbor vitae.

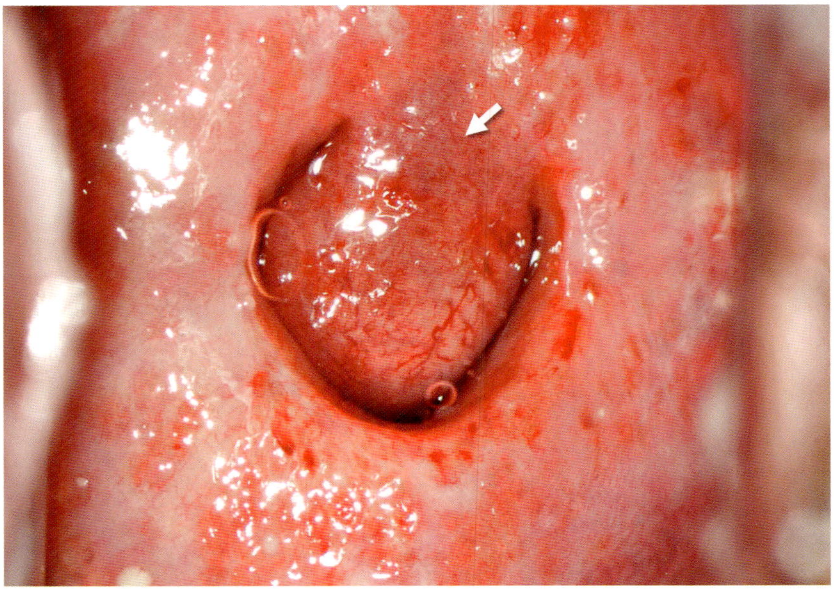

Figure 6 - The anterior stem of arbor vitae appears hypertrophic. The arrow indicates its broad anterior insertion to ectocervix.

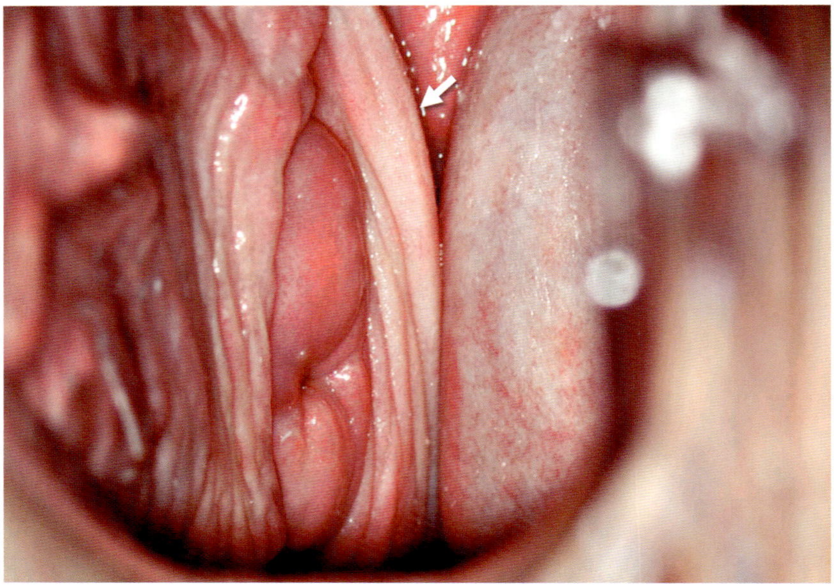

Figure 7 - Congenital stenosis of the proximal tract of vagina (arrow).

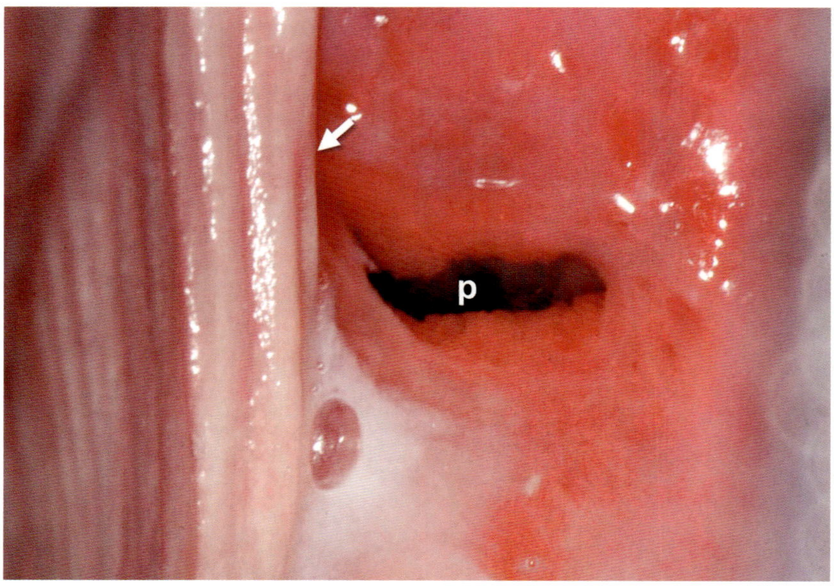

Figure 8 - A fibrous bridle (arrow) limits the complete detection of the cervix. Endocervical polyp (p).

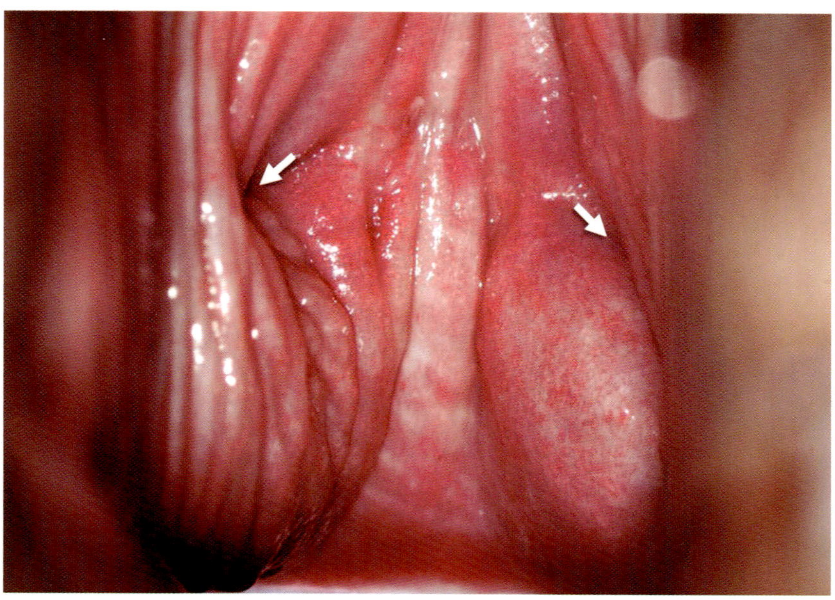

Figure 9 - Vaginal mucosal recesses at the 3 and 9 o'clock positions (arrows), usually termed as dog ears.

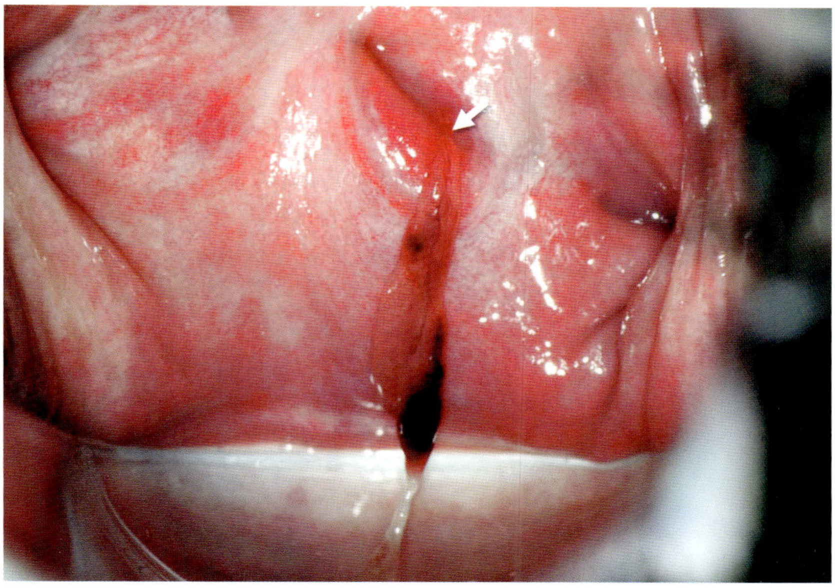

Figure 10 - Mucus mixed with blood comes out of the right vaginal recess (arrow). which hides granulation tissue following colporrhaphy.

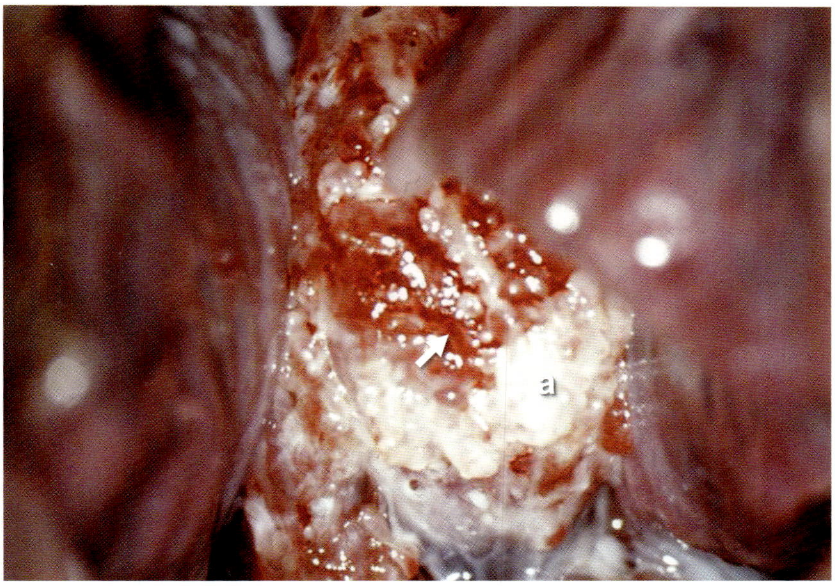

Figure 11 - The lateral vaginal recess, following hysterectomy, harbors an exophytic tissue with uneven surface, dense acetowhite area (a) and dilated atypical vessels (arrow). Excision biopsy and resultant pathology demonstrated squamous carcinoma.

Vaginal discharge is highly variable in quality and quantity among different individuals, both in physiological and pathological conditions, and even in the same individual during different periods of life. Noninfectious causes of vaginal discharge are quite rare (10% noninfectious as compared to 90% infectious causes).

In current practice, the characteristics of cervico-vaginal discharge usually direct towards a presumptive clinical diagnosis, so it may be useful to define the various types of vaginal fluid or cervical secretion frequently found in daily gynecological practice. It should be pointed out that cervico-vaginal infections may produce no discharge and that no particular discharge is pathognomonic for any infection.

During the advanced follicular phase, the mucus appears white and cloudy (Figure 12) and may feel gluey or stretchy in consistency. Immediately prior to ovulation, most women usually detect increased vaginal secretions that are slippery and may remind them of the consistency of raw egg whites. With the increasing estrogen stimulation, the endocervical mucus becomes clear and stretchy (Figure 13), and is not modified by acetic acid, which acts as an efficient mucolytic agent, so remaining limpid. An abundant and transparent cervical mucus facilitates exploration of the endocervix (Figure 14). Seminal fluid deposited in the vagina can have the same appearance as the preovulatory mucus (Figure 15). Direct microscopy can resolve doubts, by visualizing spermatozoa (Figure 16).

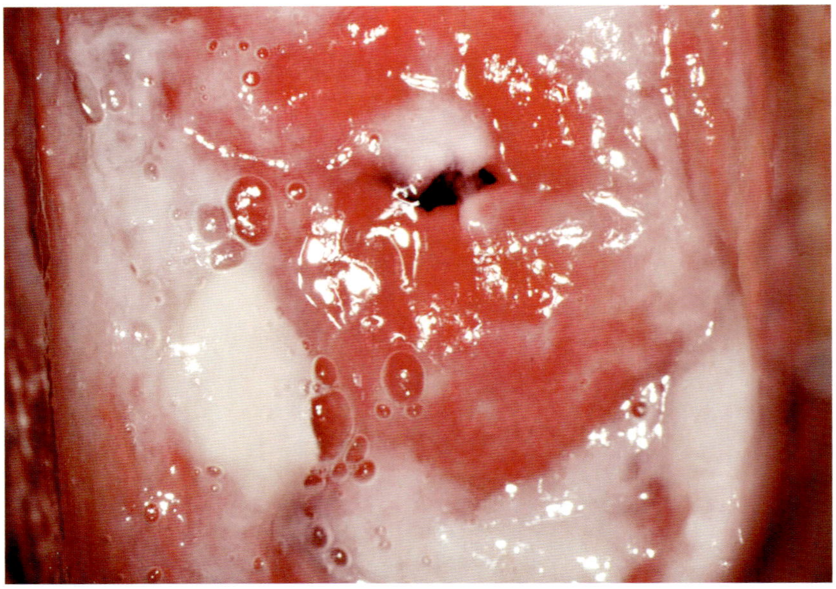

Figure 12 - Abundant white and cloudy mucus during advanced follicular phase.

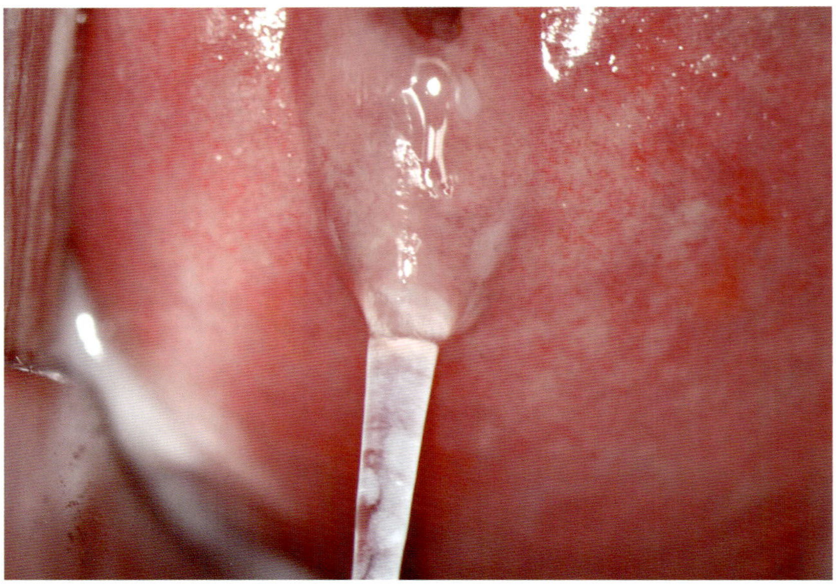

Figure 13 - The clear and stretchy mucus, induced by estrogen stimulation, is not modified by acetic acid and remains limpid.

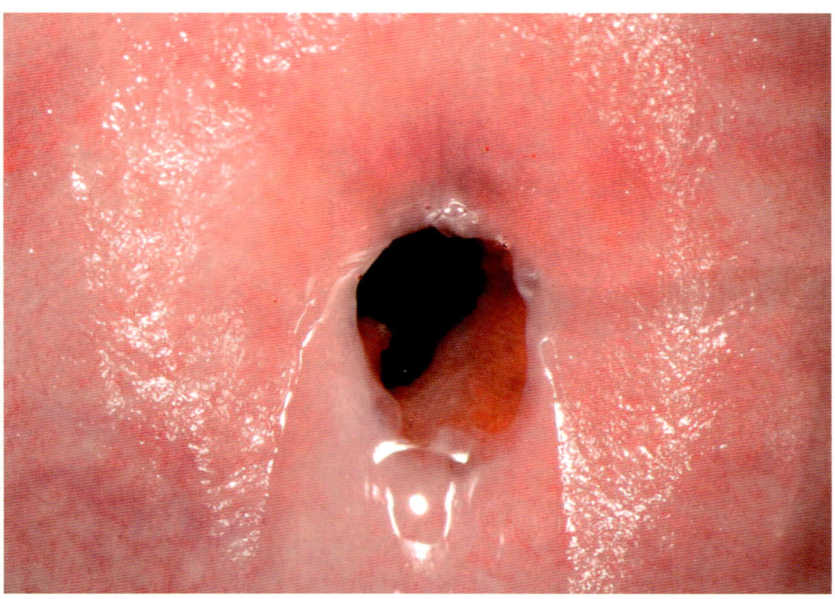

Figure 14 - The transparent cervical mucus facilitates exploration of the endocervix.

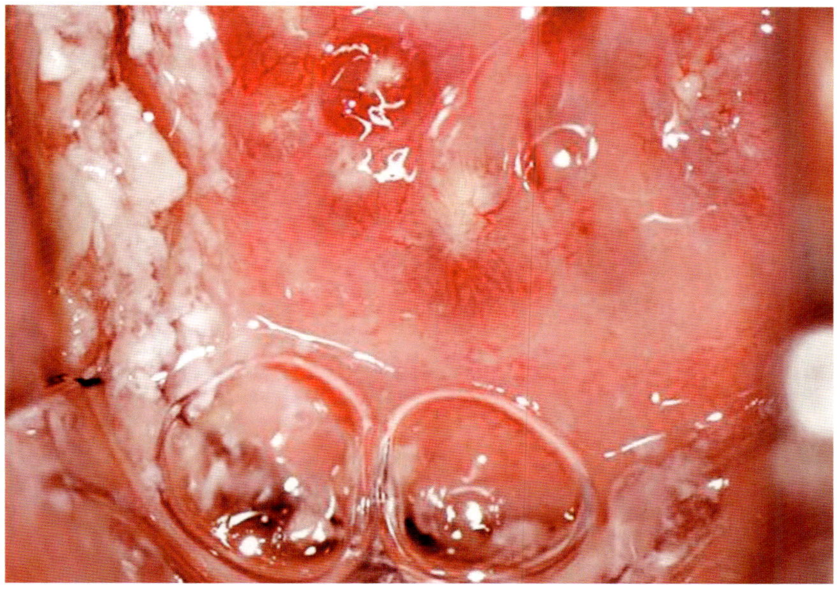

Figure 15 - Seminal fluid deposited in vagina may mimic preovulatory mucus.

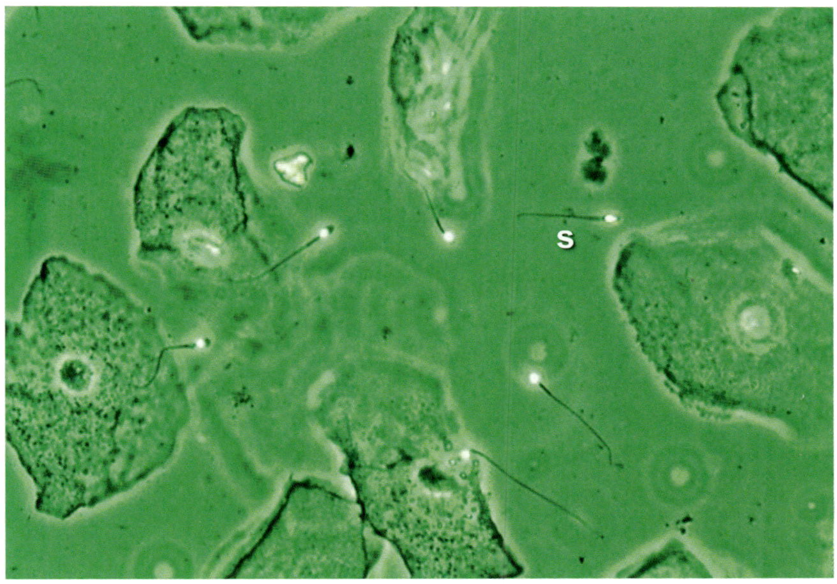

Figure 16 - Spermatozoa (s) are present in vagina.

After ovulation, there will be less discharge as it may turn thicker, cloudy, or gluey again (Figure 17). Opaque mucus may obscure the evaluation of the squamocolumnar junction; furthermore, the fine details of the endocervical canal may be clouded (Figure 18). In this case, an endocervical cytobrush may be gently twirled in the cervical canal, encouraging the viscous mucus to remain entrapped around the device. Alternatively, the thick mucus can be temporarily pushed into the cervical canal with an acetic acid-soaked cotton swab. A white, cloudy and gluey discharge is often associated with an exposed columnar epithelium (Figure 19).
Vaginal discharge may appear white creamy in normal conditions such as abundant cell discharge (Figure 20), accompanied with numerous Lactobacilli (Figure 21). Yeast infection too can produce a white and homogeneous creamy discharge, sometimes associated with erythematous macules or papules that involve both cervix and vaginal walls (Figure 22).
A homogeneous milky discharge may be observed in the presence of **bacterial vaginosis** (BV) (Figure 23). However, this infection which is the most common cause worldwide of vaginal discharge in women of childbearing age, accounting for 40 to 50 percent of cases, usually shows a malodorous white and frothy discharge (Figure 24). Microscopically BV which is often sub-clinical and remains asymptomatic in, at least, half of all cases, is characterized by adherence of pleomorphic bacteria on the so-called *clue cell* (Figure 25). A white and frothy discharge, undistinguishable from that produced by bacterial vaginosis,

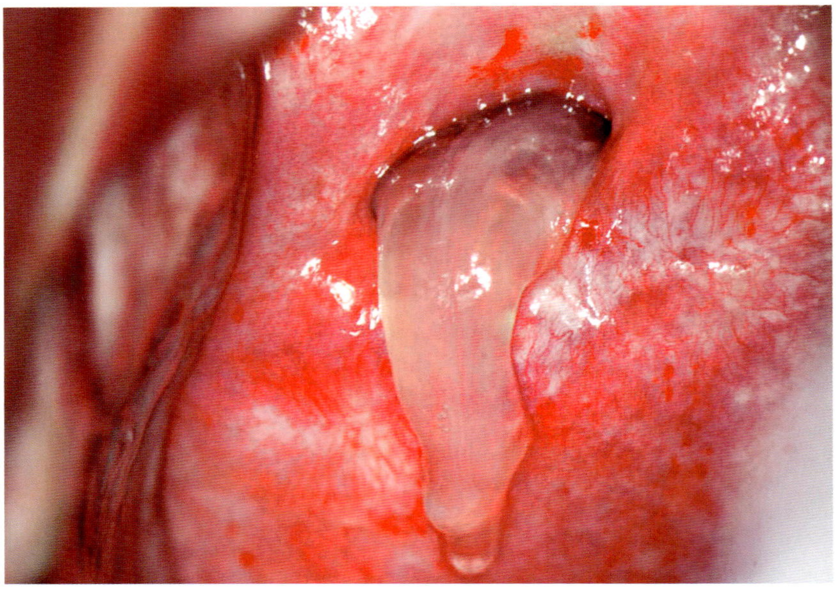

Figure 17 - Thick, cloudy and gluey cervical secretion after ovulation.

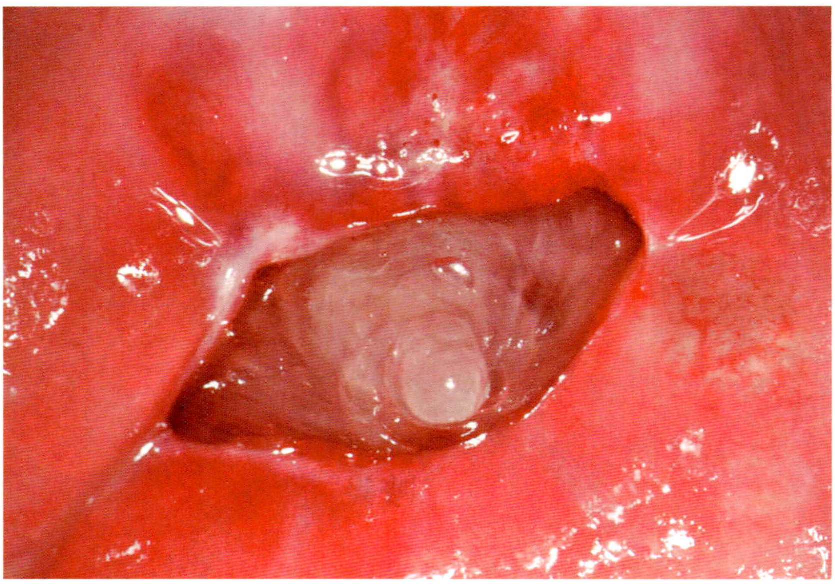

Figure 18 - Opaque mucus may obscure the evaluation of the squamocolumnar junction and the fine details of the endocervical canal.

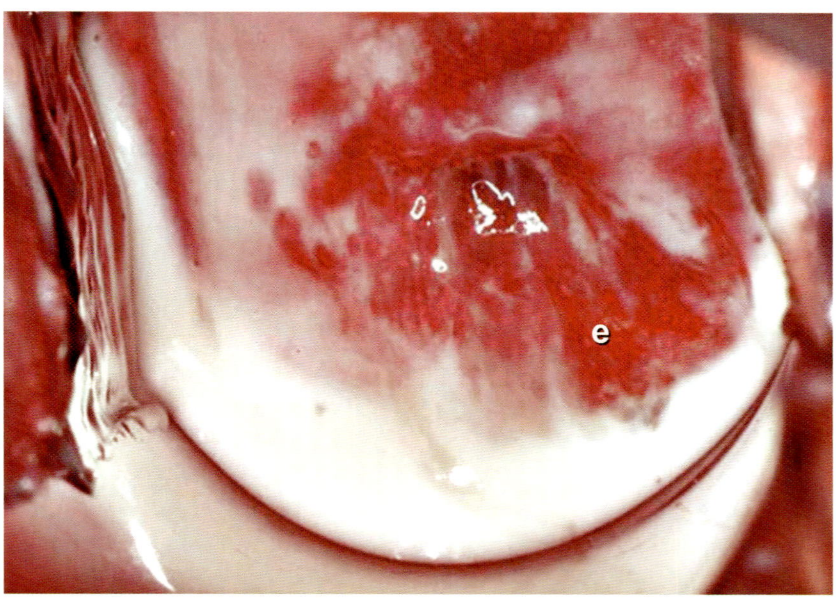

Figure 19 - White, cloudy and gluey discharge associated with an exposed columnar epithelium (e).

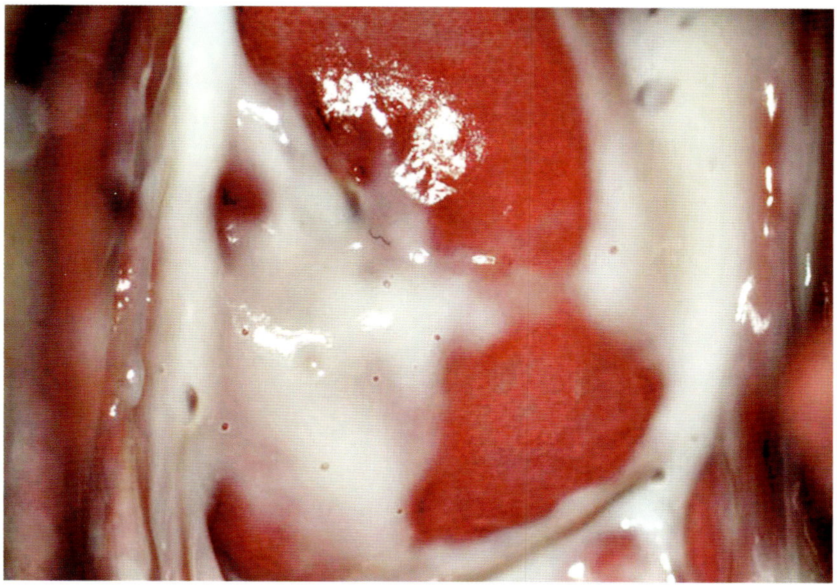

Figure 20 - In normal conditions, abundant cell discharge may be responsible for a white creamy and homogeneous discharge.

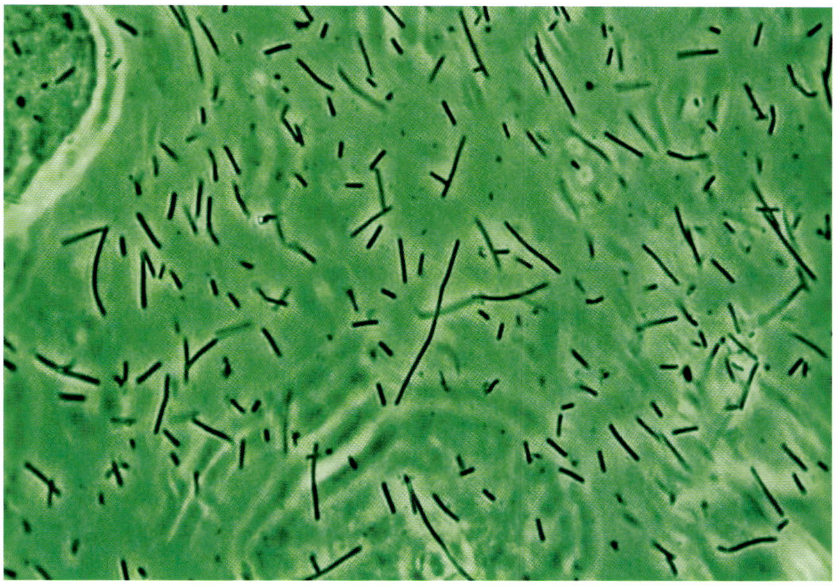

Figure 21 - Microphotograph of Lactobacilli (wet mount microscopy).

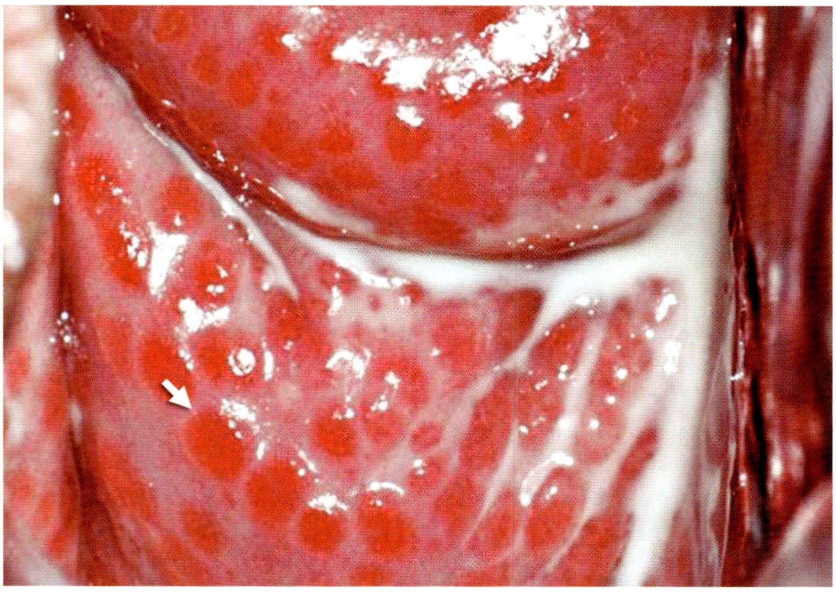

Figure 22 - White and homogeneous creamy discharge in candidiasis. Large erythematous papules (arrow) involve both cervix and vaginal walls.

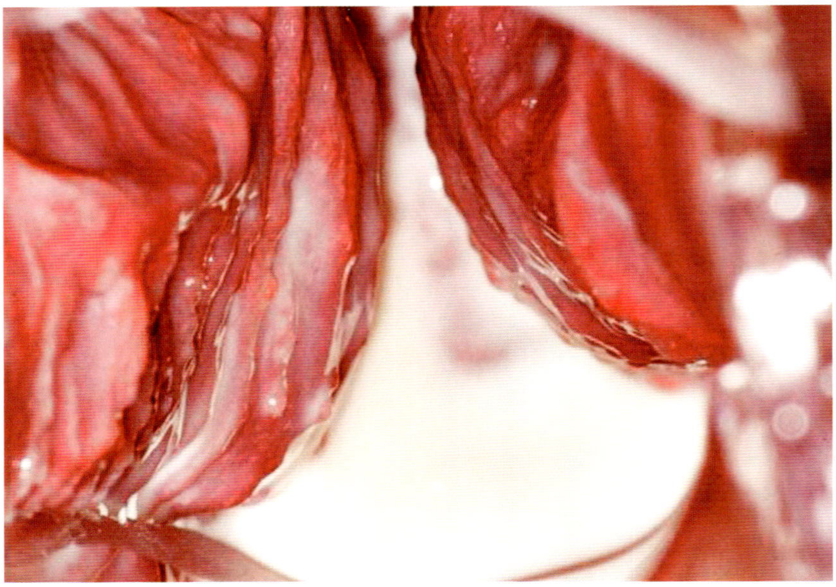

Figure 23 - The copious homogeneous and white discharge in bacterial vaginosis resembles a cup of milk that has been poured into the vagina.

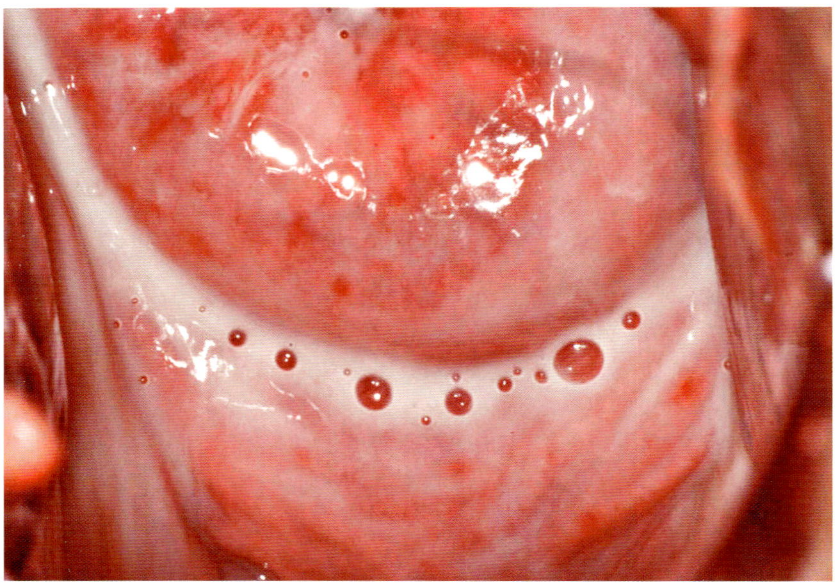

Figure 24 - White and frothy discharge in bacterial vaginosis.

can be observed in the presence of exposed columnar epithelium (Figure 26) and trichomoniasis (Figure 27). Wet mount microscopy may assist in reaching a correct diagnosis. **Trichomonas vaginalis** has an offensive cytolytic effect on cervical epithelium with resulting erosion of superficial and intermediate layers. Capillaries are dilated and surrounded by crowded, activated leukocytes. The colposcopic translation of these histologic changes is represented by easy epithelial abrasion and contact bleeding during scraping to carry out a smear or with only the insertion of a speculum.

In the acute phase, the cervix may show diffuse fine capillary hairpin loops and a punctate and papilliform appearance, resulting from the congested stromal papillae and microscopic, punctate hemorrhages. With severe inflammation, both vagina and cervix are studded by multiple, patchy red spots (Figure 28), whose coalescence in large, irregular patches gives the characteristic aspect of *macular colpitis*. This colposcopic pattern, however, is not pathognomonic. A diagnosis is confirmed with the aid of direct microscopy by the visualization of motile trichomonads.

Trichomonas vaginalis is a flagellated protozoan possessing five flagella, four of which protrude from its front end (Figure 29). The parasite propels itself using the four whip-like flagella (Figure 30). The fifth flagellum extends rearward and is incorporated within the undulating membrane of the parasite, supported by a slender noncontractile costa. The functionality of the fifth flagellum is not known. The

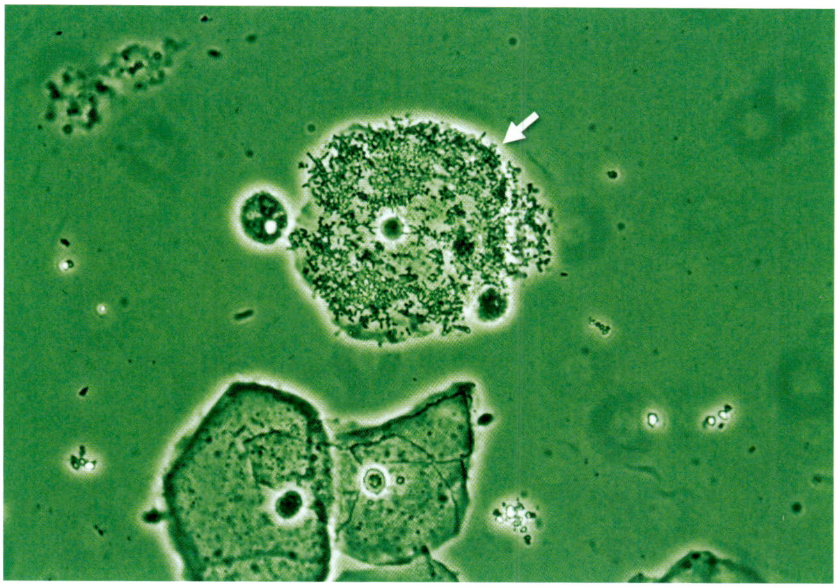

Figure 25 - Wet mount preparation showing a clue cell (arrow), characterized by a diffuse adhesion of pleomorphic bacteria (bacterial vaginosis).

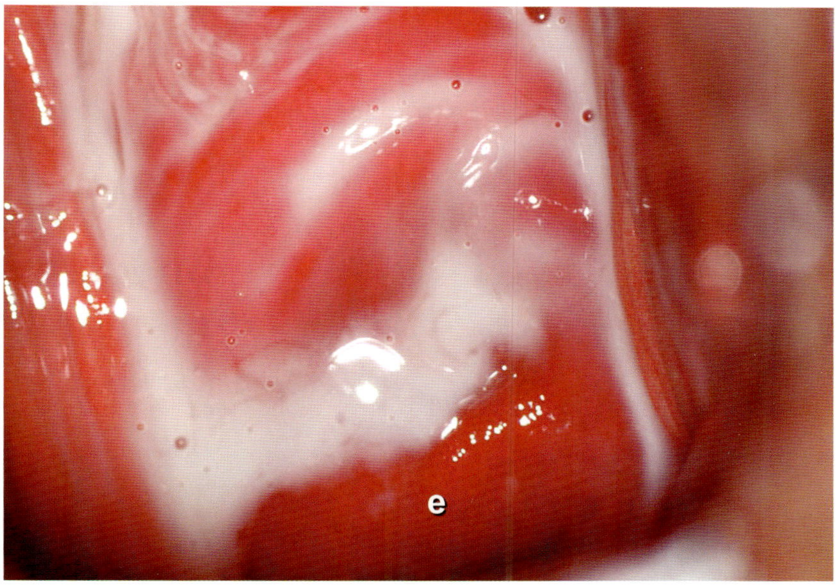

Figure 26 - White and frothy discharge associated with exposed columnar epithelium (e).

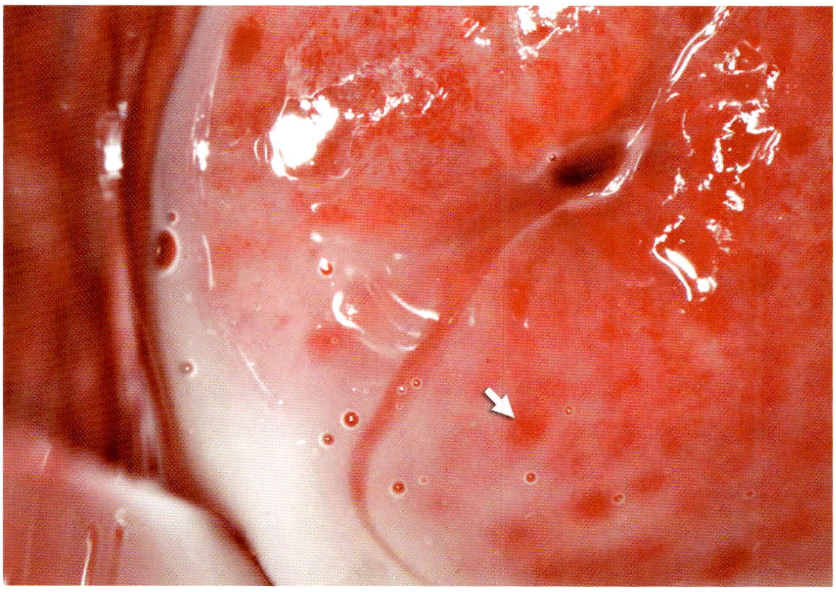

Figure 27 - White and frothy discharge and multiple, patchy red spots (arrow) in trichomoniasis.

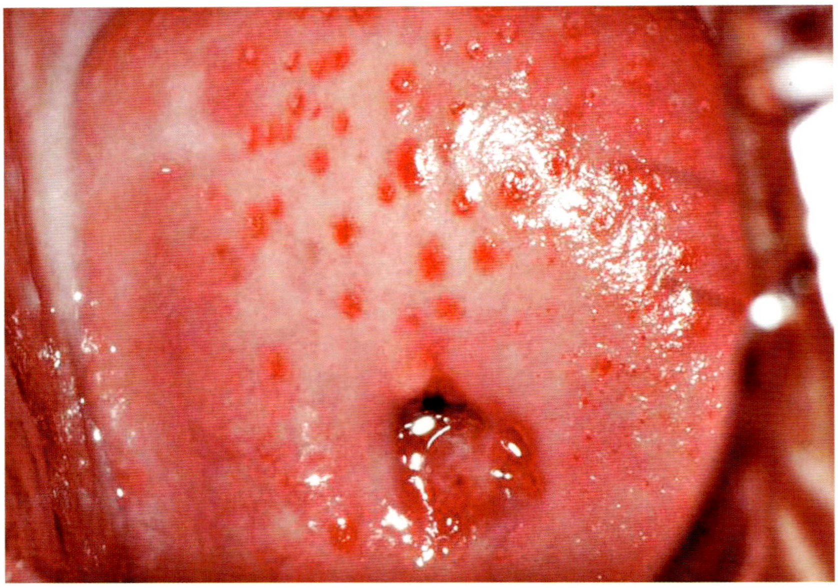

Figure 28 - Colpitis macularis in trichomoniasis (strawberry cervix).

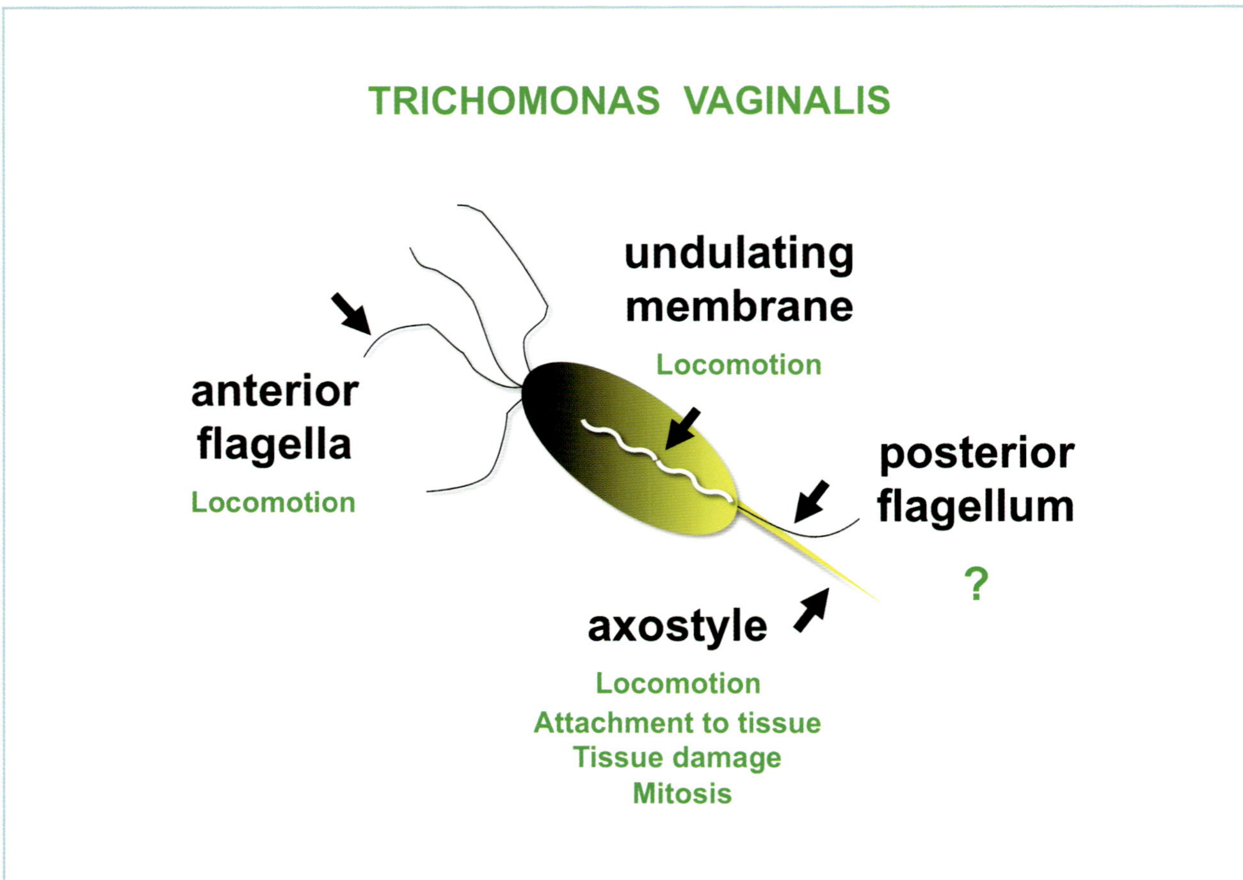

Figure 29 - Diagrammatic representation of Trichomonas vaginalis.

undulating membrane gives T. vaginalis a characteristic quivering motility. A barb-like axostyle (Figure 31) projects opposite the four-flagella bundle, as a posterior prolongation of cyto-skeleton. The axostyle participates in locomotion, attachment to tissue and host cell damage, and also in mitosis during cell division. Currently, wet prep is a quick and easy test that can be done in real time and is commonly used to diagnose trichomoniasis. It can easily be recognized by its jerky, swaying, or tumbling motion.

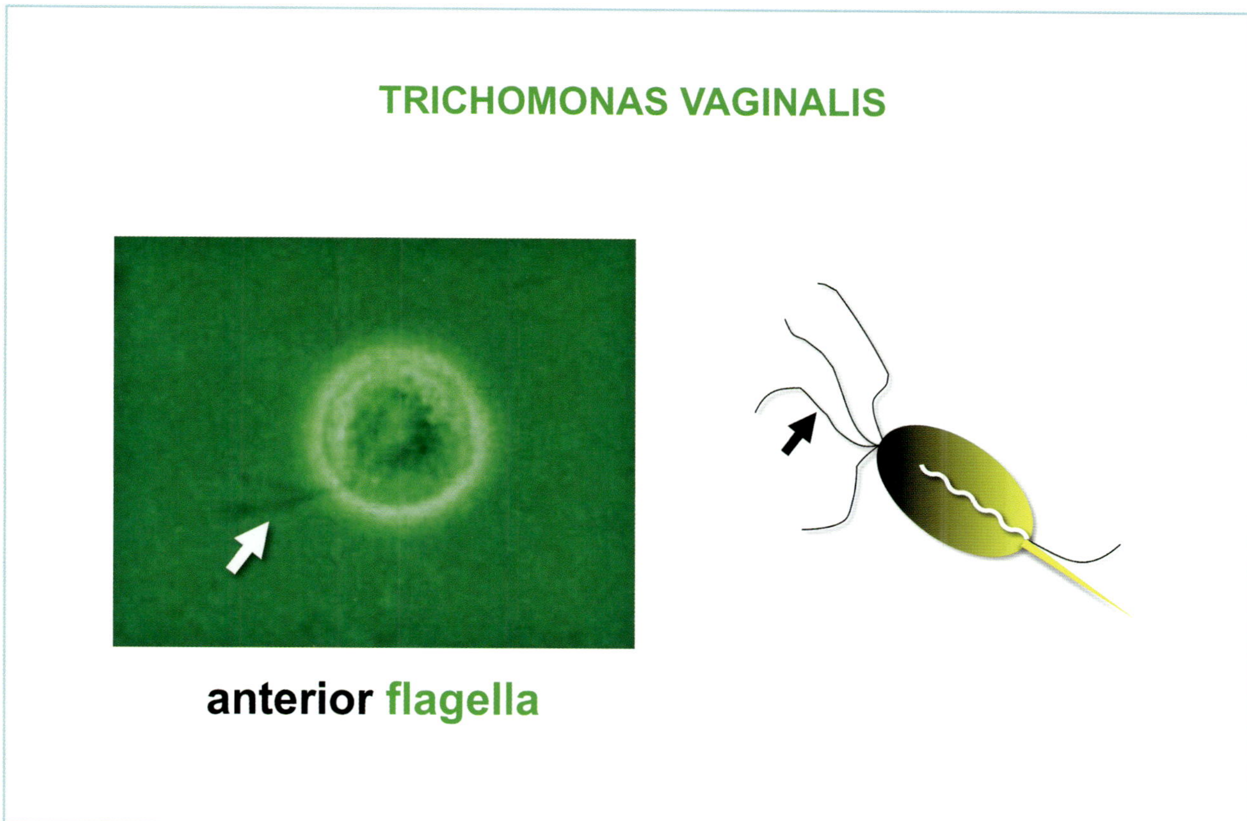

Figure 30 - Diagrammatic representation and microphotograph of anterior flagella (arrows) of Trichomonas vaginalis.

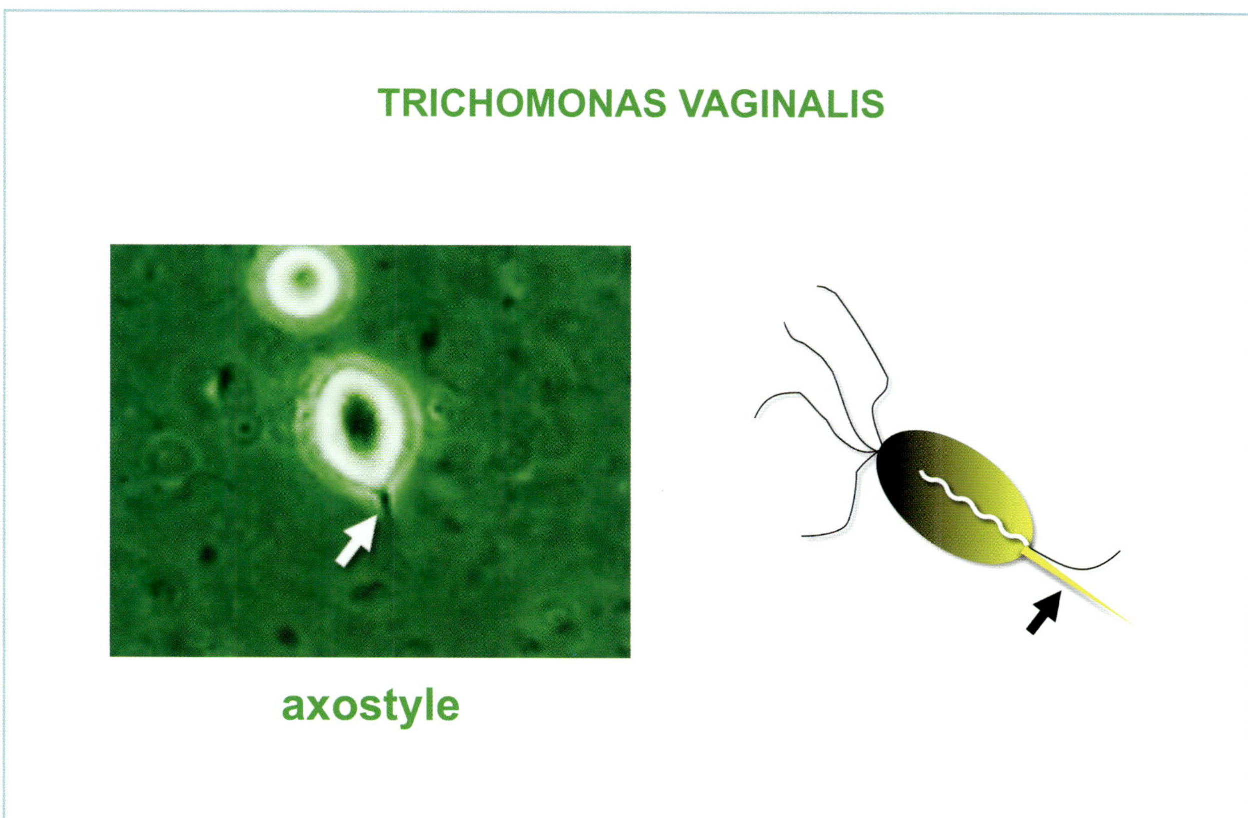

Figure 31 - Diagrammatic representation and microphotograph, showing the axostyle of a trichomonad (arrows).

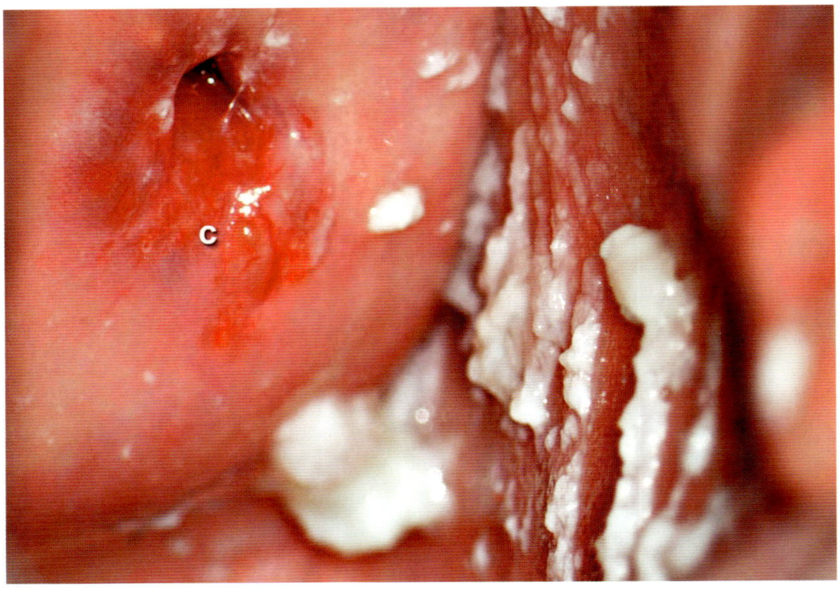

Figure 32 - White and lumpy discharge in vagina and congested cervix (c) (candidiasis).

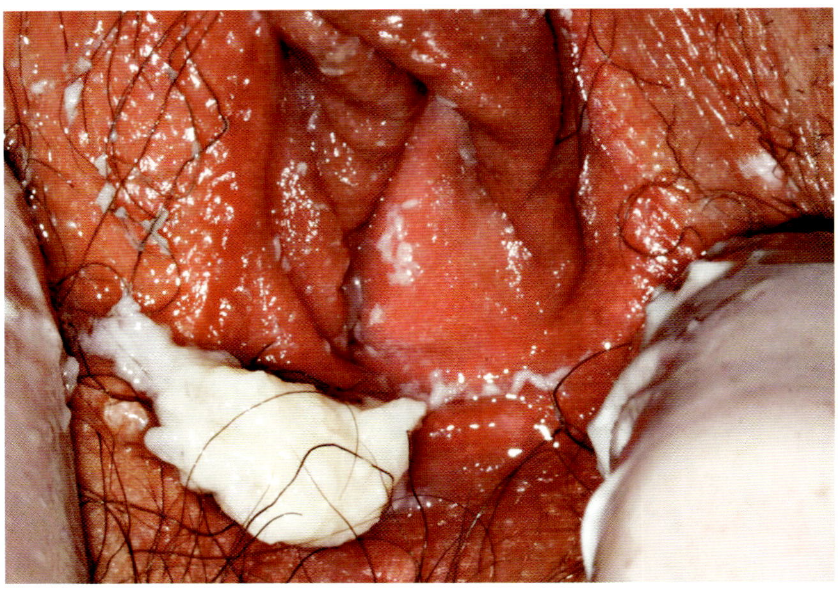

Figure 33 - White and lumpy discharge on the vulva (candidiasis).

Usually, **Candida albicans** causes a white, lumpy discharge in the vagina (Figure 32) and on the vulva (Figure 33). Candida species produces both blastospores and hyphae, easily observable in wet mount preparations (Figure 34). More and more frequently, despite symptoms consistent with candidal vaginitis, fungal yeast cells and hyphae are not visible under direct microscopic observation and cultures may yield false negative results. Furthermore, vaginal specimens are too often inappropriately submitted for bacterial cultures that inevitably reveal bacteria which play no role in the pathogenesis of vaginitis. This diagnostic failure depends on Candida penetration into vaginal cells by means of several proteases produced by hyphae (Figure 35). Estrogen promote blastospore adhesion to epithelial cells, and hypha development. Hyphae may be observed while penetrating epithelium, showing a characteristic diaphanous aspect when they are in the intracellular space (Figure 36).

In 1994, the author described a pathognomonic cell change induced by Candida due to its penetration through the vaginal epithelium, defined as *Candida cytopathy*.

This cytopathic effect can be clearly observed in different forms: cytoplasmic holes (Figures 37, 38), grooves (Figure 39), marginal erosions (Figure 40) and tunnels (Figure 41). In all of its forms, Candida cytopathy is characterized by a sharply condensed border.

When bacterial vaginosis and Candida infection are simultaneously present, vaginal frothy discharge may

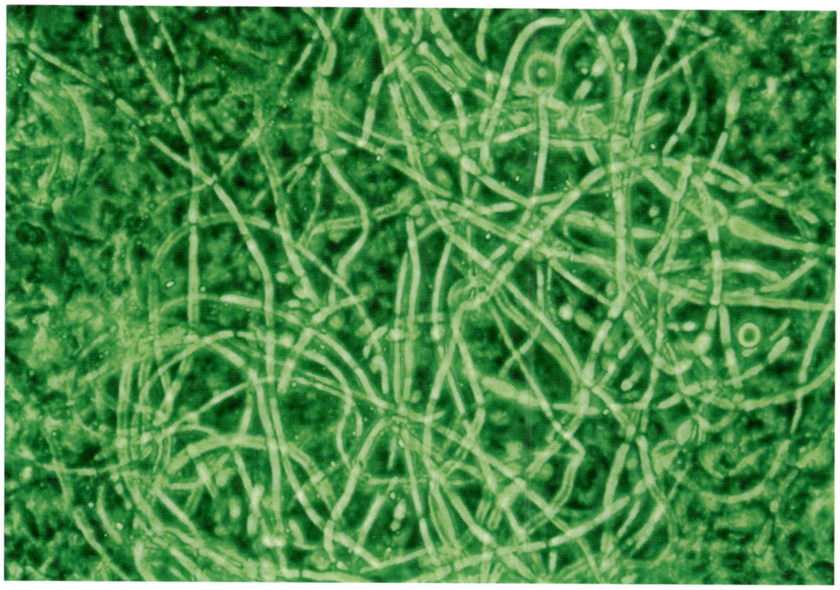

Figure 34 - Branching and budding hyphae of Candida albicans.

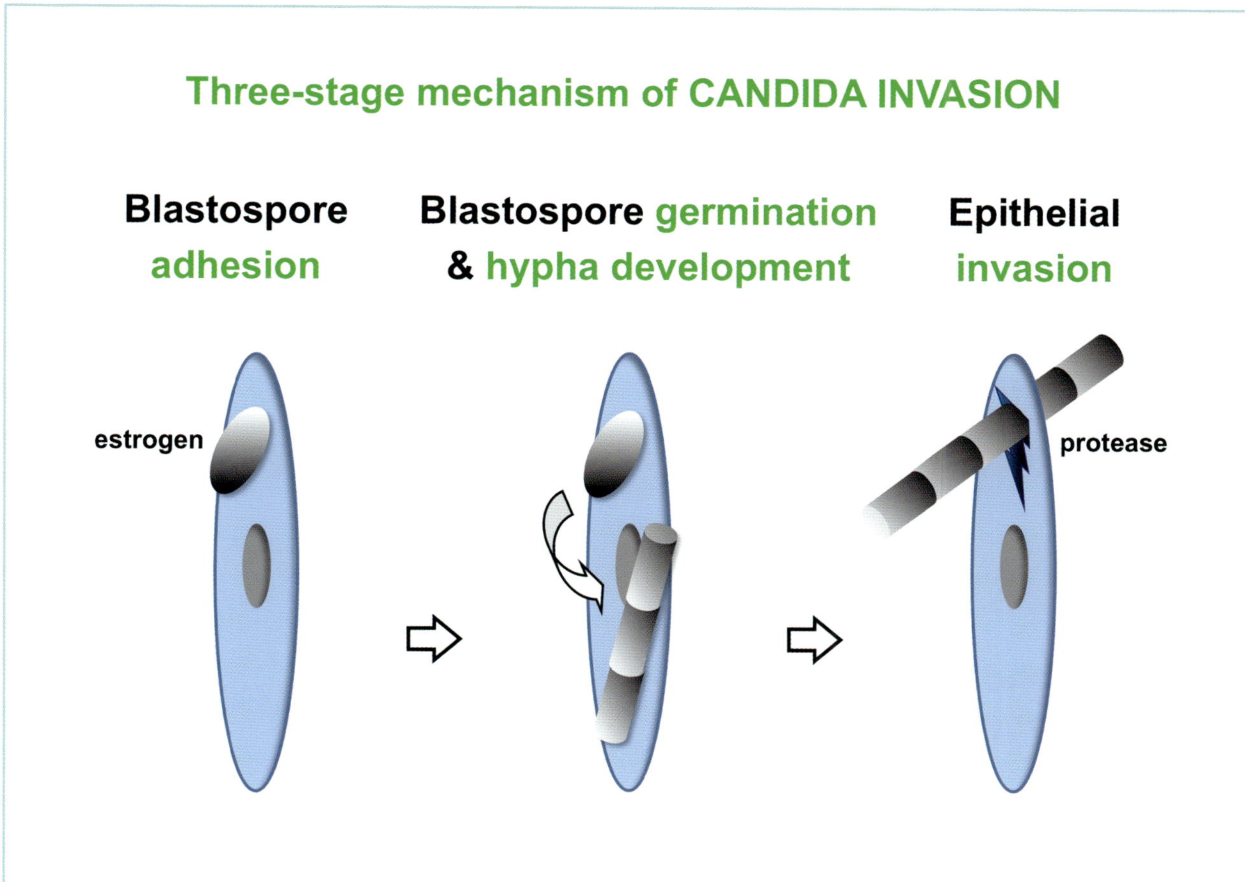

Figure 35 - Diagrammatic representation of the three-stage mechanism of Candida epithelial invasion.

be associated with erythematous macules (Figure 42), and wet mount microscopy can disclose both clue cells and fungal hyphae (Figure 43).
A clumpy discharge is characteristic of candidiasis but not pathognomonic. In fact, **vaginal lactobacillosis** can produce an annoying, profuse creamy-white or clumpy discharge (Figure 44), with the sensation of incessantly having wet oneself. Vaginal lactobacillosis is not a vaginal infection as it is caused by a lactobacillus overgrowth but it can mimic a

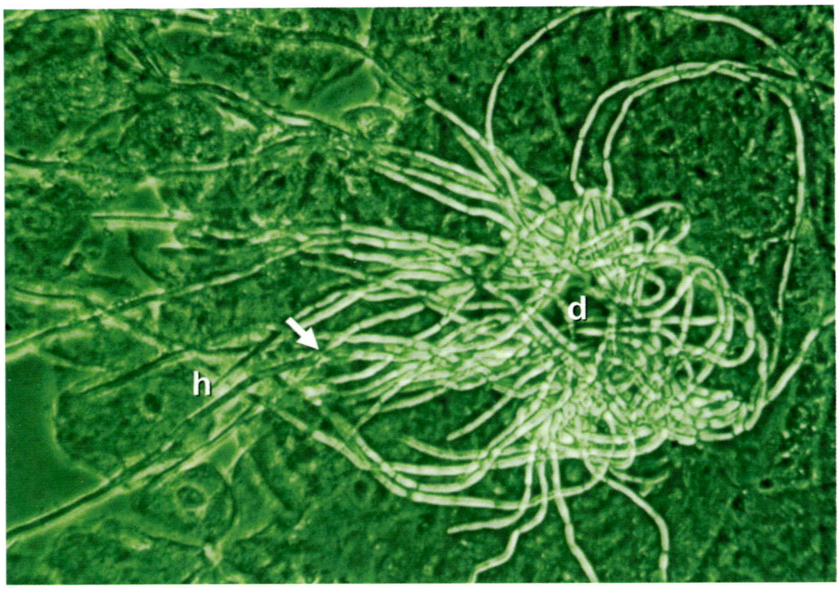

Figure 36 - The microphotograph shows a distinct hypha (h) penetrating (arrow) into the cell. Intraepithelial hyphae have a diaphanous appearance (d).

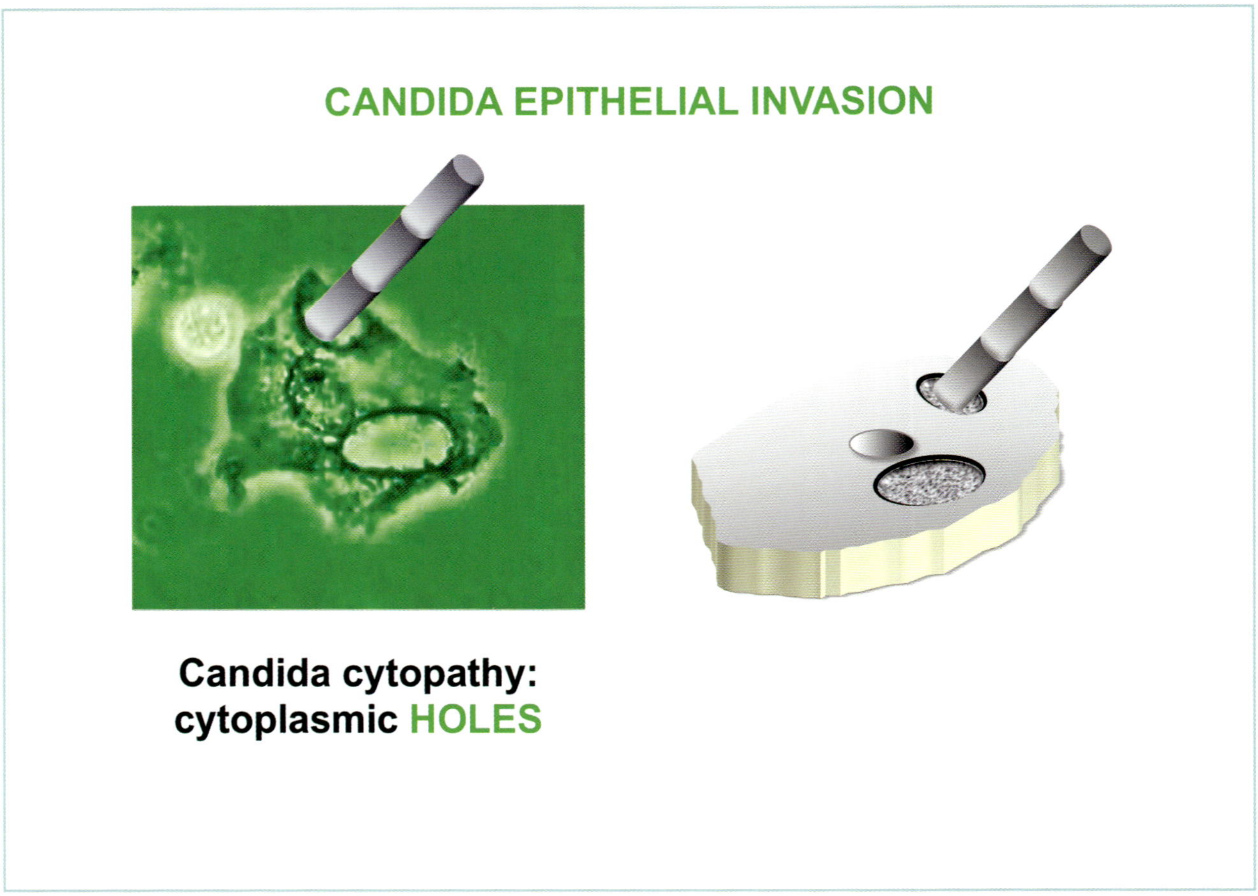

Figure 37 - Microphotograph and diagrammatic representation of Candida cytopathy: cytoplasmic holes.

fungal infection because it is often associated with vulvar and vaginal itching.
In patients who have signs and symptoms of vaginal candidiasis, but unresponsive to antifungal drugs, a diagnosis of vaginal lactobacillosis must be envisaged.

Vaginal lactobacillosis is also known as lactobacillus overgrowth syndrome or cytolytic vaginosis. Its etiology is unknown and its prevalence is approximately 15%. Lactobacillosis is characterized by the presence in vaginal wet mount preparations of abundant and

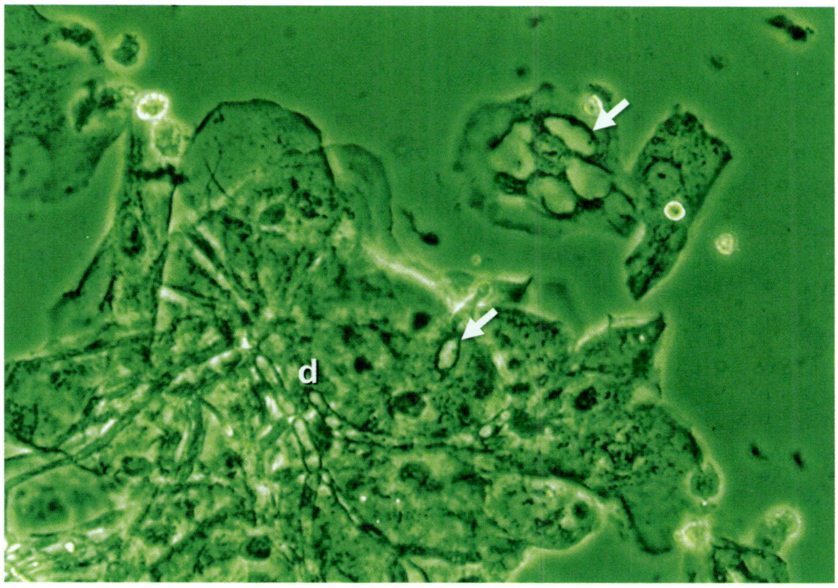

Figure 38 - Diaphanous aspect of intraepithelial hyphae (d) and cytoplasmic holes (arrows) (Candida cytopathy).

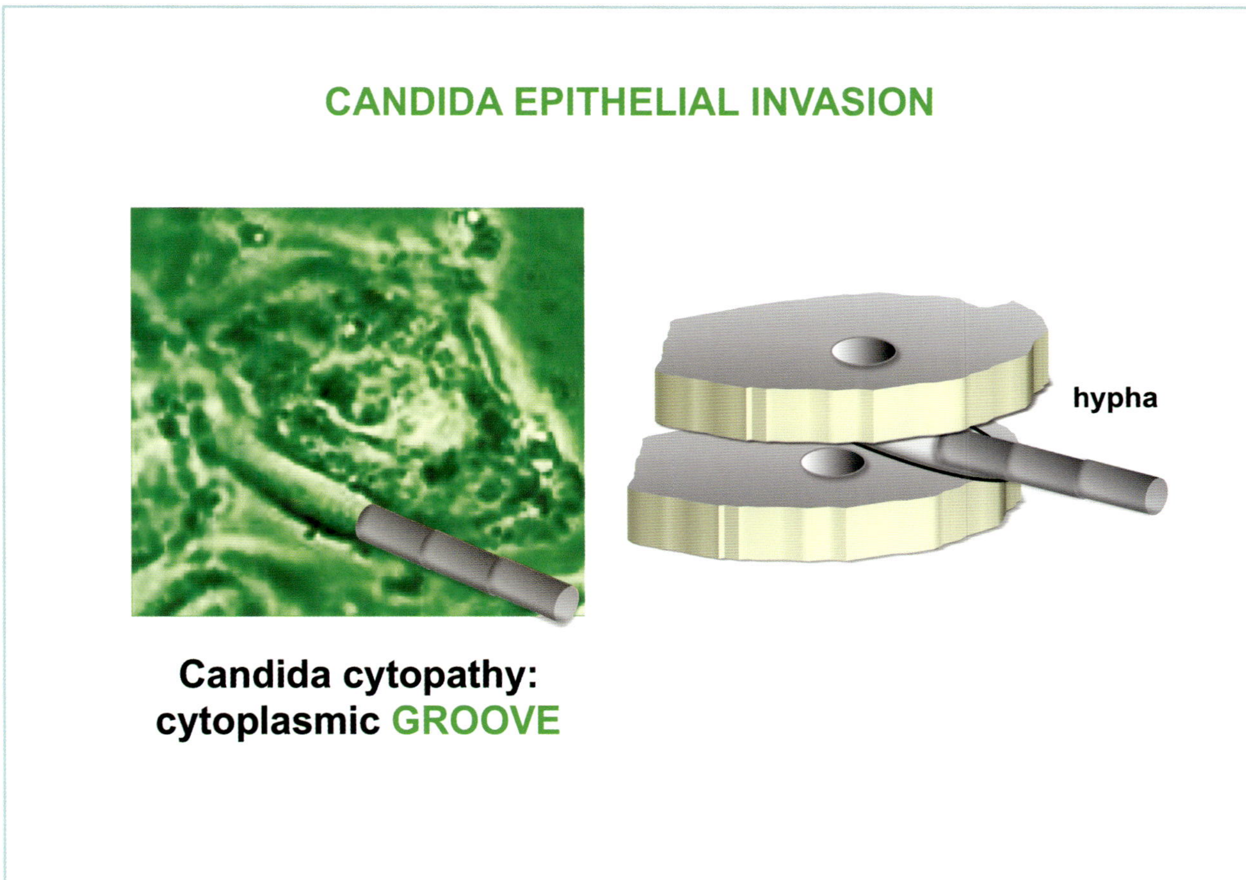

Figure 39 - Microphotograph and diagrammatic representation of Candida cytopathy: cytoplasmic groove.

much longer (filamentous) than normal lactobacilli, often adhered to squamous cells (Figure 45), resulting in lysis of vaginal epithelial cells. If lactobacillosis is misinterpreted as a fungal infection, allergic reactions to antimycotic therapy may result in a continuation of symptoms that are incorrectly thought to be caused by yeast. Wet mount microscopy offers an immediate distinction between the two opposite conditions and enables to avoid unnecessary and even harmful pharmacological treatments.

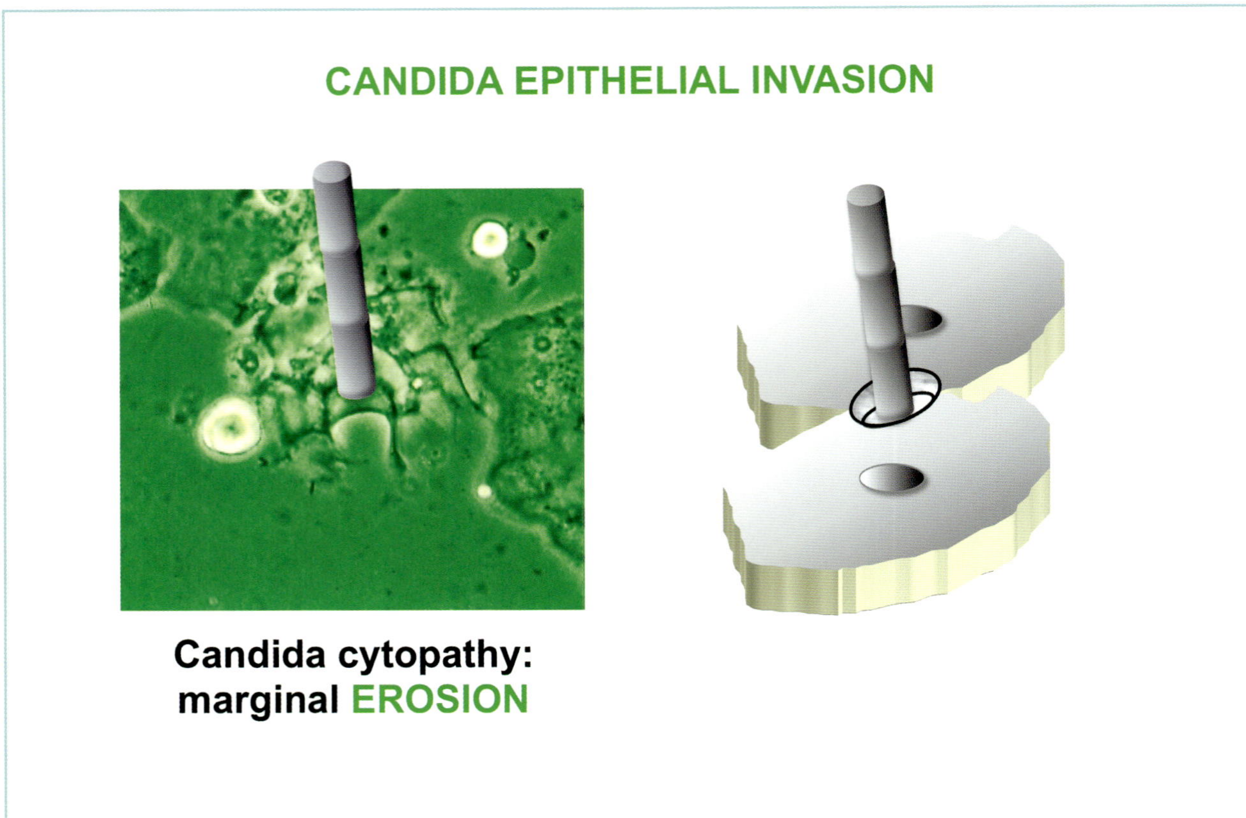

Figure 40 - Microphotograph and diagrammatic representation of Candida cytopathy: cytoplasmic marginal erosion.

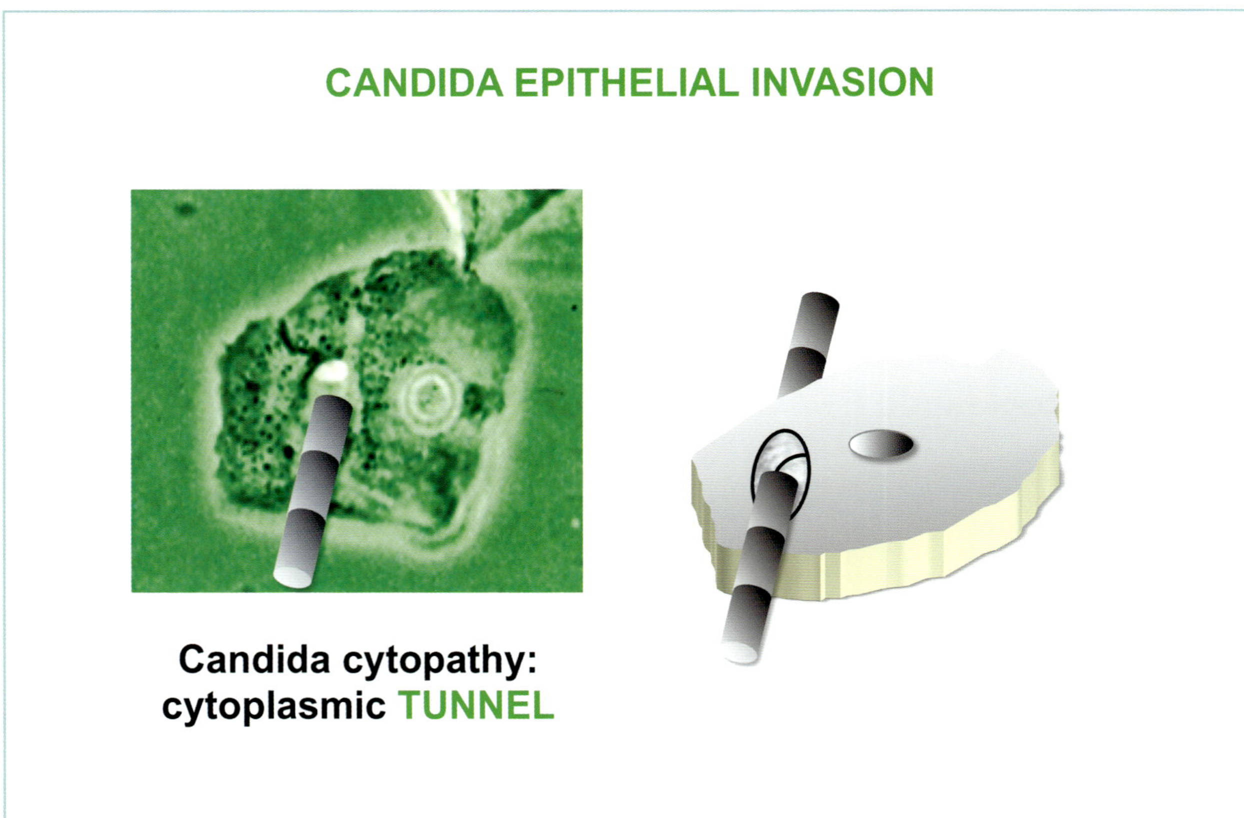

Figure 41 - Microphotograph and diagrammatic representation of Candida cytopathy: cytoplasmic tunnel.

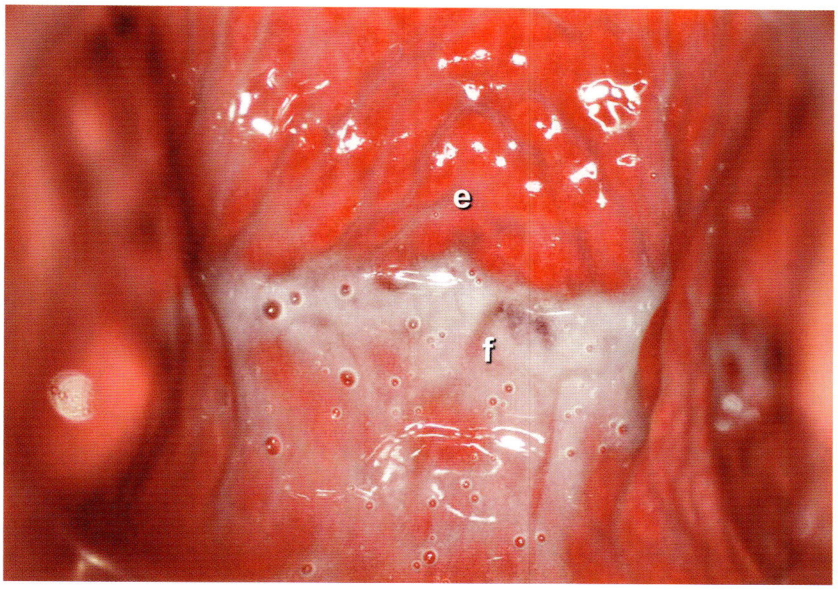

Figure 42 - Frothy discharge (f) due to bacterial vaginosis is seen together with erythematous papules (e), induced by candidiasis.

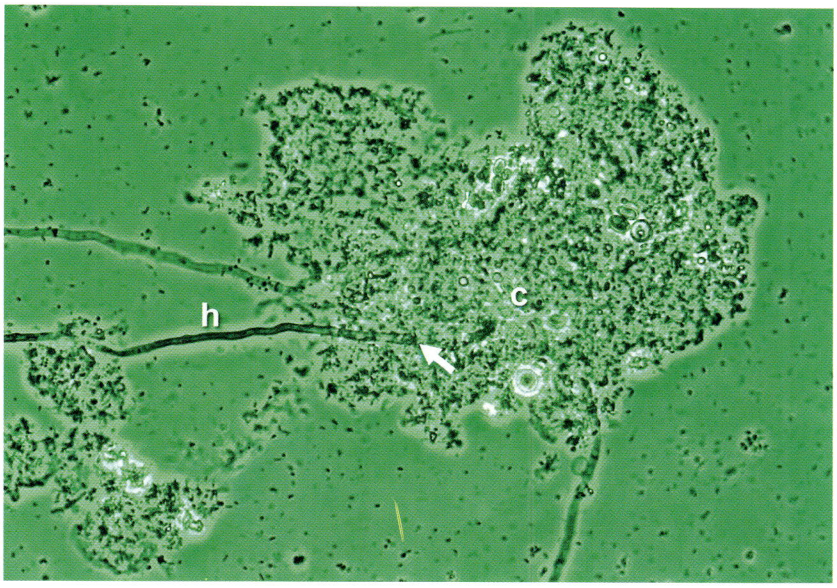

Figure 43 - Fungal hyphae (h) (Candida albicans) penetrate (arrow) into a clue cell (c) (bacterial vaginosis).

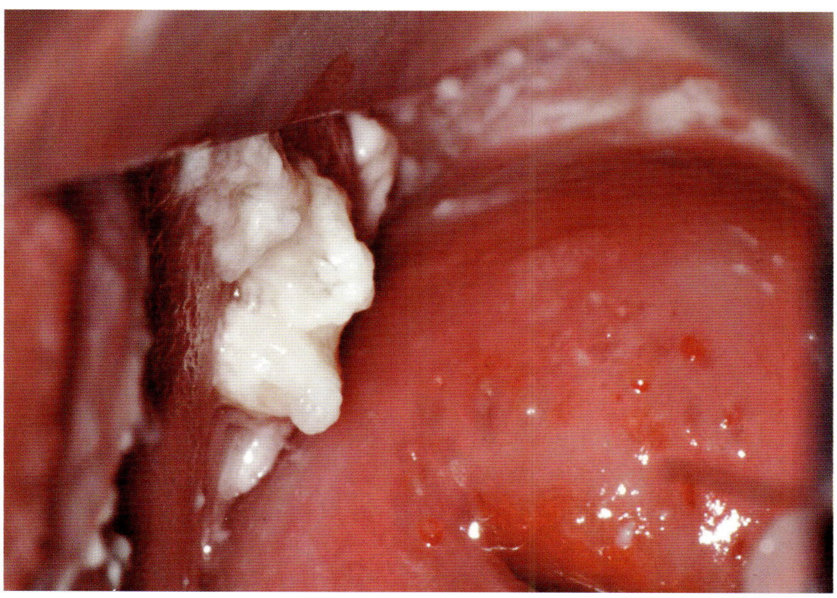

Figure 44 - Clumpy discharge in vaginal lactobacillosis.

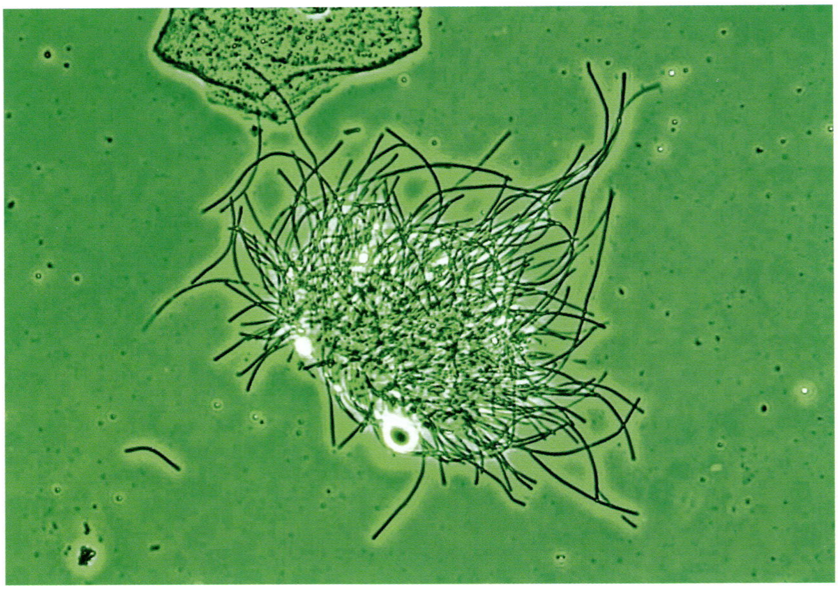

Figure 45 - Filamentous Lactobacilli adhered to a squamous cell in wet mount preparation.

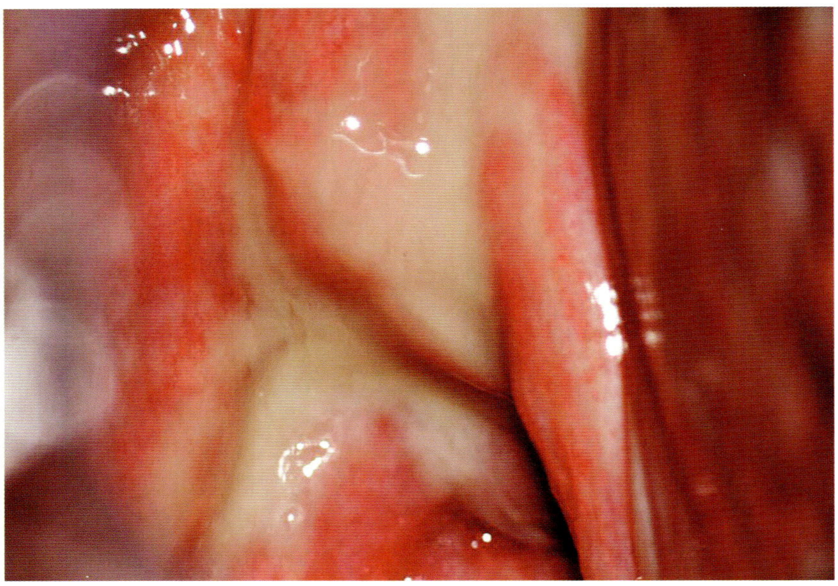

Figure 46 - Grey-yellowish and cloudy discharge in aerobic vaginitis.

A grey-yellowish and cloudy discharge may be observed in the presence of **aerobic vaginitis** (Figure 46), but it is not rare to find a frank yellow discharge (Figure 47).
Aerobic vaginitis (AV) is a new unclassifiable pathology that is neither specific vaginitis nor bacterial vaginosis. Although many studies state that the frequency of AV is still unknown, it is found in 25% of pregnant women and is with an increased risk of preterm delivery, chorioamnionitis and funisitis of the fetus. *Escherichia coli* is cited as one of the most common causes of this type of vaginitis and sometimes is isolated alone, even though *Enterococcus faecalis*, *Staphylococcus sp.* and *group B streptococcus* are also involved. It should be pointed out that the mere presence of an organism in the culture does not denote causation. Therefore, how can we distinguish an infection that requires treatment from vaginal contamination that is not necessary to treat? Aerobic vaginitis is accompanied by an increased localized inflammatory reaction (Figure 48), as opposed to the suppressed immune response that is characteristic of bacterial vaginosis (Figure 49). The diagnosis of "aerobic vaginitis" is essentially based on microscopic examinations using a phase contrast microscope.
Other cervico-vaginal infections can produce a mucopurulent discharge, such as Chlamydia trachomatis infection, gonorrhea and desquamative inflammatory vaginitis (DIV).
In cervical **chlamydial infection** exudate is characteristically seen coming out from the cervical canal (Figure 50). Microscopy observation enables to easily

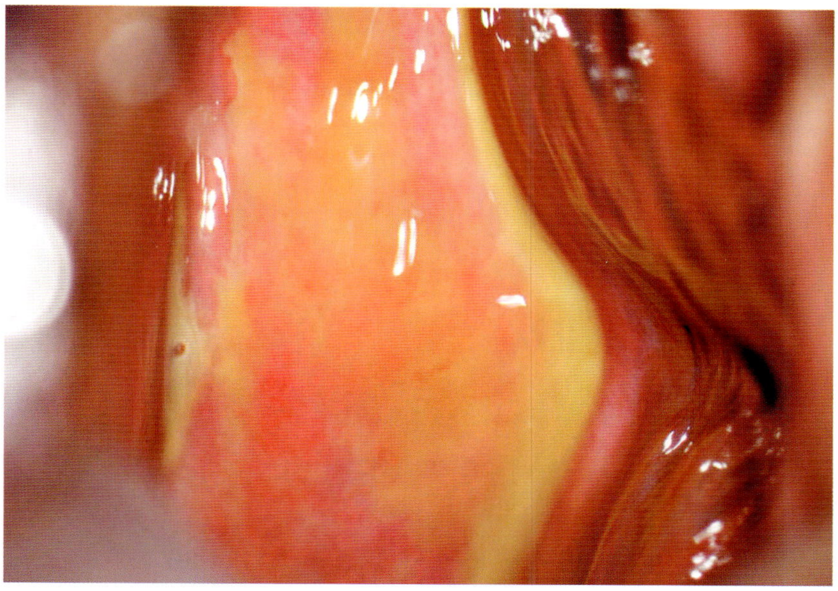

Figure 47 - Frank yellow discharge in aerobic vaginitis.

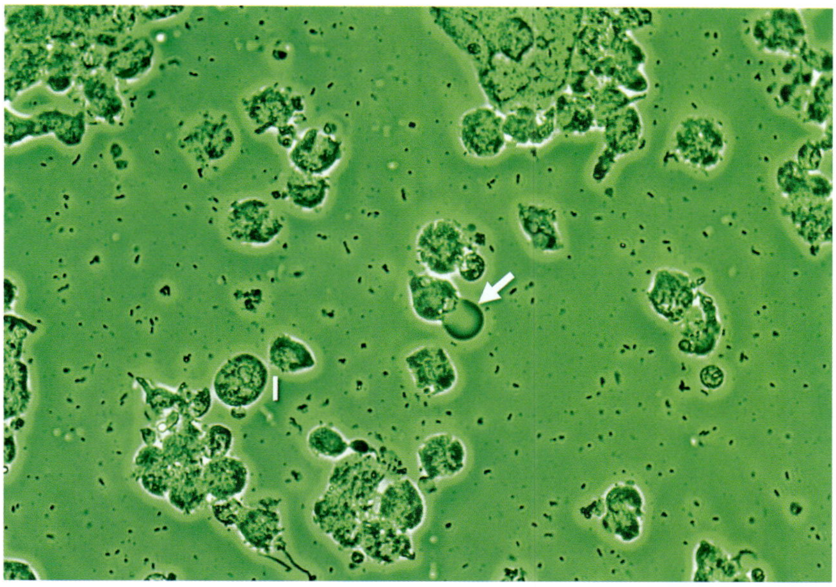

Figure 48 - Free floating bacteria are associated with numerous leukocytes (I) (aerobic vaginitis). The arrow indicates a vesicle of exocytosis, where digested bacteria are expelled.

detect a large cytoplasmic inclusion which expands to accommodate the increasing number of C. trachomatis, pushing the nucleus progressively towards the periphery of the infected cell (Figure 51).

Women with **gonorrhea** may experience a burning sensation during urination, yellowish vaginal discharge (Figure 52), vaginal bleeding between periods, and/or pelvic pain. Gonococci appear in coffee bean-shaped pairs, as typical intracellular diplococci upon microscopic examination of endocervical secretions from women (Figure 53).

Desquamative inflammatory vaginitis is a rare chronic clinical syndrome of unknown etiology, frequently unrecognized, characterized by vaginal rash and purulent discharge (Figure 54). Postmenopausal women are more likely than premenopausal women to be diagnosed with desquamative inflammatory vaginitis (DIV). The vestibule (Figure 55) and the inside of the vagina itself are usually red. Irritation, burning, soreness, as well as, pain during sexual activity, are the usual presenting complaints. Vulvar and vaginal erythema induced by Candida infection must be differentiated from the similar finding associated with DIV. On colposcopy, the different aspect of discharge provides helpful diagnostic hints whereas direct microscopy detects, in real time, the etiologic agent. Desquamative inflammatory vaginitis is a diagnosis of exclusion, and other causes of purulent vaginitis should be excluded. Although etiology and pathogenesis remain unknown, the favorable response to anti-inflammatory agents suggests that the etiology is immune mediated. Through

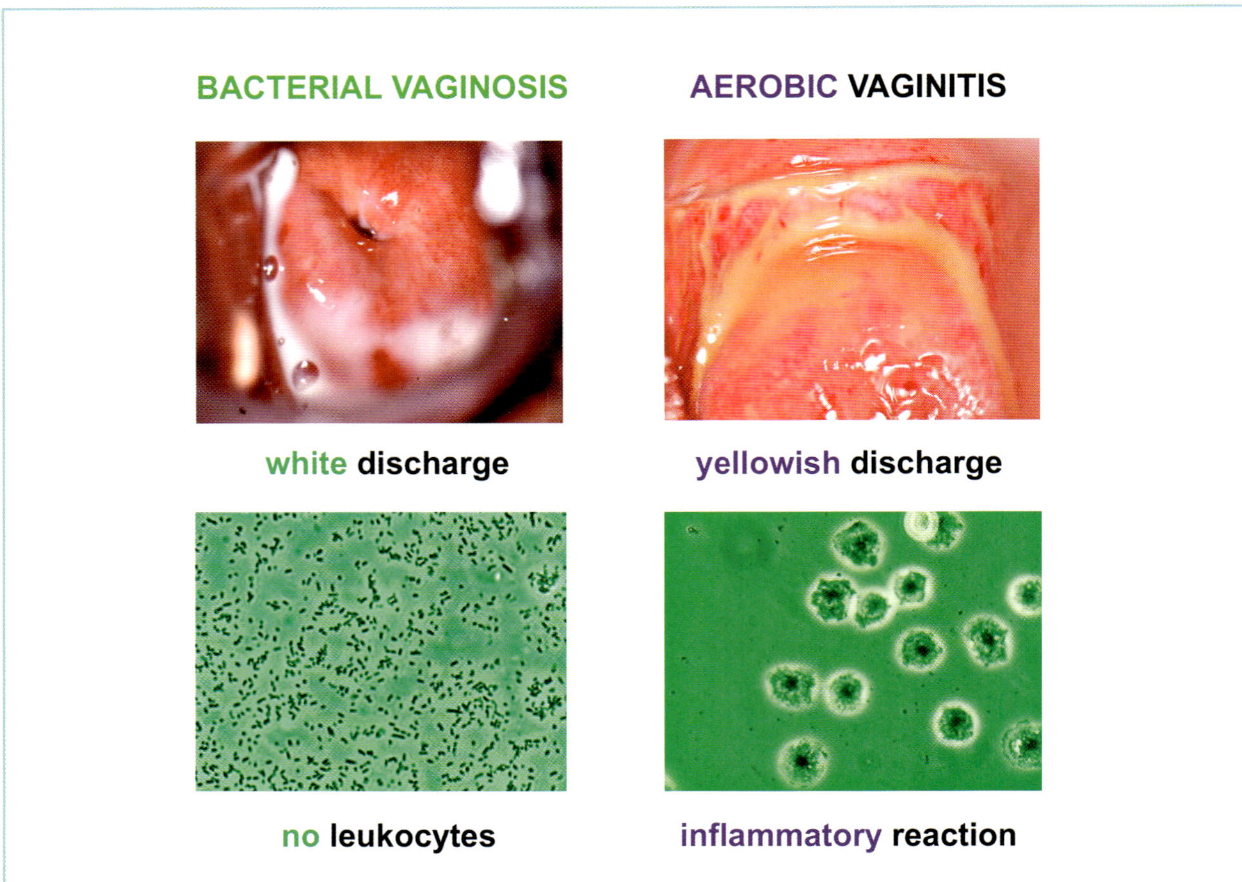

Figure 49 - Colposcopic and wet mount microscopy appearances of bacterial vaginosis and aerobic vaginitis showing the differences in the discharge aspect, and presence of leukocytes.

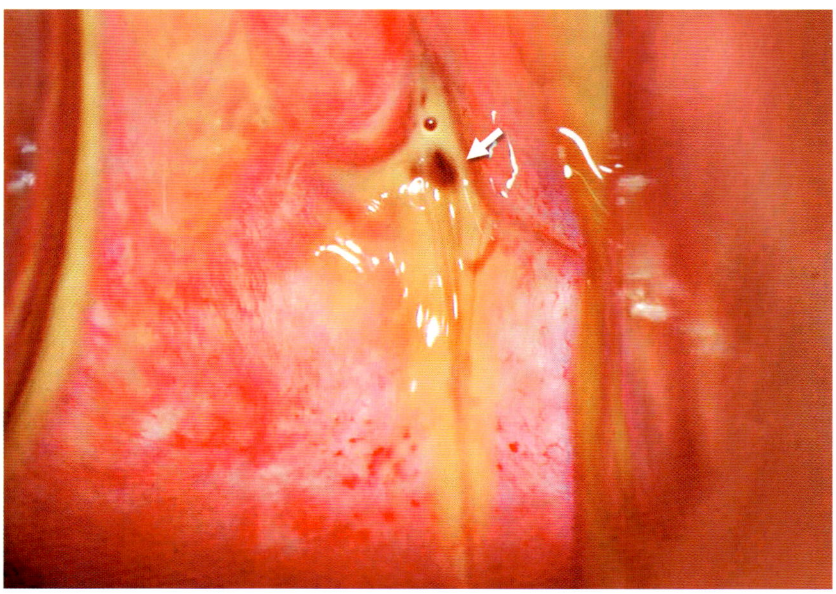

Figure 50 - Mucopurulent discharge comes from the endocervical canal (arrow) in Chlamydia trachomatis infection.

wet mount of the vaginal secretions, DIV is defined by an increase in inflammatory cells and parabasal epithelial cells (Figure 56).
Candidiasis represents one of the most frequent causes of **vulvar erythema** (Figures 57, 58). Ano-vulvar indurated erythema (Figure 59) induced by Candida albicans may pose diagnostic problems but the detection of Candida cytopathy (Figure 60) in pre-keratotic cells and horny cells may assist in reaching a correct diagnosis.

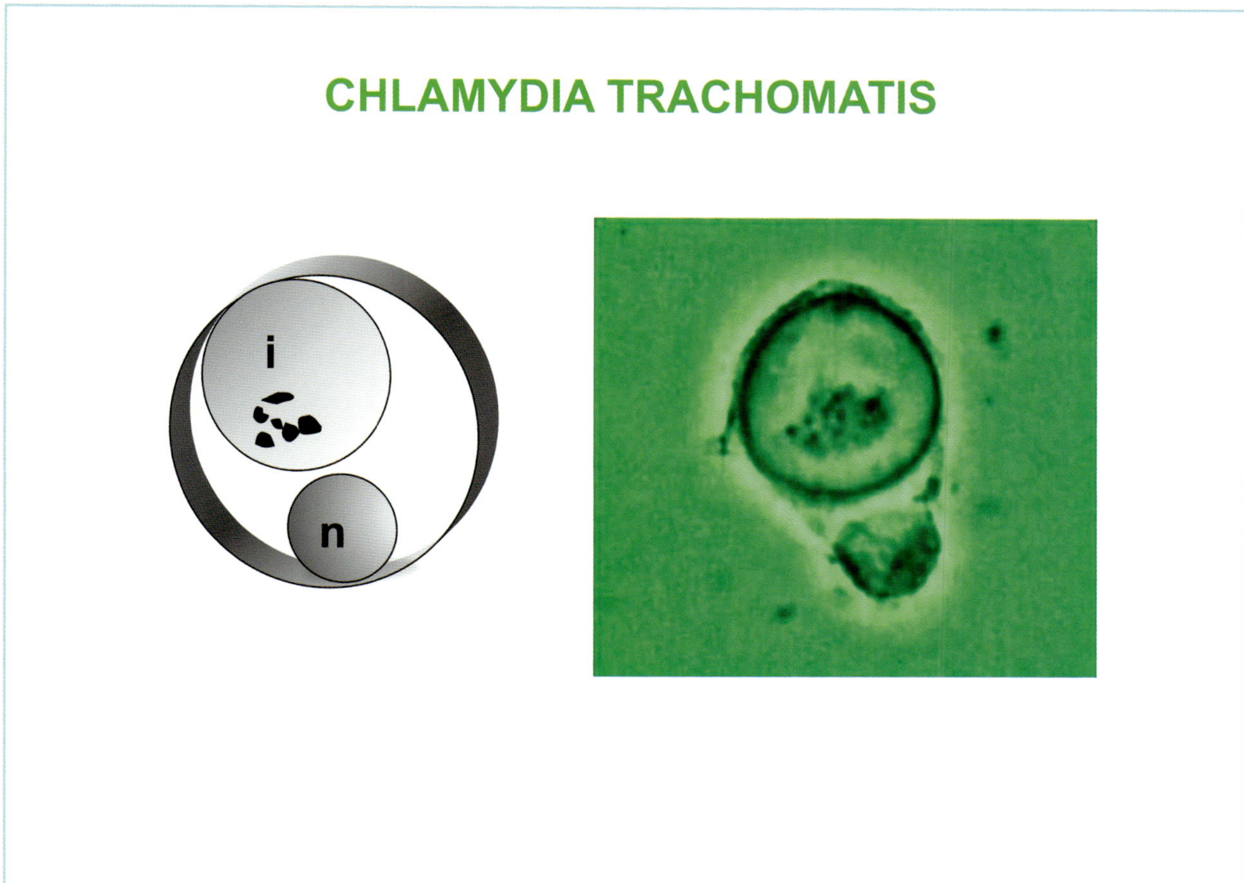

Figure 51 - Diagrammatic representation and microphotograph of the inclusion (i) containing a fragmented body (hot-air balloon feature). Nucleus (n).

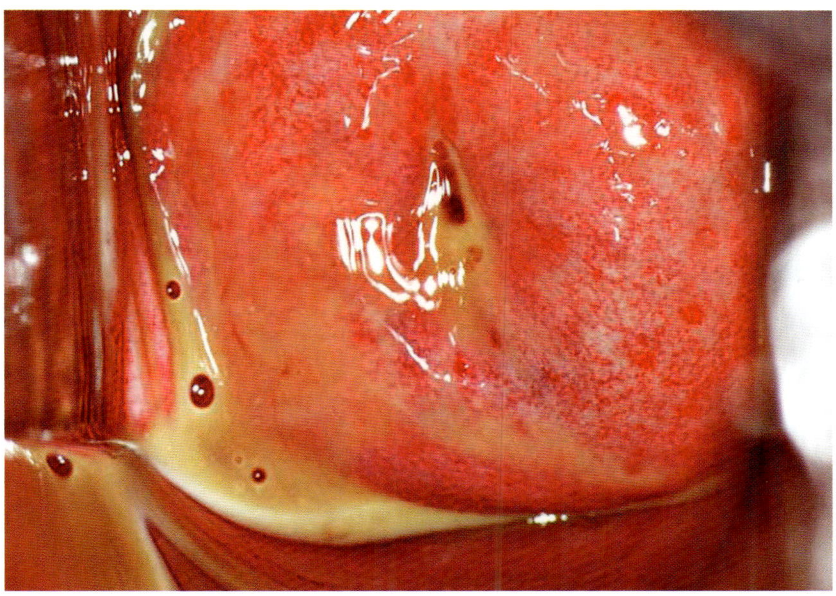

Figure 52 - Abundant mucopurulent discharge in gonorrhea.

Intense vulvar erythema can be observed also in the presence of exposure to hyperosmotic lubricants (Figure 61), erythematous psoriasis and lichen planus. Erythematous psoriasis (Figure 62) exhibits a bright erythema that may extend to the perianal skin, shows a sharp outline and often characteristic satellite lesions.

Lichen planus may cause vulvar erythema (Figure 63). The final diagnosis of lichen planus is only histological and is characterized by irregular acanthosis

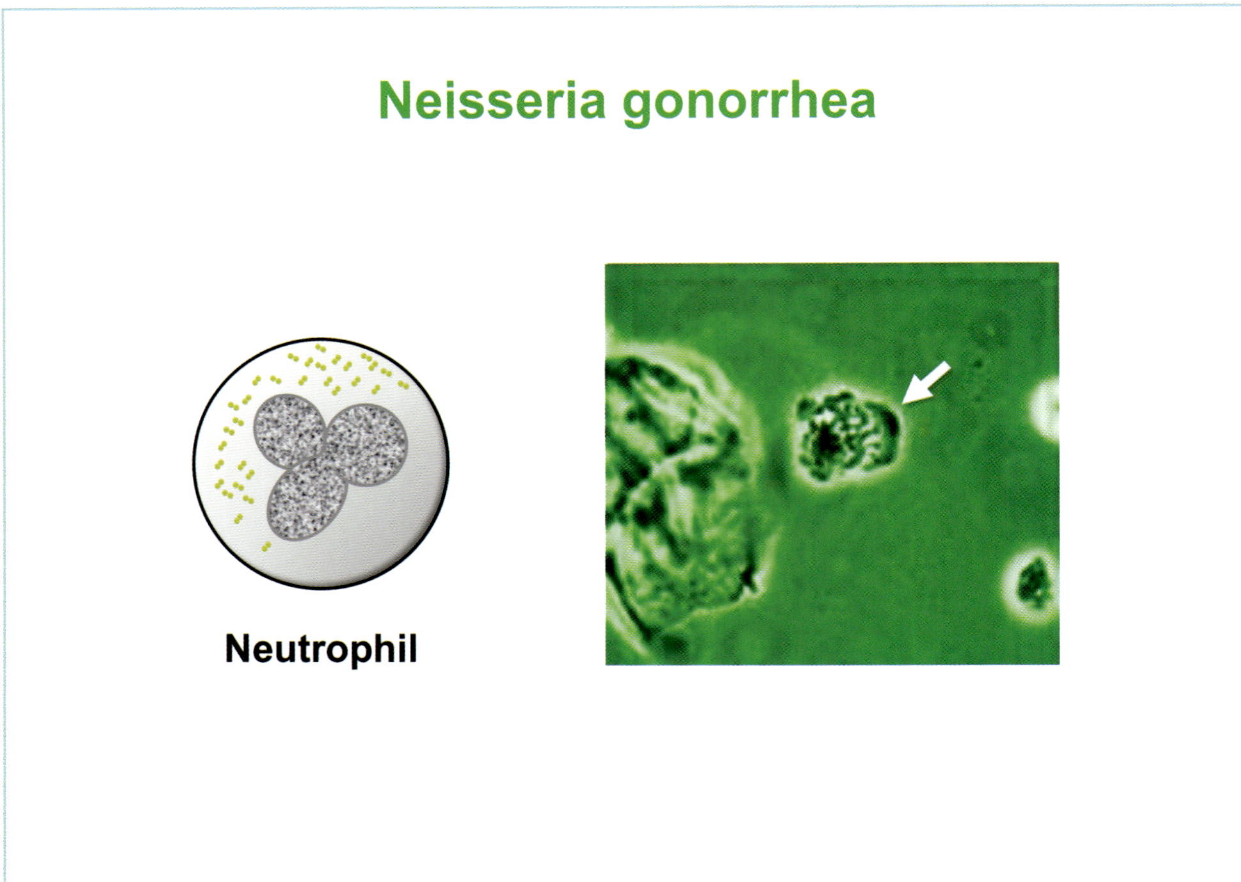

Figure 53 - Diagrammatic representation and wet mount microphotograph of a neutrophil (arrow) full of diplococci.

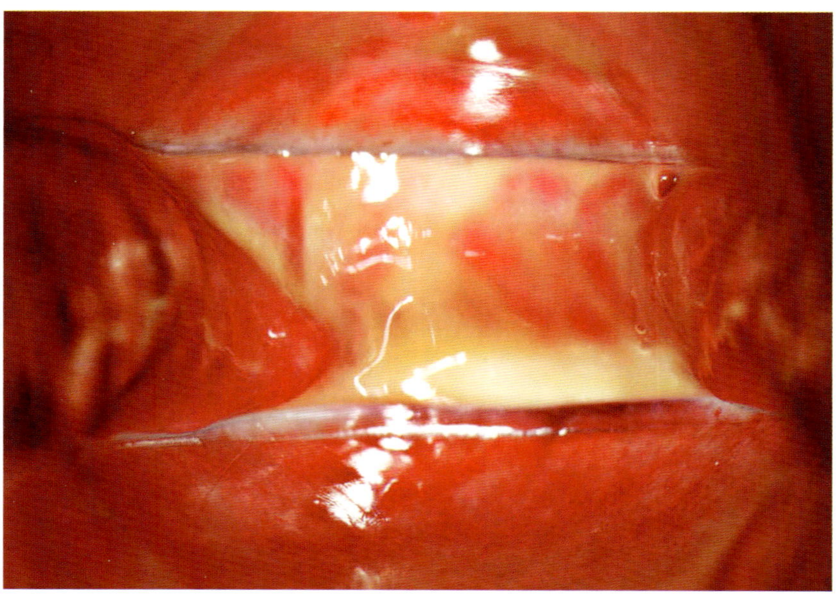

Figure 54 - Vaginal rash and purulent discharge in desquamative inflammatory vaginitis (DIV).

of the epidermidis, liquefative degeneration of the basal cell layer and band-like infiltrate of lymphocytes in the upper epidermidis.
In the presence of **Human Papillomavirus** infection (HPV), no discharge is detectable, unless other concomitant vaginal infections are present. Human Papillomavirus infection is the most common sexually transmitted infection. HPV is so common that nearly all sexually active men and women get the virus at some point in their life. Although the majority of

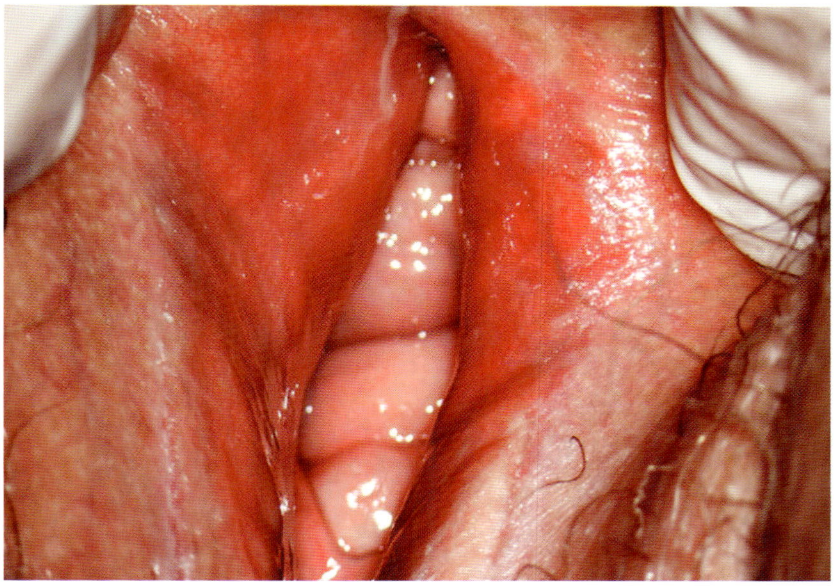

Figure 55 - Intensely red vaginal vestibule in DIV.

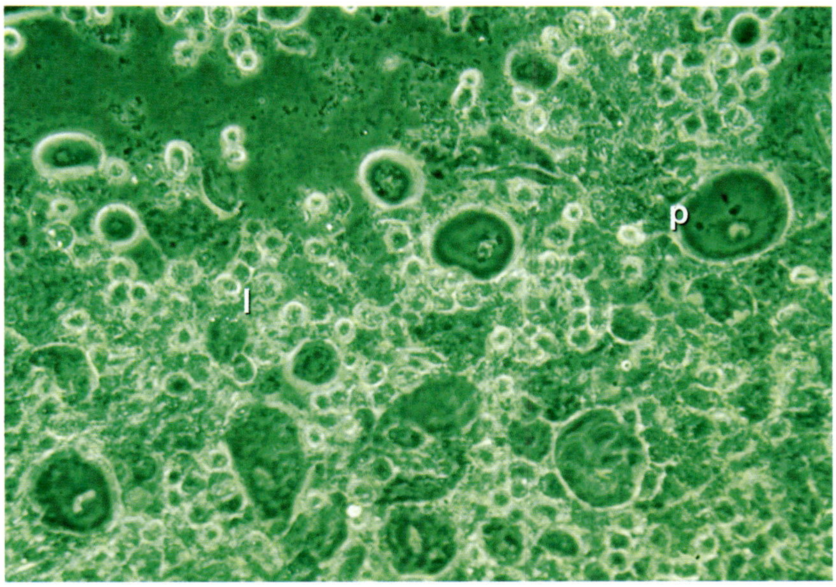

Figure 56 - Parabasal cells (p) and increased leukocytes (l) characterize the microscopic finding of DIV.

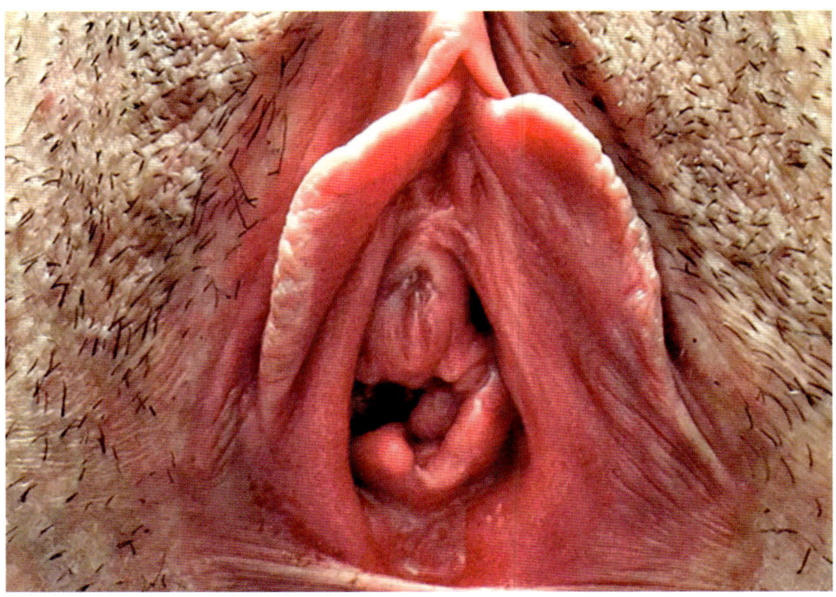

Figure 57 - Vulvar erythema in vaginal candidiasis.

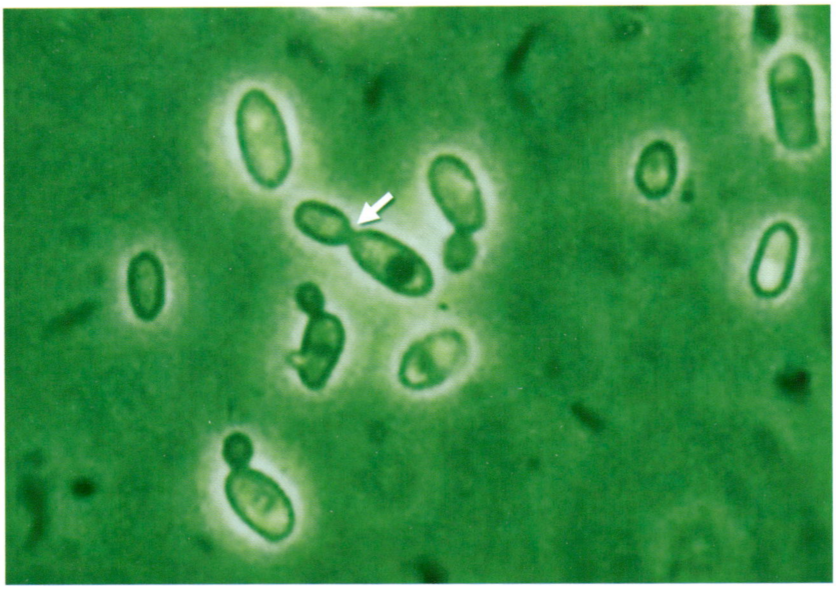

Figure 58 - Single and budding (arrow) blastospores of Candida albicans.

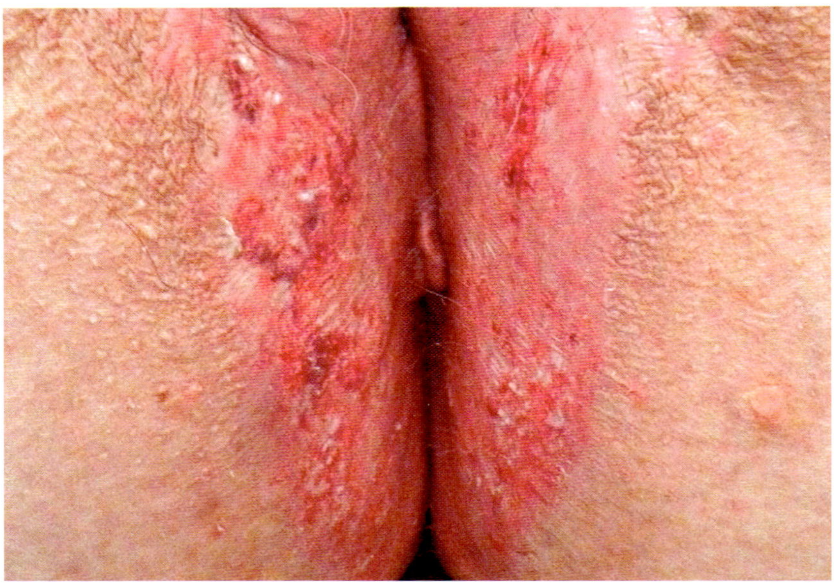

Figure 59 - Vulvar and perianal indurated erythema.

sexually active adults will be infected with HPV at least once in their lives, the highest rates of infection are found in sexually active women under 25. Colposcopic features induced by HPV infection may be divided into two groups: exophytic or productive lesions and flat lesions or Subclinical Papillomavirus Infections (SPI):

- exophytic lesions
  - exophytic condyloma
  - micropapillary lesions
- flat lesions (SPI)
  - flat condyloma
  - white punctation

The former group includes macroscopic lesions, like exophytic condyloma and early micropapillary lesions, that are visible to the naked eye. Flat lesions may be seen as flat, acetowhite lesions or as white punctation.

Exophytic or *papillary condyloma* are usually easy to diagnose colposcopically, particularly when they show typical elongated finger-like processes (Figure 64). The vessels within the papillae may take a comma, staghorn or corkscrew shape. After application of acetic acid, the majority of these vessels are masked, whereas the papillae whiten, retract and separate, thus, becoming more easily recognized. Sometimes, the coarseness of these exophytic lesions gives the colposcopic suspicion of atypicality. Exophytic condyloma may involve labia majora and labia minora, vestibule (Figure 65), clitoris (Figure 66), vagina (Figure 67) and cervix (Figure 68).

Condyloma acuminata or warts refer to an epider-

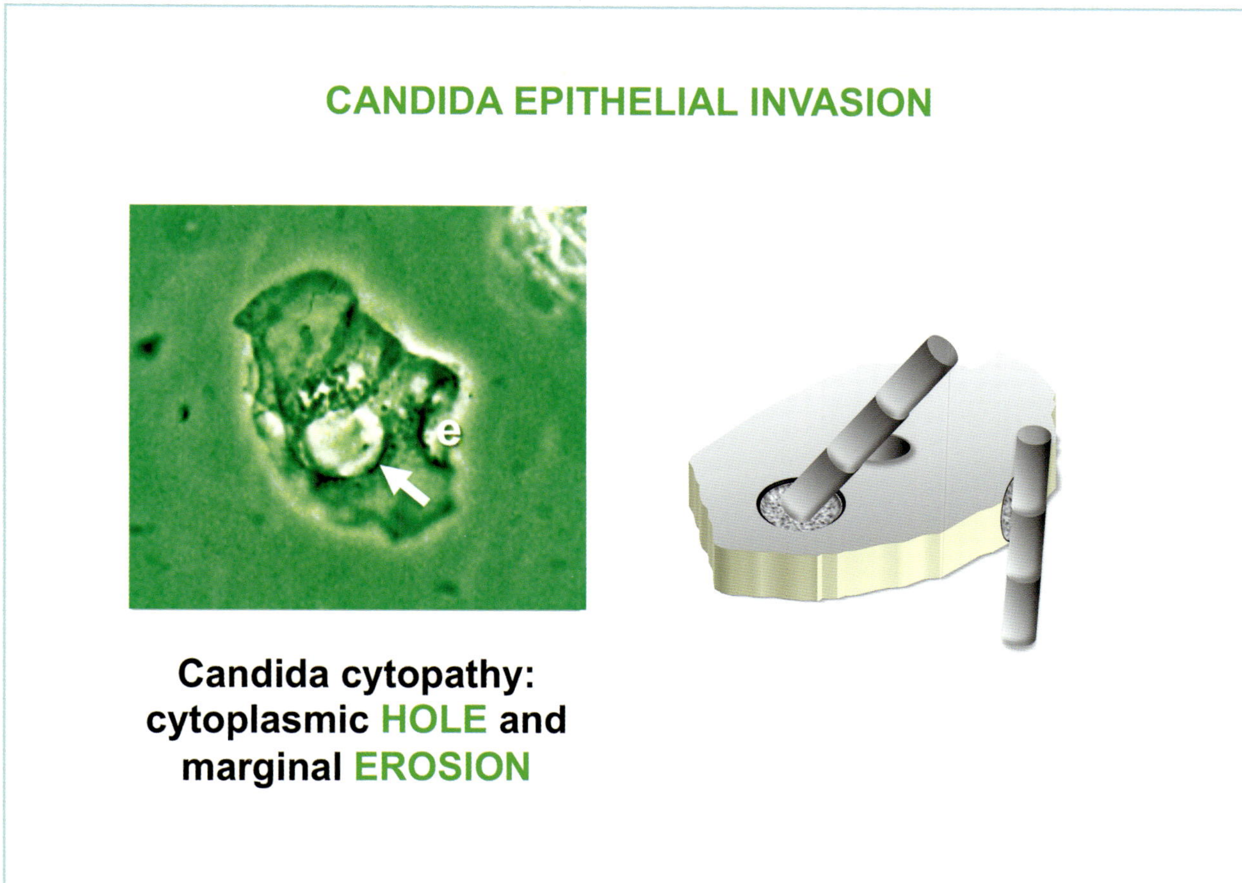

Figure 60 - Microphotograph and diagrammatic representation of Candida cytopathy: cytoplasmic hole (arrow) and marginal erosion (e) in a horny cell from the vulvar skin.

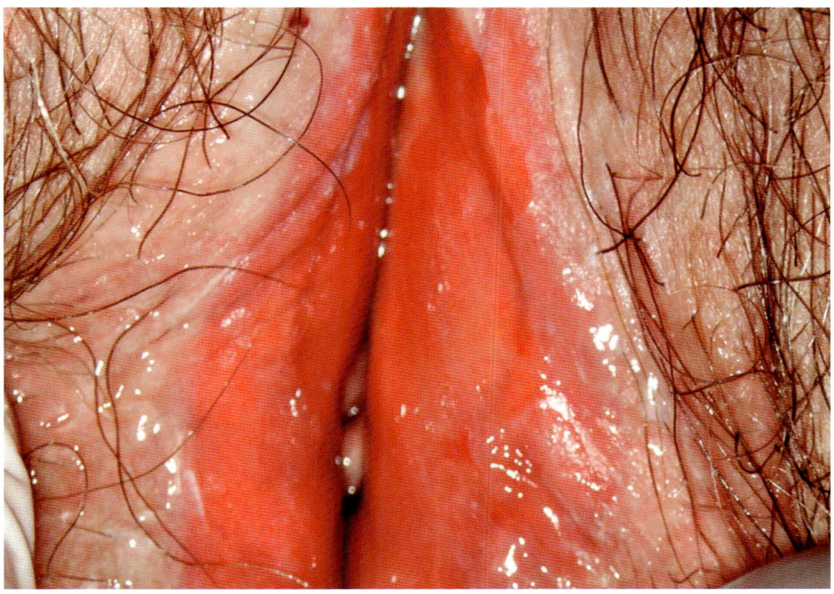

Figure 61 - Intense vulvar erythema due to exposure to hyperosmotic lubricants.

mal manifestation of exophytic condyloma. Warts appear as small to large soft, flesh-colored lumps. Condyloma acuminata may occur in clusters and some of these clusters have a cauliflower-like appearance. In the presence of anal warts (Figure 69), it is advisable to inspect the lower rectum (Figure 70). Genital and anal warts can spread, even when no warts seem to be present. The incubation period after exposure ranges from three weeks to eight months.

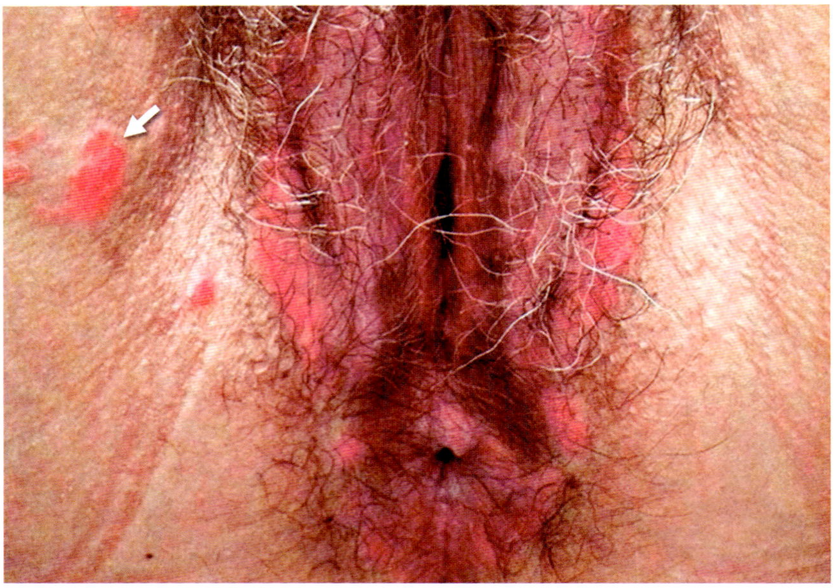

Figure 62 - Erythematous psoriasis involves both vulva and perianal skin. The arrow indicates a characteristic satellite lesion.

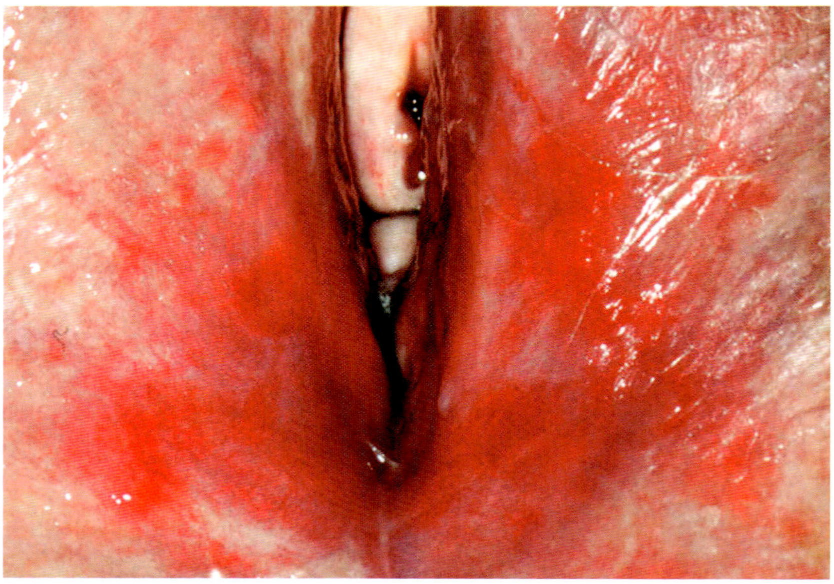

Figure 63 - Vulvar erythema in lichen planus.

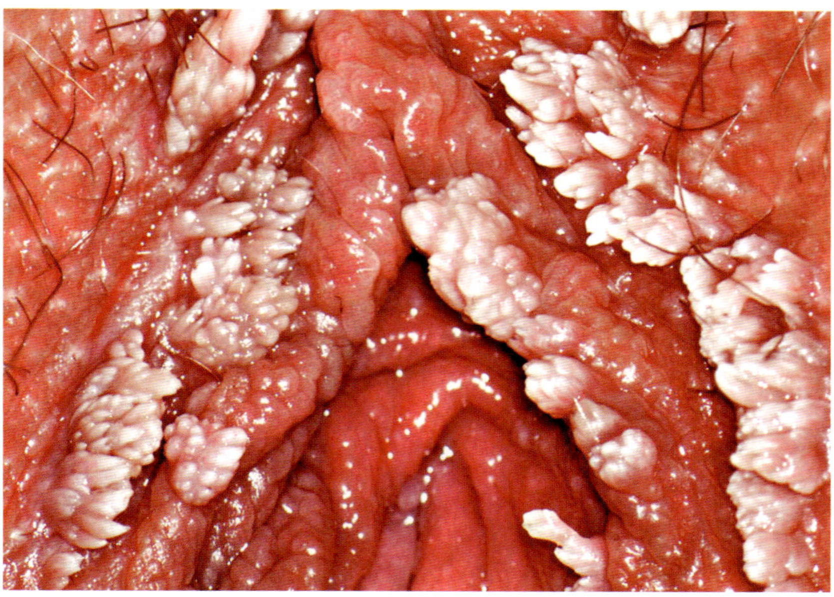

Figure 64 - Vulvar exophytic condyloma. After application of acetic acid, vessels are masked, whereas the finger-like processes whiten, retract and separate, so becoming more easily recognizable.

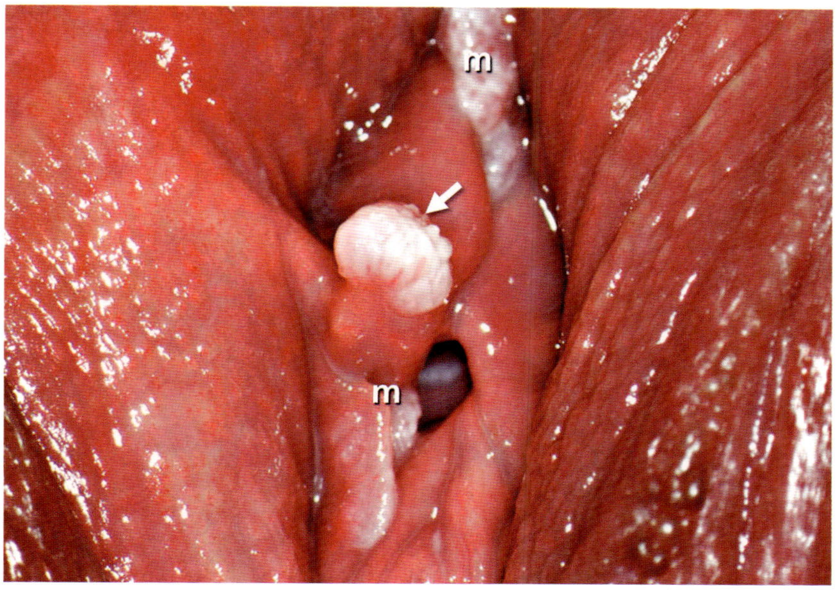

Figure 65 - Vestibular florid condyloma (arrow) and HPV micropapillary lesions (m).

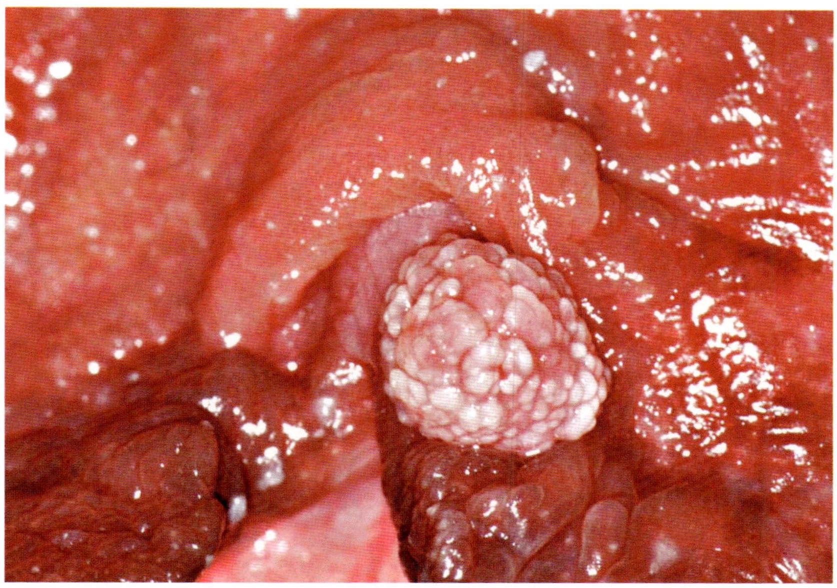

Figure 66 - Clitoral florid condyloma.

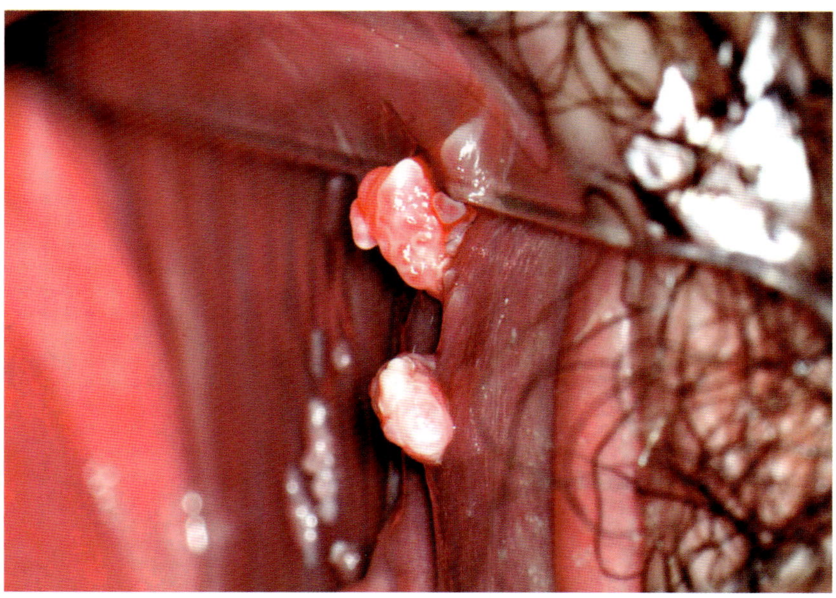

Figure 67 - Florid condylomas involve the vaginal wall.

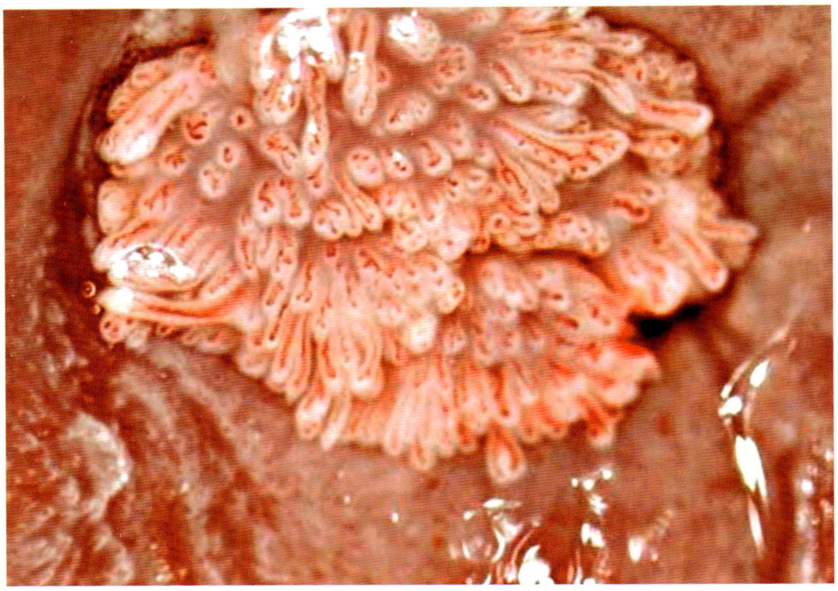

Figure 68 - Cervical exophytic condyloma with typical elongated finger-like processes containing dilated axial capillaries.

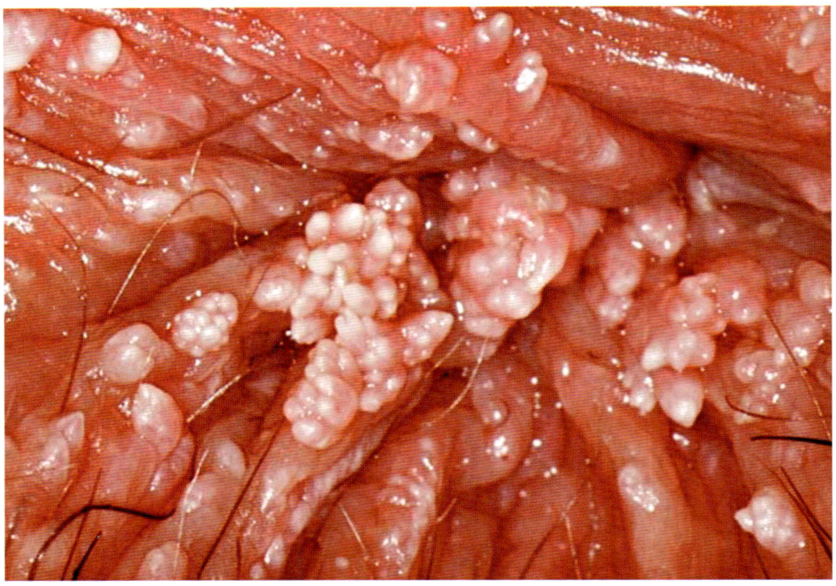

Figure 69 - Anal warts.

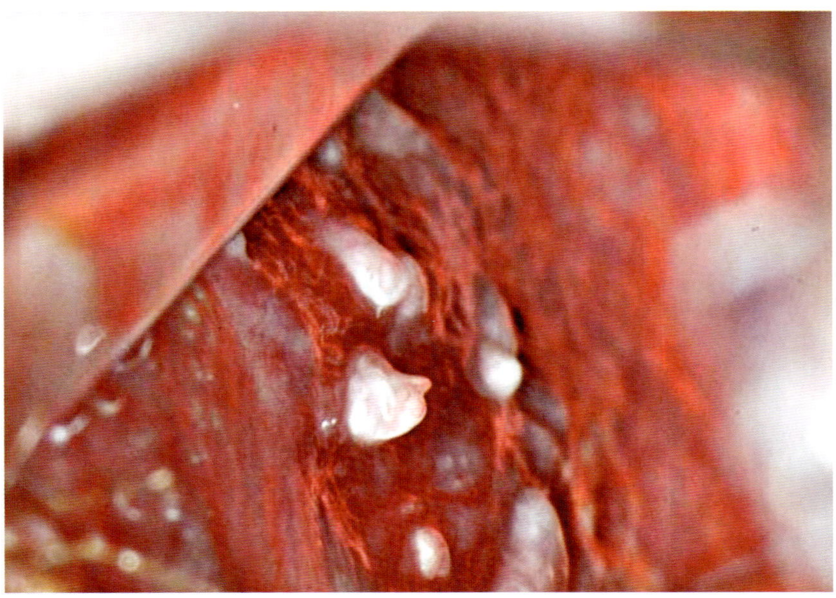

Figure 70 - Rectal exophytic condylomas.

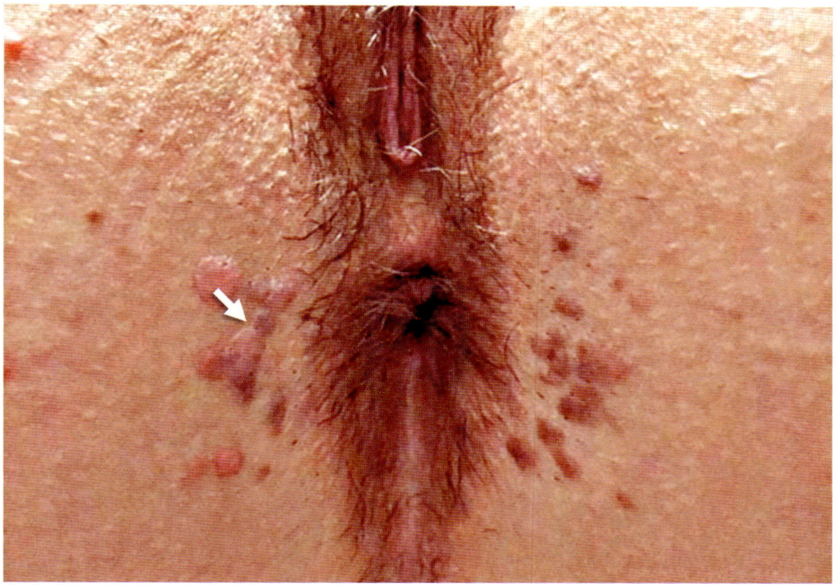

Figure 71 - Perianal Bowenoid Papulosis. The lesions may be confluent (arrow).

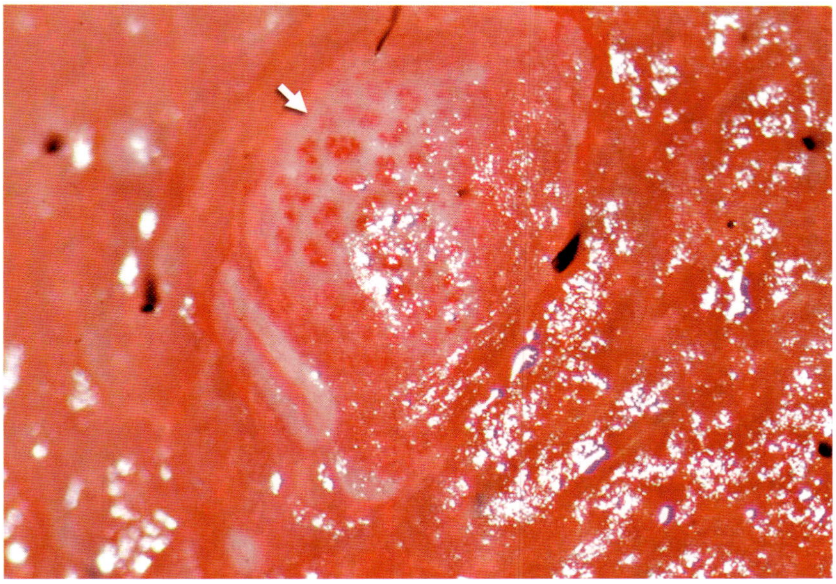

Figure 72 - HPV micropapillary lesion of the genital skin (arrow).

Bowenoid papulosis (Figure 71) is a rare form of intraepithelial neoplasia that can mimic genital or anal warts. It has single or multiple small, red, brown or flesh-colored spots or patches on the genitals and perianal region. The diagnosis is usually made by skin biopsy.

Micropapillary lesions show a micropapillary surface appearance and a fine vascular arrangement similar to a miniature condyloma. They are not easily detected without a special examination of the skin (Figure 72), vaginal vestibule (Figure 73), vagina (Figure 74), cervix (Figure 75) and perianal region (Figure 76). Sometimes, especially on the everted columnar epithelium, and even in the presence of surface excrescences, the epithelium affected by HPV and containing koilocytes can involve columnar crypts. This particular histologic type of lesion is known as *inverted condyloma*.

Human Papillomavirus can induce specific cytopathic effects that are easily detectable by microscopy: koilocyte, dark nuclei and multinucleation. *Koilocyte* (Figure 77) shows a characteristic wide perinuclear halo with a sharply condensed border. The nucleus may exhibit an irregular membrane contour and usually appears enlarged (two to three times the normal size) with abnormal chromatin distribution. A darker than normal staining pattern in the nucleus known as *hyperchromasia* can be observed in HPV infection. As wet mount microscopy does not recur to staining, the term *dark nuclei* (Figures 78, 79) is preferred to hyperchromasia.

Multiple nuclei all derive from one nucleus (Figure 80).

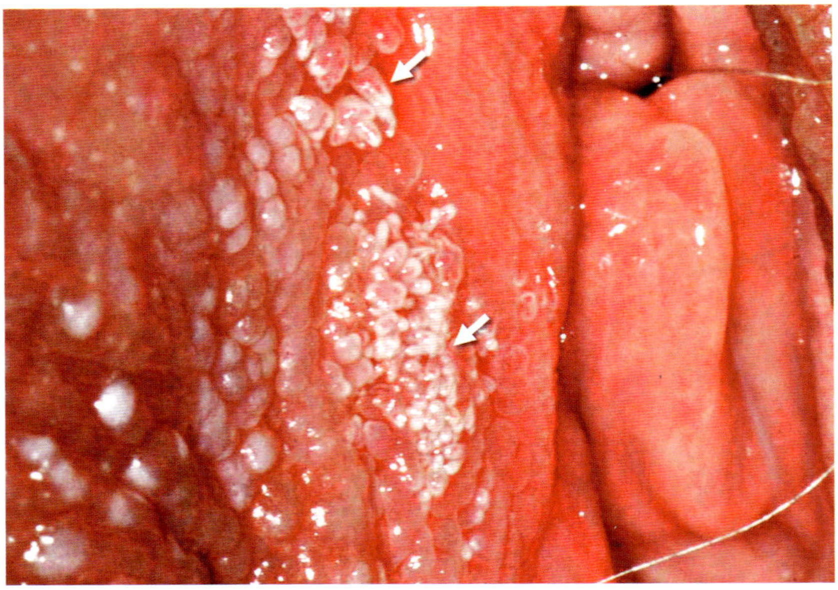

Figure 73 - HPV micropapillary lesions of the vestibule (arrows).

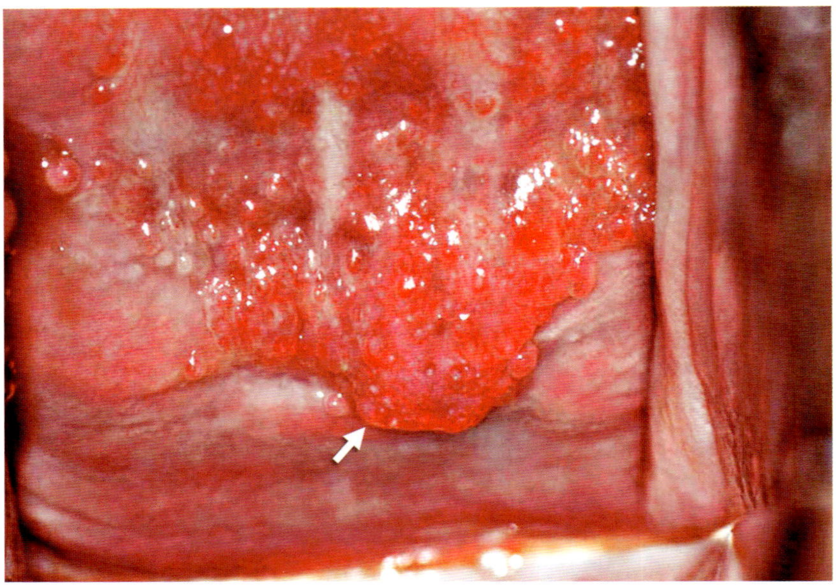

Figure 74 - HPV micropapillary lesion of the posterior vaginal fornix (arrow).

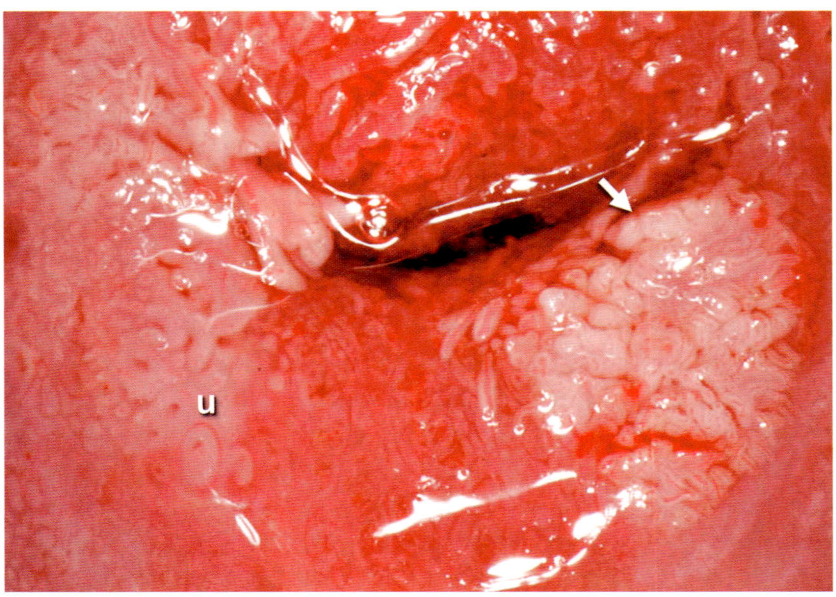

Figure 75 - HPV micropapillary lesion of the posterior lip of the cervix (arrow) and umbilication (u).

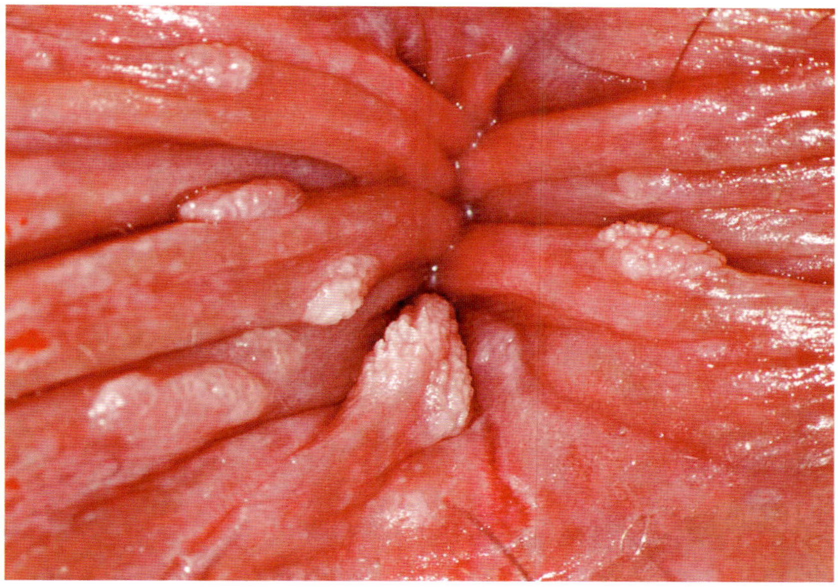

Figure 76 - Perianal HPV micropapillary lesions.

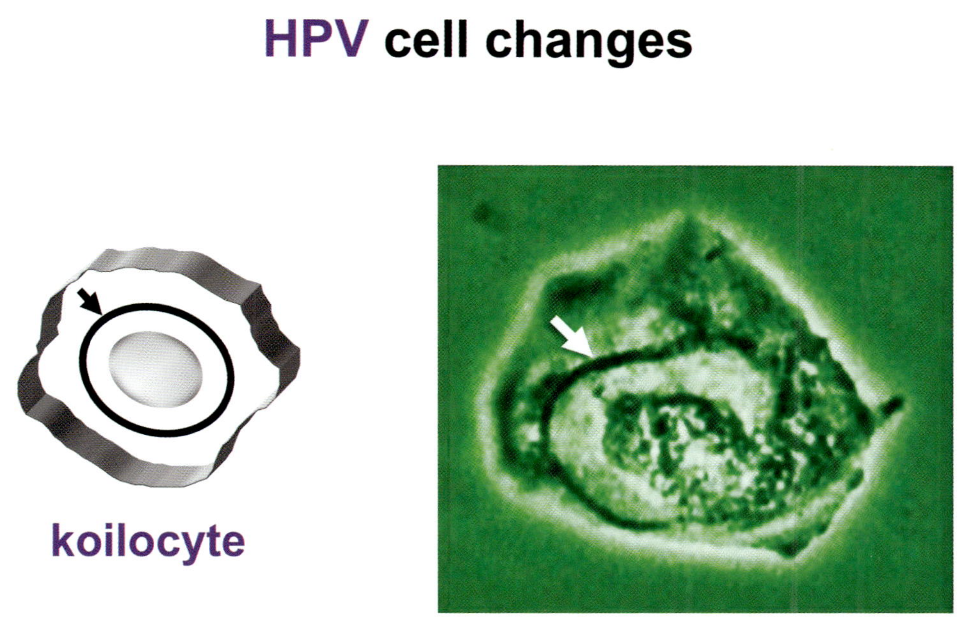

Figure 77 - Diagrammatic representation and wet mount appearance of a koilocyte with the sharply condensed border (arrows) delimiting the wide perinuclear halo.

When multinucleation is present, nuclei are dispersed in the cytoplasm, or at least appear overlapping, but they are never gathered and molded as in polykaryocyte by Herpes simplex virus (HSV) (Figure 81). Furthermore, nuclei affected by HSV often contain coarse intranuclear inclusions (Figure 82) and always appear pale, with a "ground glass" aspect.

Micropapillary lesions induced by HPV must be distinguished from vestibular papillae (Figure 83) which represent a variant in normal epithelium and

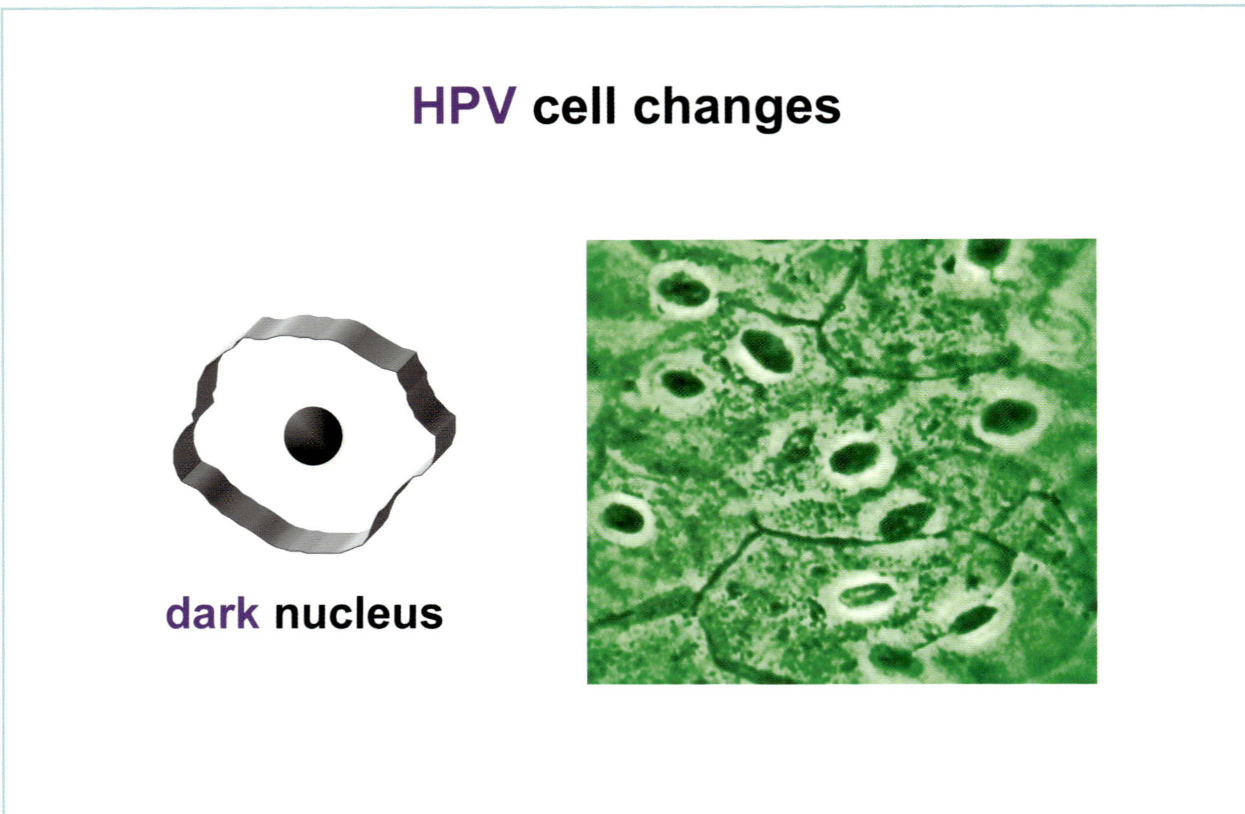

Figure 78 - Diagrammatic representation and wet mount appearance of dark nuclei, due to condensed chromatin.

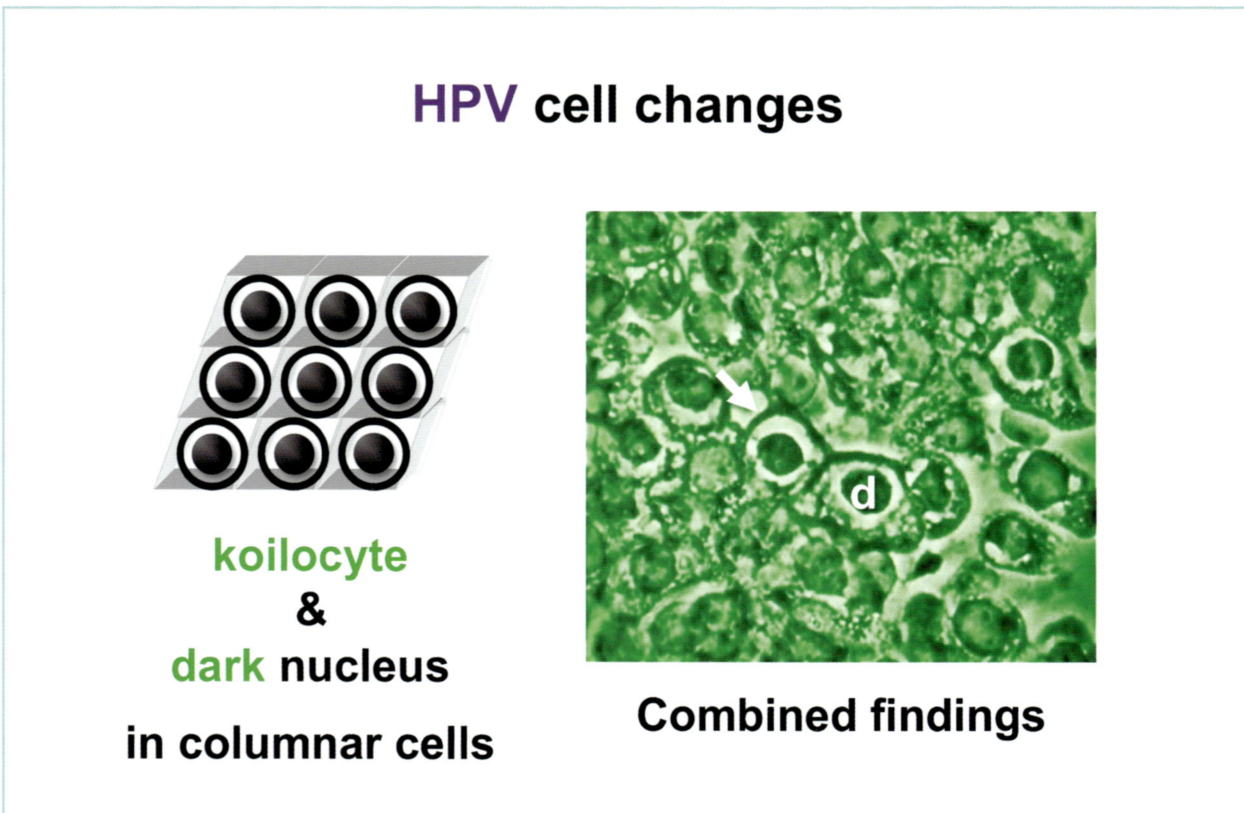

Figure 79 - Diagrammatic representation and wet mount appearance of columnar cells seen end on, showing the characteristic sharp border (arrow) around the perinuclear halo, and dark nuclei (d).

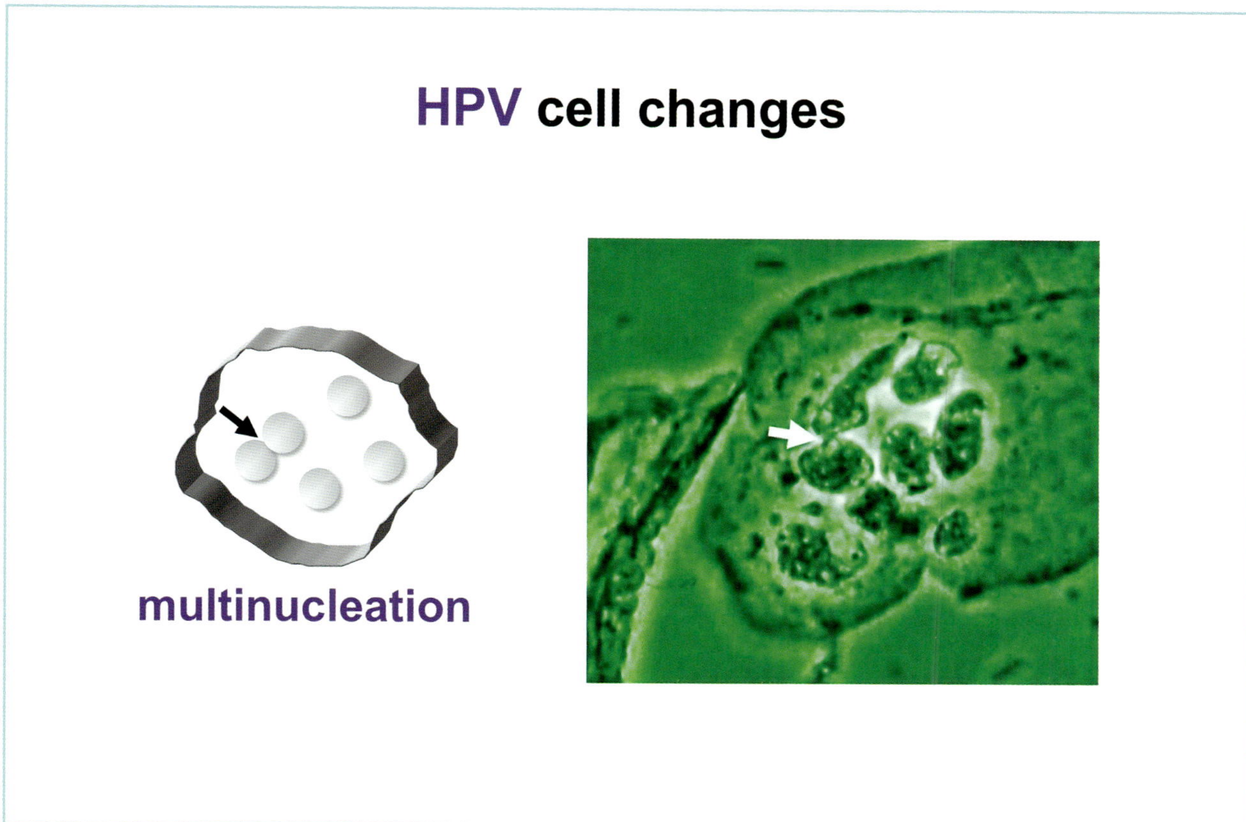

Figure 80 - Diagrammatic representation and wet mount appearance of multinucleation. The arrows indicate the dividing nucleus which generates the other nuclei.

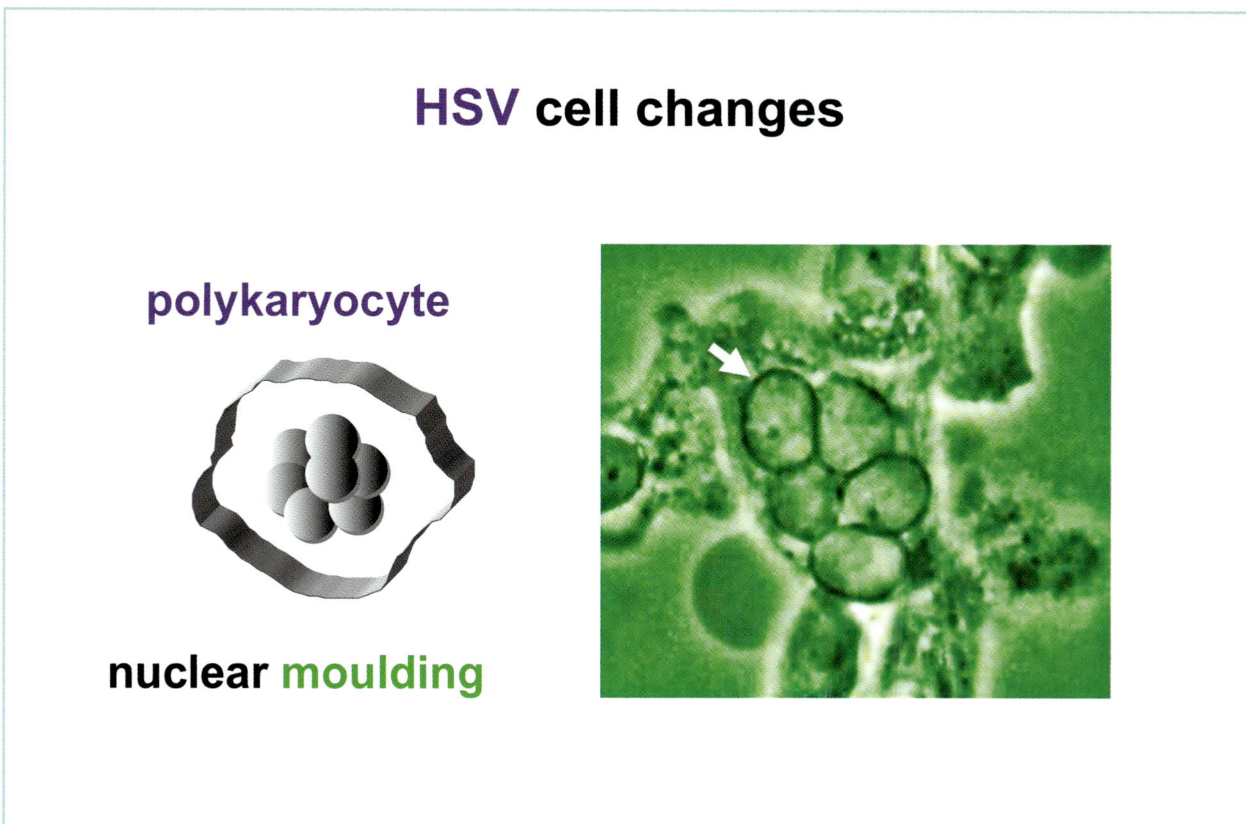

Figure 81 - Diagrammatic representation and wet mount appearance of a polykaryocyte (arrow) in HSV infection. Ground glass nuclei appear molded, resembling a blackberry.

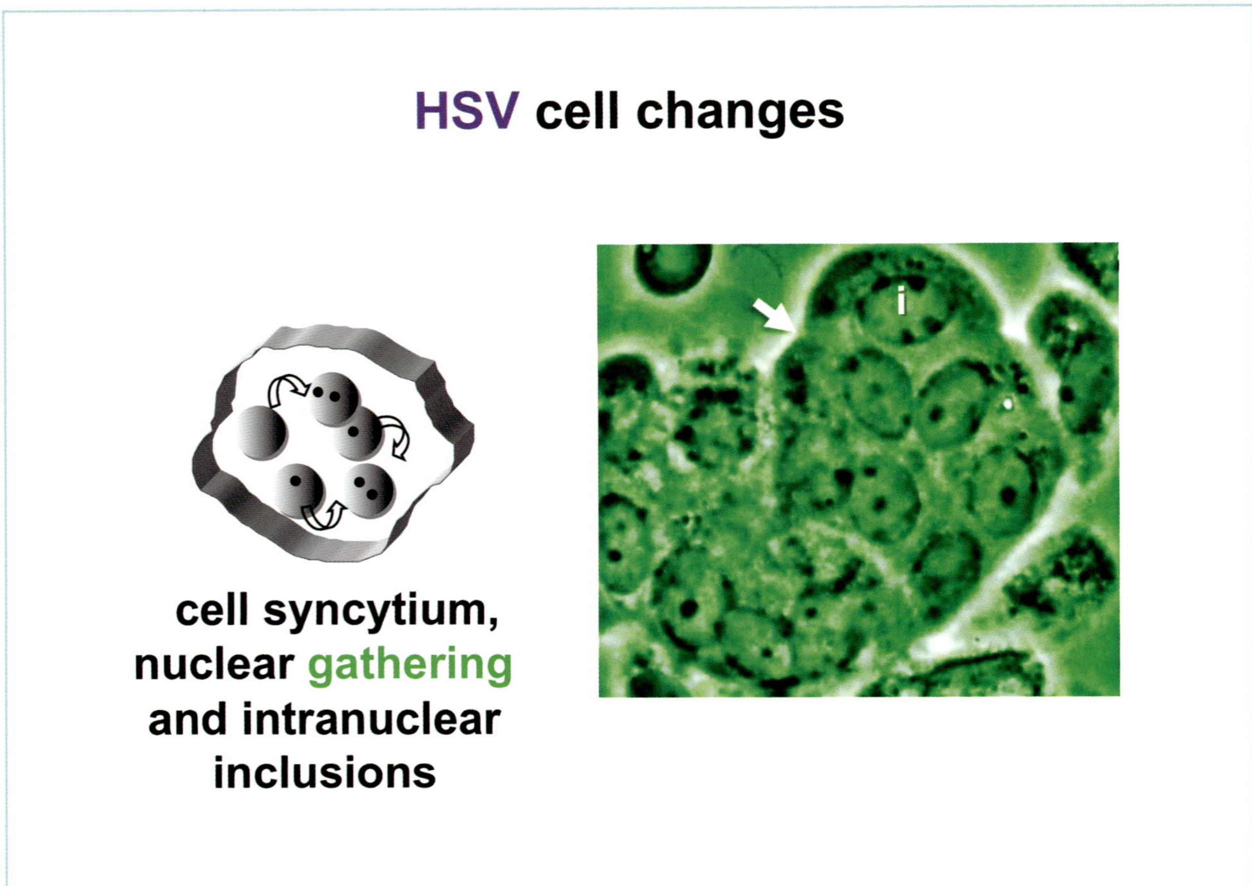

Figure 82 - Diagrammatic representation and wet mount appearance of a cell syncytium (arrow), where nuclei tend to gather. Intranuclear inclusions (i).

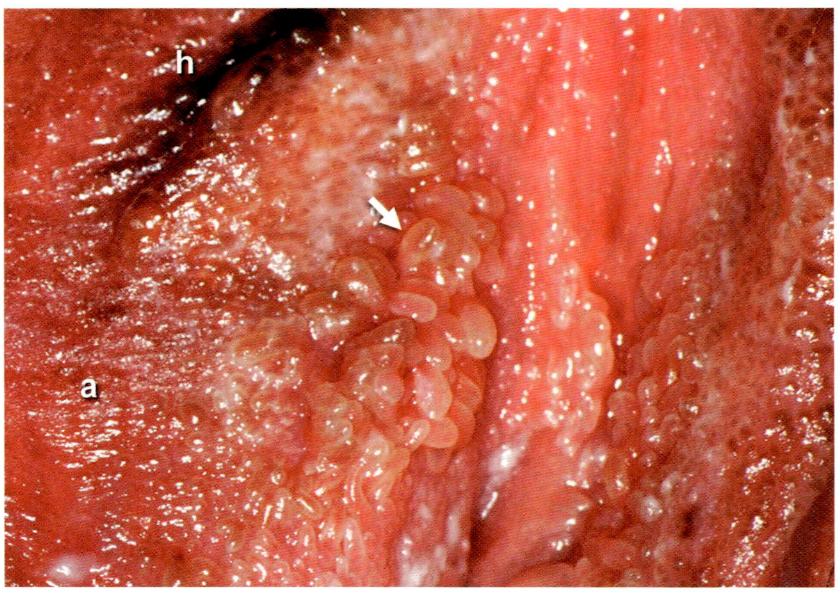

Figure 83 - Normal vestibular papillae. Agenesis (a) of the right labium minus and hyperpigmentation (h) in correspondence of the hypotrophic superior portion of the labium.

may be caused by constant rubbing. Vestibular papillae correspond to the small protuberances that may form on the ridge of penile glans in hirsuties coronae glandis (Figure 84). Sometimes, vestibular papillae appear particularly hypertrophic and elongated (Figure 85). Vestibular and hymenal (Figure 86) papillae look like finger-like smooth, soft projections which can be several millimetres long. Unlike HPV induced lesions, normal papillae show a regular shape and distribution and no tendency to

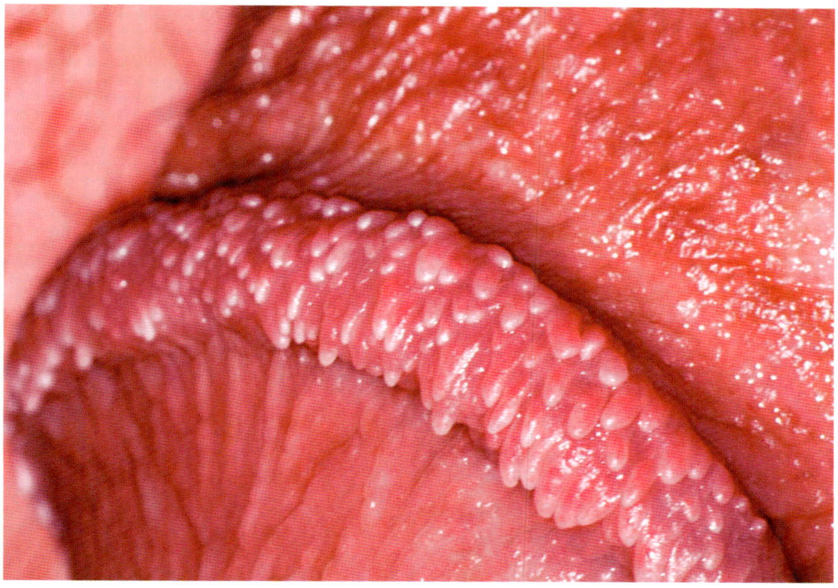

Figure 84 - Vestibular papillae correspond to the small protuberances present in hirsuties coronae glandis in male.

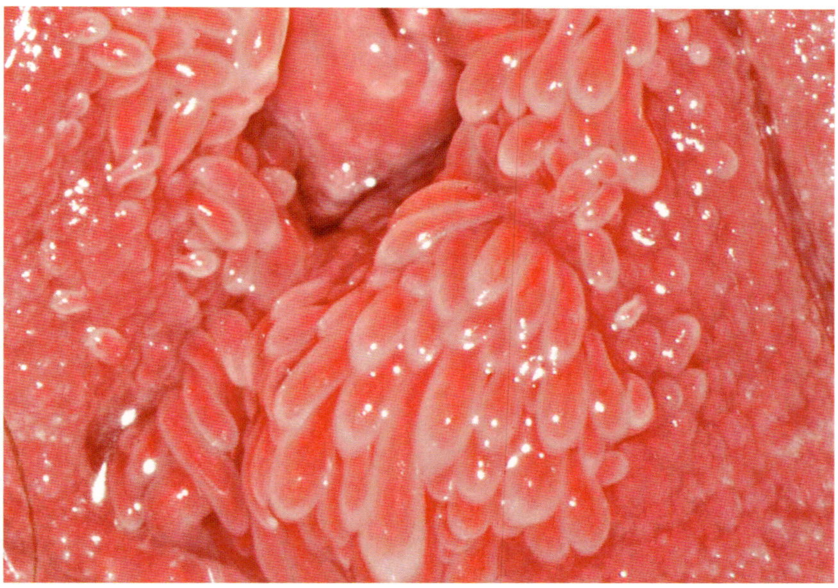

Figure 85 - Hypertrophic and elongated vestibular papillae.

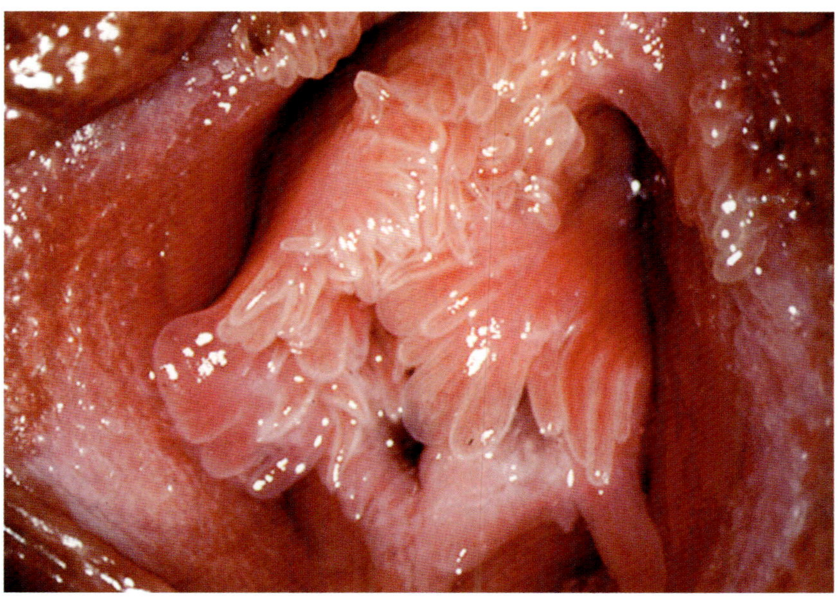

Figure 86 - Hypertrophic hymenal papillae.

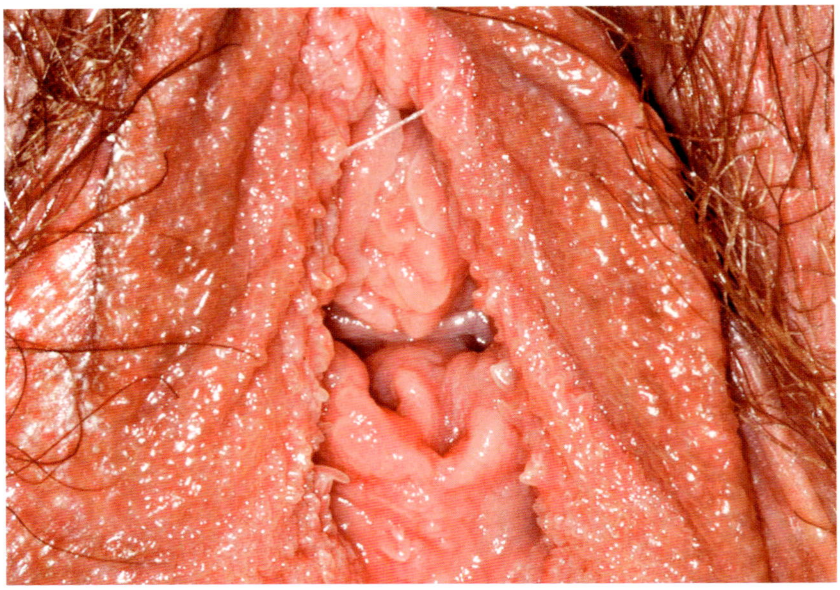

Figure 87 - Numerous and largely diffused vestibular papillae define the so called vestibular papillomatosis.

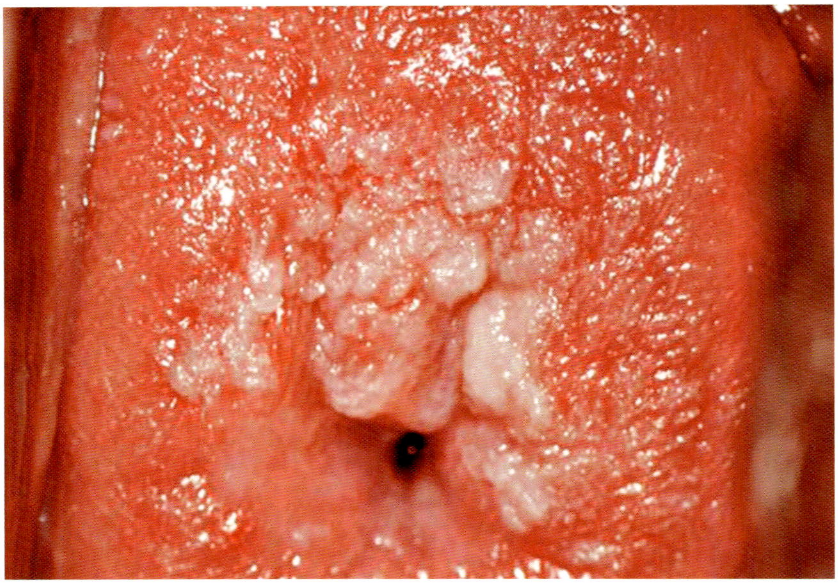

Figure 88 - Thick keratosis.

fuse. When they are numerous and largely diffused, the anatomical appearance is termed vestibular papillomatosis (Figure 87), even if this term may generate confusion.

Thick **keratosis** or leukoplakia (Figure 88) may mimic micropapillary lesions but keratosis is an epithelium that appears white before application of acetic acid, due to the presence of keratin. Keratosis is usually idiopathic, but may be caused by estrogen stimulation, inflammatory conditions, recurrent vaginal infections, chronic foreign body irritation, HPV infection and even squamous neoplasia.

The term keratosis is preferred to leukoplakia because keratosis is not always observed in the form of a well-demarcated white area, but may show a white epithelium with diffuse margins or may be seen in the form of scattered fine granules on the cervix (Figure 89) or on the vagina (Figure 90). Keratosis does not involve only the cervix, but also the vagina (Figure 91), vulva (Figure 92) and anus (Figure 93). Keratosis involving anus must be differentiated from anal lichen sclerosus (Figure 94).

Histologically, leukoplakia is due to hyperkeratosis and parakeratosis, both characterized by a highly keratinized cytoplasm of the cells (Figure 95). Hyperkeratosis is represented by horny cells which are anucleate or show only a nuclear shadow (Figure 96). Parakeratosis is characterized by parakeratotic cells which like horny cells show a highly keratinized cytoplasm but still contain a viable nucleus (Figure 97). Histologically, keratosis is often associated with acanthosis, an increase in the number of cells in the

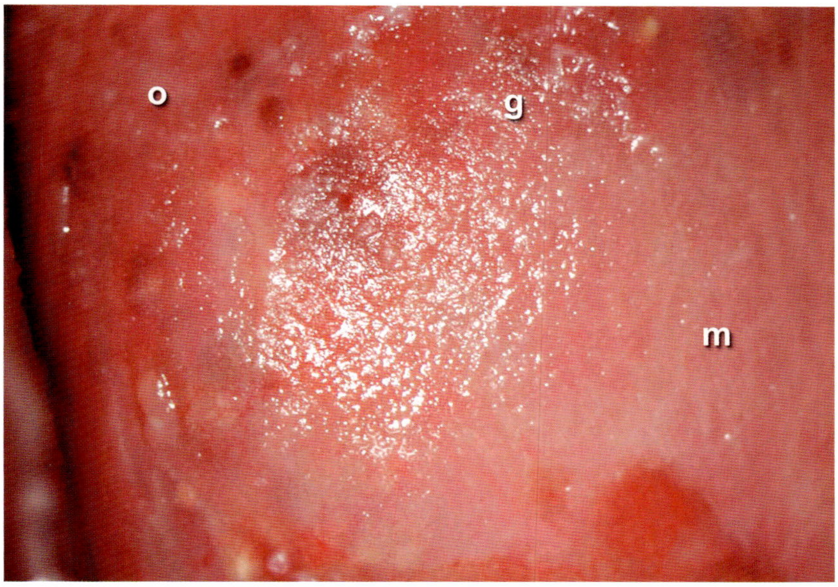

Figure 89 - Scattered keratotic granules (g) on a mature squamous metaplastic epithelium (m) which appears whitish-pink, in contrast with the darker pink original squamous epithelium (o).

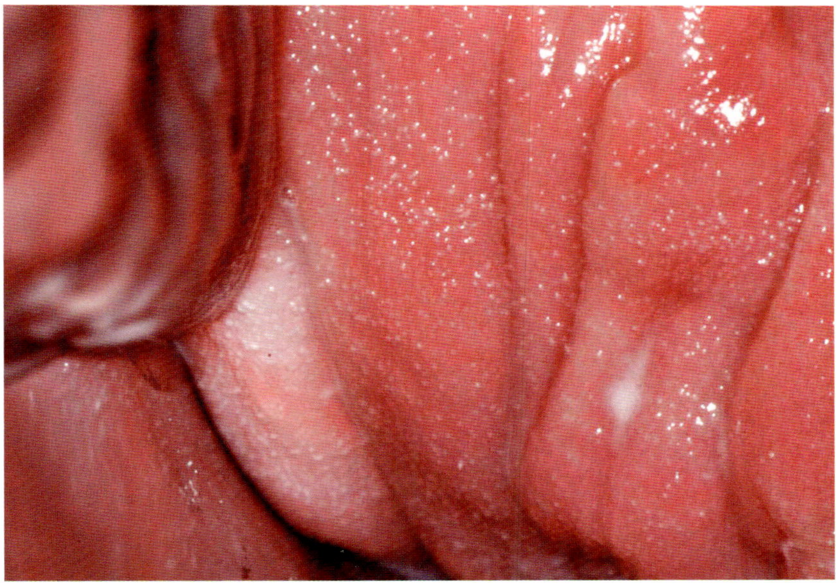

Figure 90 - Scattered vaginal keratotic granules.

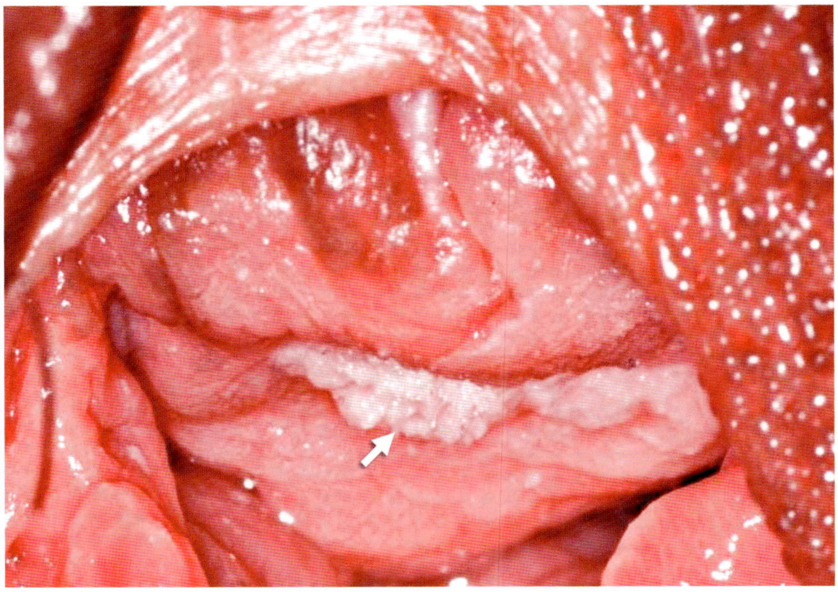

Figure 91 - Thick and irregular keratosis on the anterior vaginal wall (arrow).

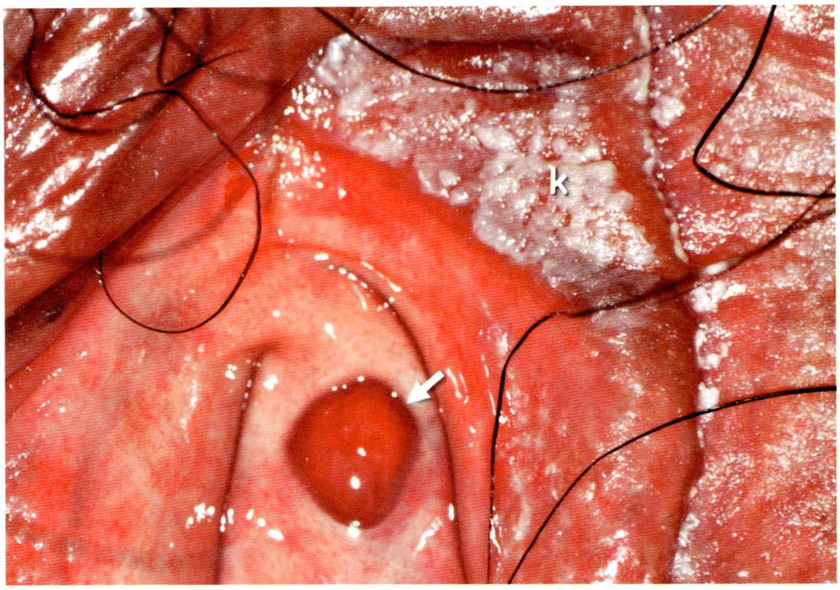

Figure 92 - Thick keratosis (k) involving vulvar labia in a post-menopausal woman affected by lichen sclerosus. The arrow indicates a benign red, congested outgrowth of the posterior lip of the urethral meatus (urethral caruncle).

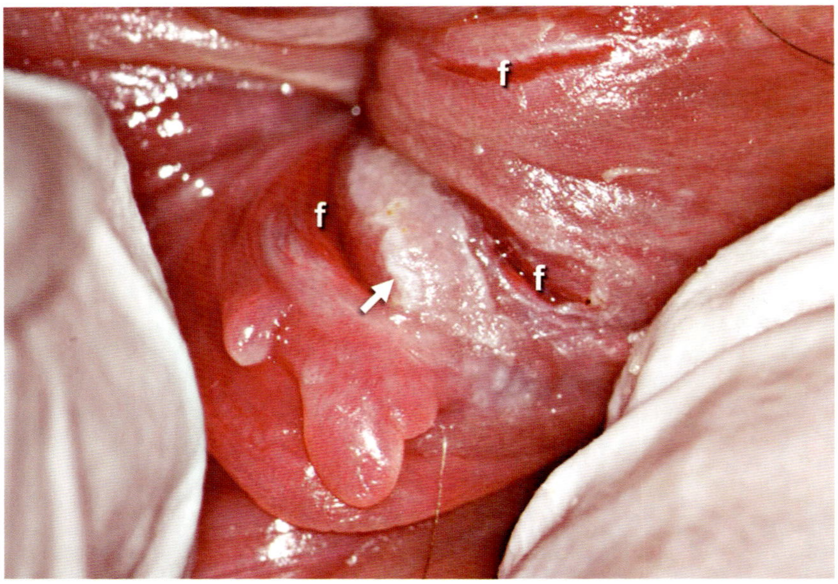

Figure 93 - Anal keratosis of varying grade (arrow). Perianal fissures (f).

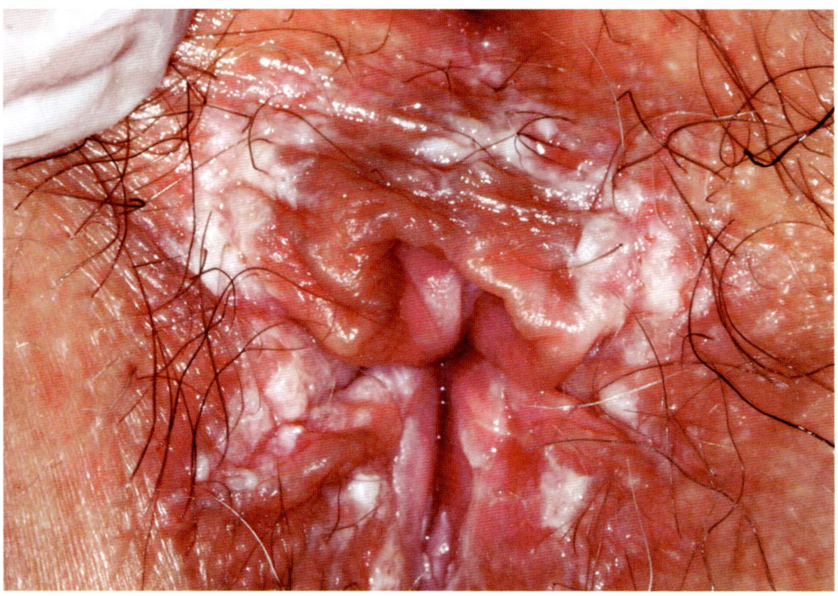

Figure 94 - Lichen sclerosus involving only the anus in a 28-year-old woman.

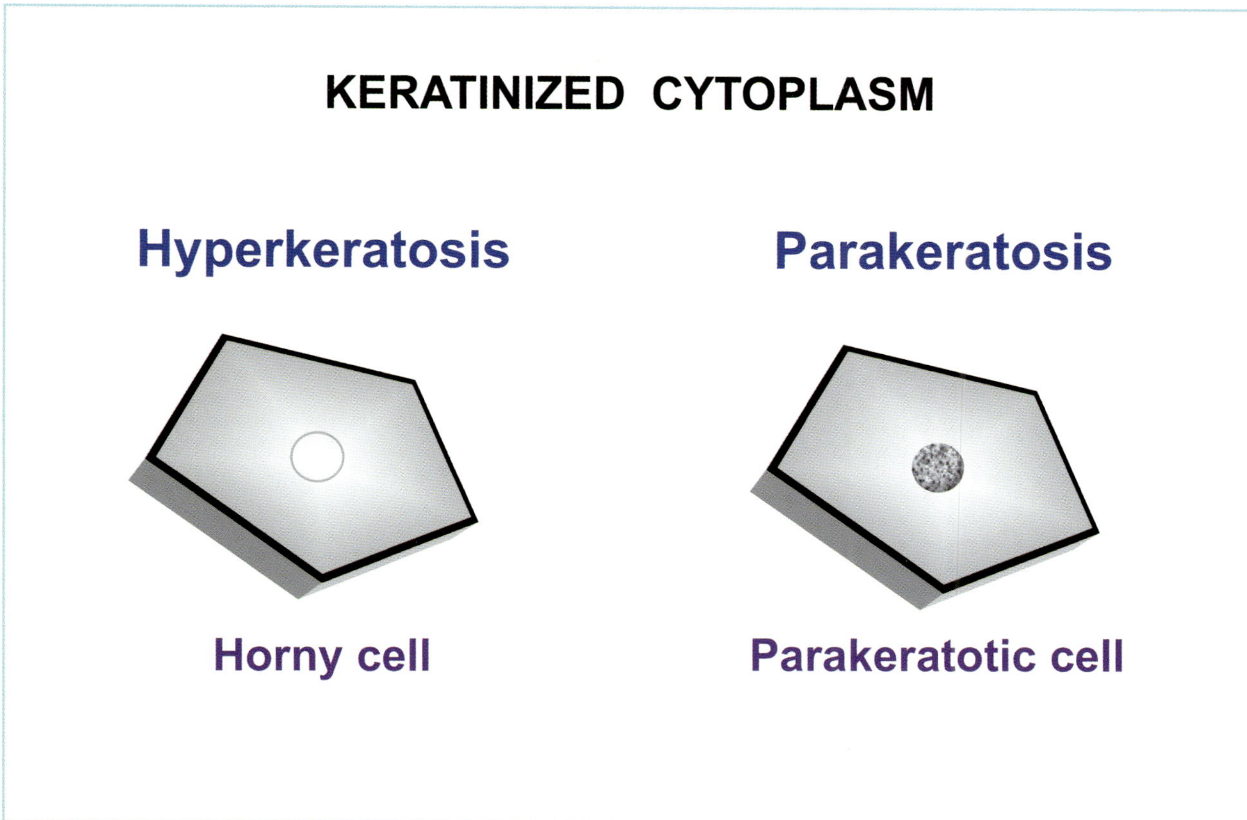

Figure 95 - Diagrammatic representation of keratinized cytoplasm.

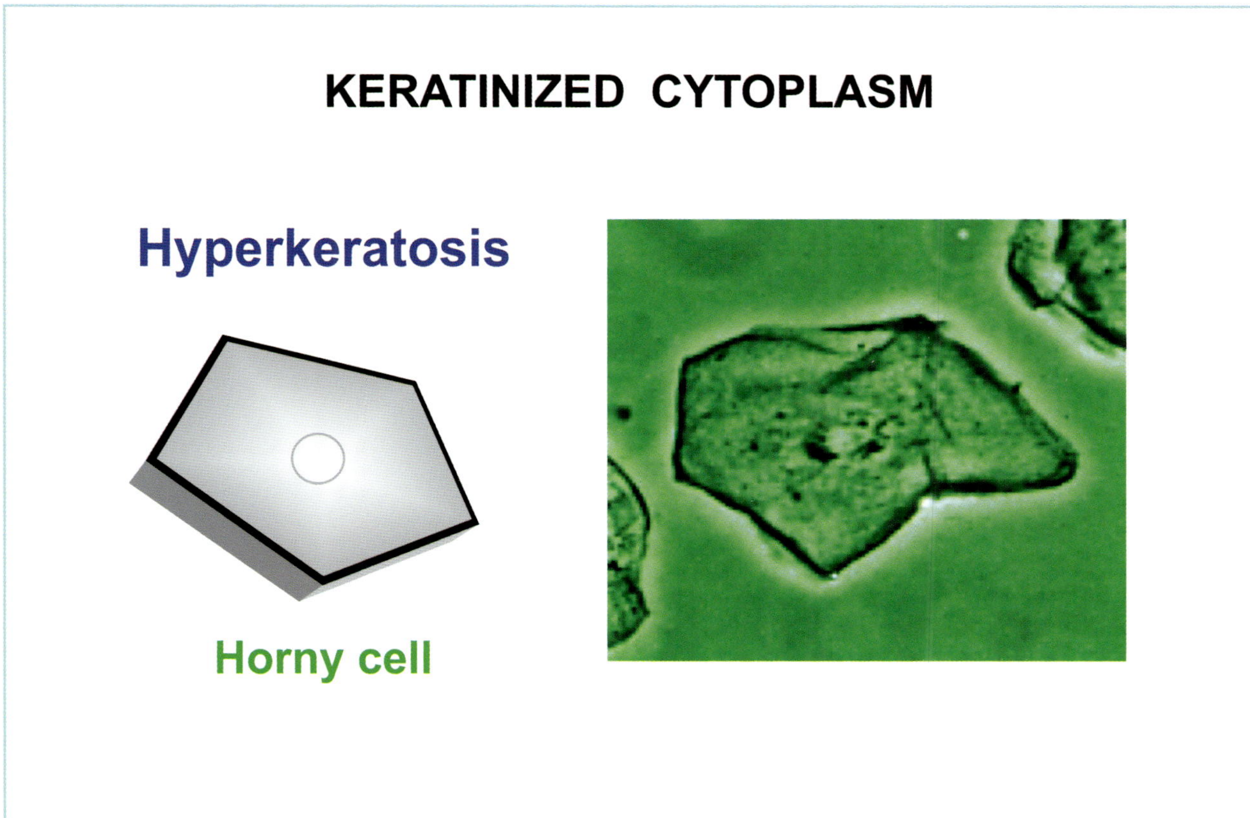

Figure 96 - Diagrammatic representation and microphotograph of an anucleate horny cell.

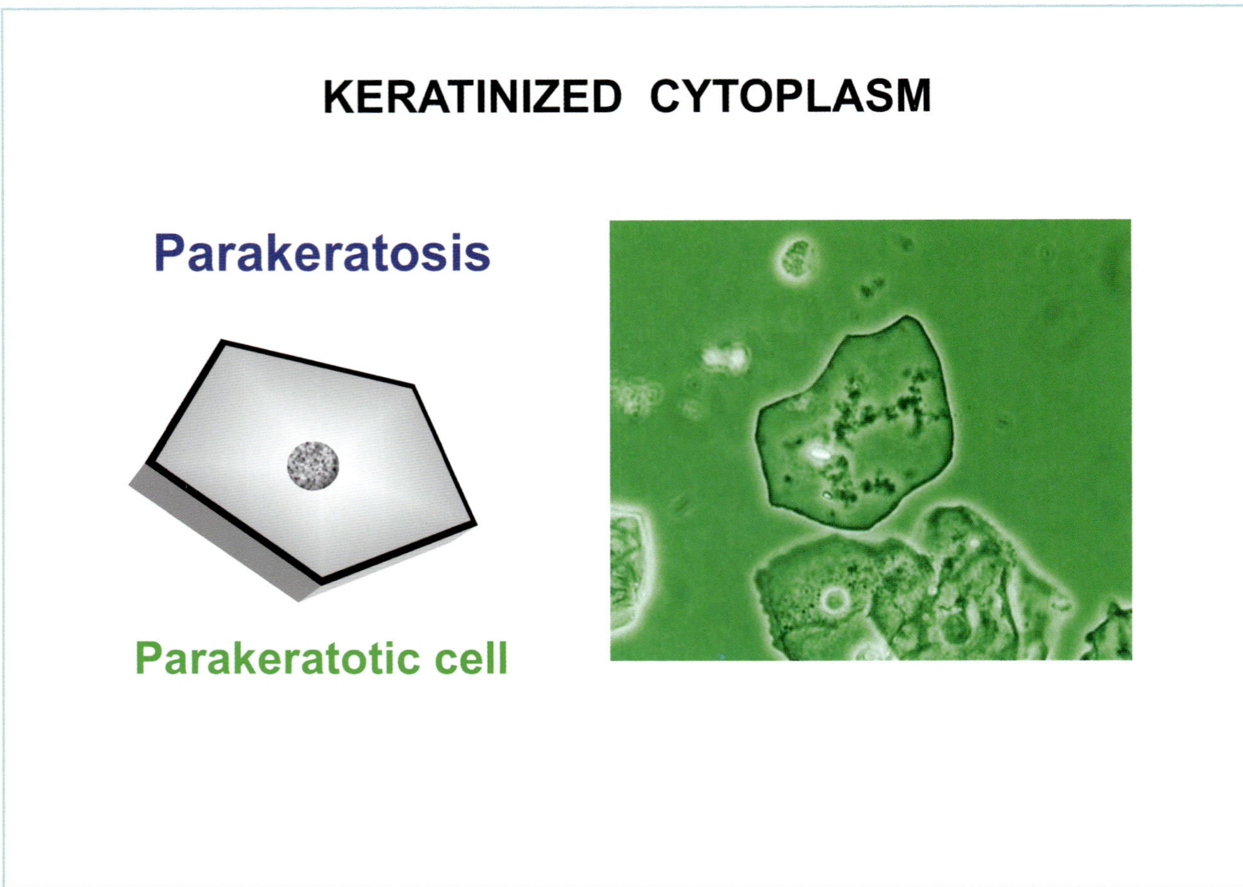

Figure 97 - Diagrammatic representation and microphotograph of a parakeratotic cell with a viable, pyknotic nucleus.

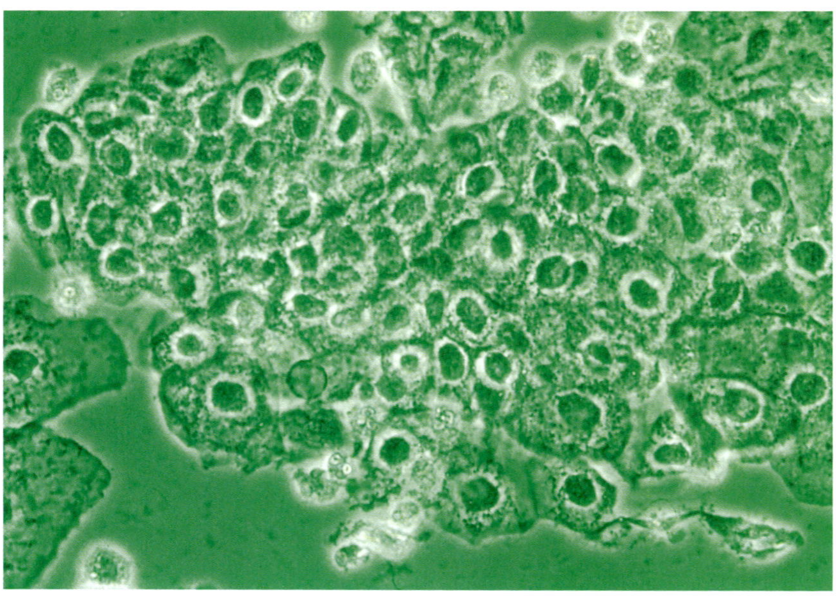

Figure 98 - Direct microscopy appearance of a sheet of akantotic prickle-cells, containing characteristic crowded nuclei.

prickle cell layer of stratified squamous epithelium, with crowding of the nuclei (Figure 98).
Leukoplakia may be thin, which is usually not significant (Figure 99), or thick with an uneven surface (Figure 100). All degrees of keratosis, including keratotic granules, may be simultaneously present on the cervix (Figure 101). When the keratin layer is peeled off, red punctation appears (Figure 102).
Any thick leukoplakia should be biopsied to rule out pronounced atypical lesions such as high-grade

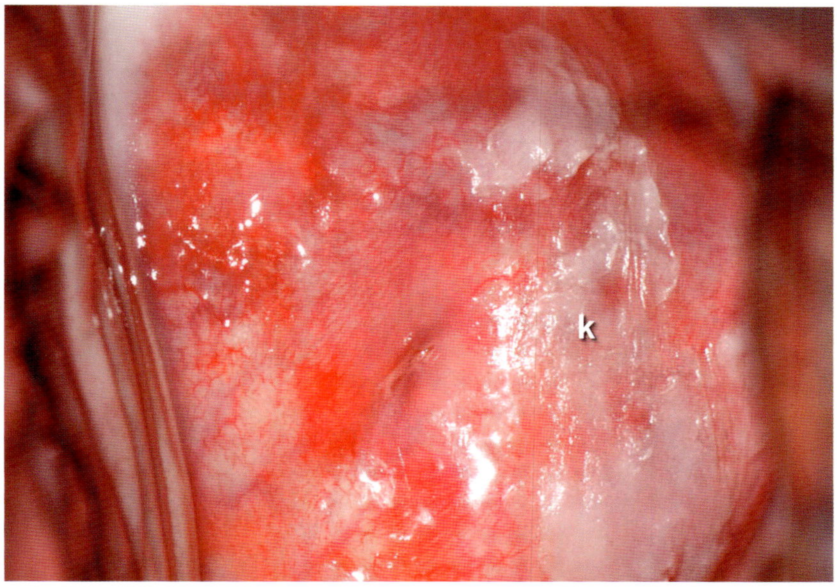

Figure 99 - Extended thin keratosis (k).

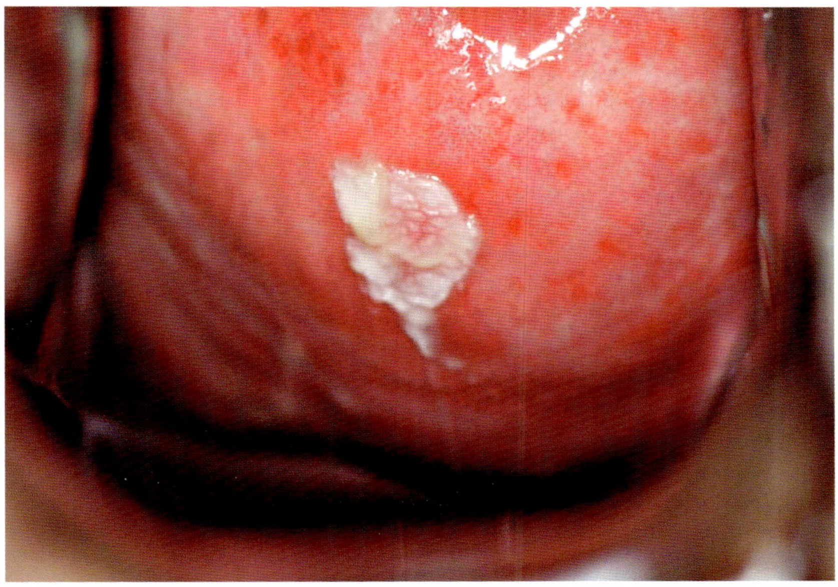

Figure 100 - Thick keratosis.

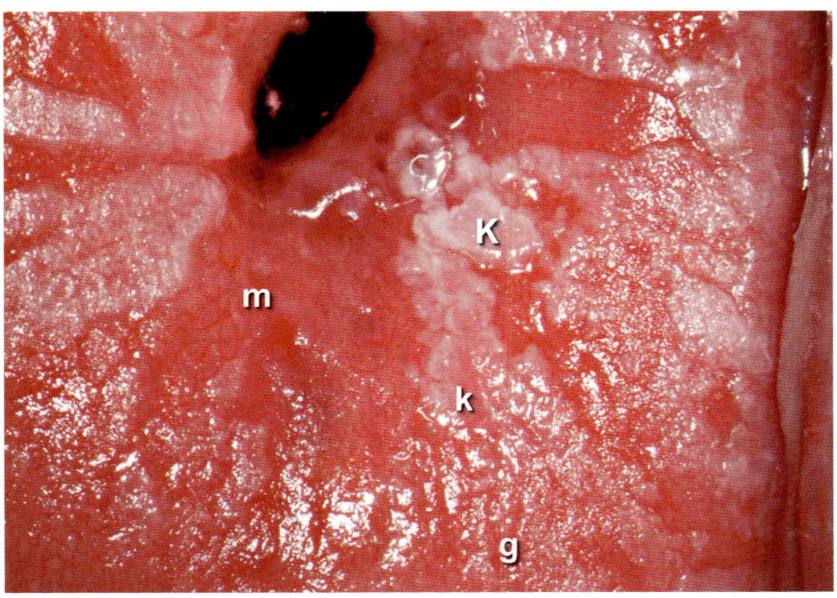

Figure 101 - Thick keratosis (K), thin (k) keratosis, and keratotic granules (g) are concurrently present on the cervix. A small area of mosaic base (m) can be observed.

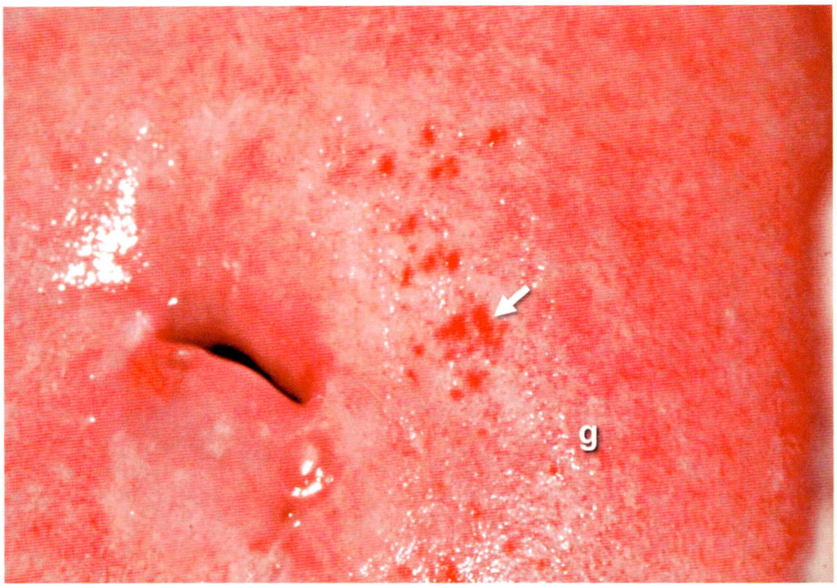

Figure 102 - When the keratin layer is peeled off, red punctation appears (arrow). Persistent keratotic granules (g).

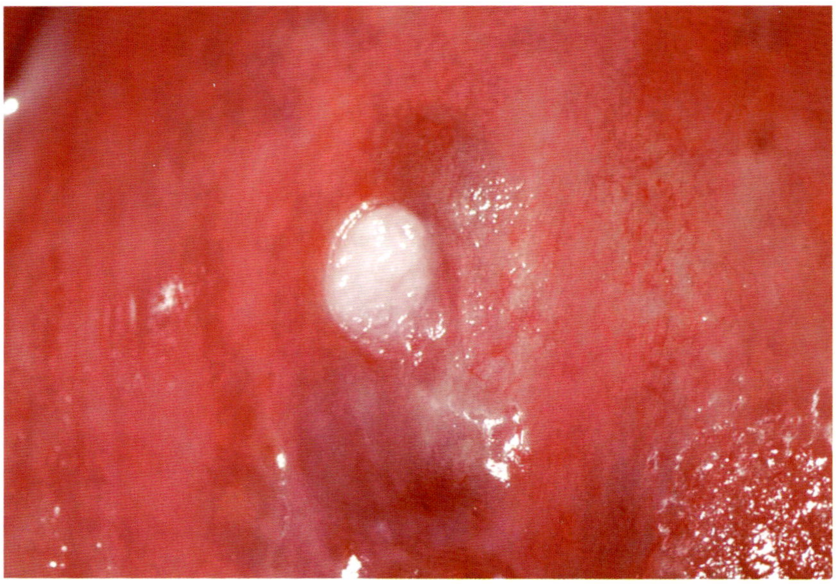

Figure 103 - Well circumscribed area of thick keratosis. The keratin covered an underlying carcinoma in situ.

CIN or malignancy (Figure 103). Sometimes thick, irregular keratosis can be seen overlying neoplastic lesions (Figure 104).

HPV flat lesions are diagnosed colposcopically or by visual inspection with acetic acid (VIA), and hence are termed Subclinical Papillomavirus Infections (SPI).

Flat condylomas may show a finely granular or a distinctive pearly surface as a result of hyperkeratosis observable on the cervix (Figure 105), vestibular introitus (Figure 106), hymen (Figure 107), clitoris (Figure 108), vaginal walls (Figure 109), and perianal skin (Figure 110). These flat lesions can display a punctation (see Figure 105) or mosaic, depending on whether the supporting stroma produces papillae or ridges. The thickness of epithelium and the stromal architecture render the surface of flat condylomas coarser of similar colposcopic lesions due to atypical epithelia, even if the difference based on colposcopic is sometimes difficult. On histology, nuclear atypia must be present to make a diagnosis of HPV-related lesion.

Scattered cervical (Figure 111) and vaginal (Figure 112) flat condylomas must be differentiated from centrally depressed erythematous papules induced by Candida infection (Figure 113). Once acetic acid has been applied, fungal papules remain reddish or may appear faint white with a red contour (Figure 114), and disappear after a proper therapy based on a correct diagnosis with wet mount microscopy.

During pregnancy, cervical (Figure 115) or vaginal (Figure 116) decidual polyps may be misinterpreted

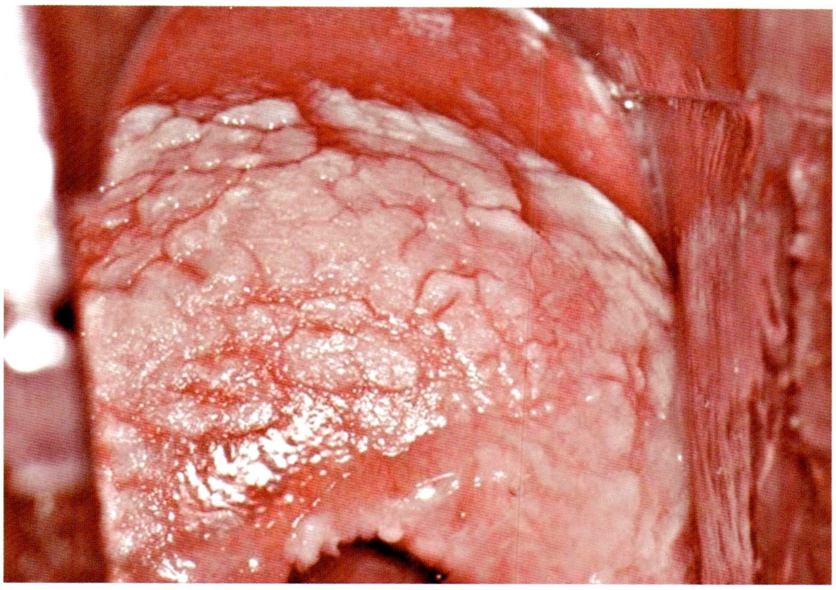

Figure 104 - Extensive and intense thick keratosis. Biopsy disclosed a small area of frank invasive squamous cell carcinoma.

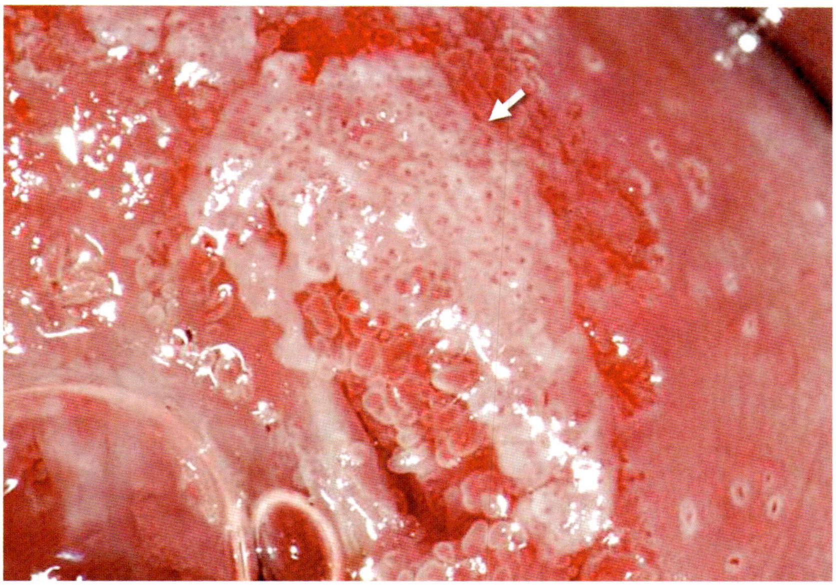

Figure 105 - Cervical HPV flat condyloma (arrow) with coarse punctation.

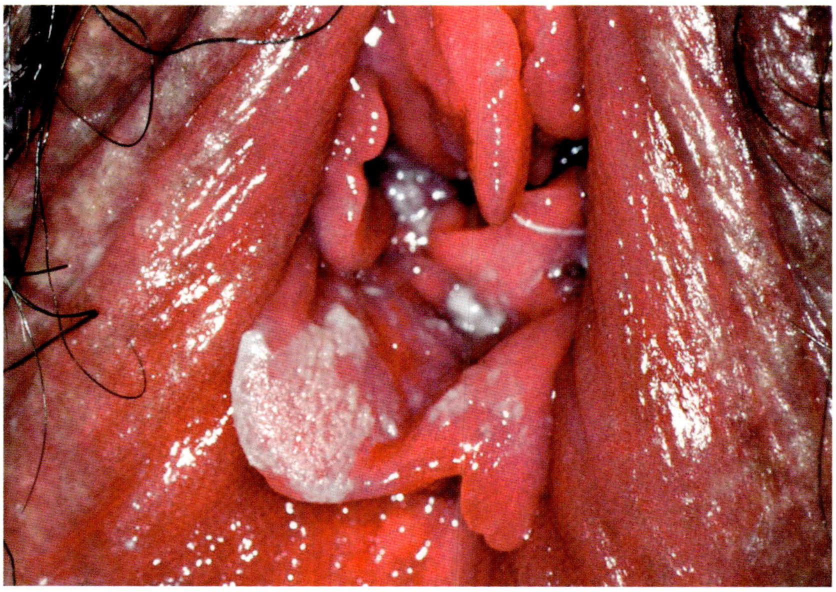

Figure 106 - Vestibular HPV flat condyloma.

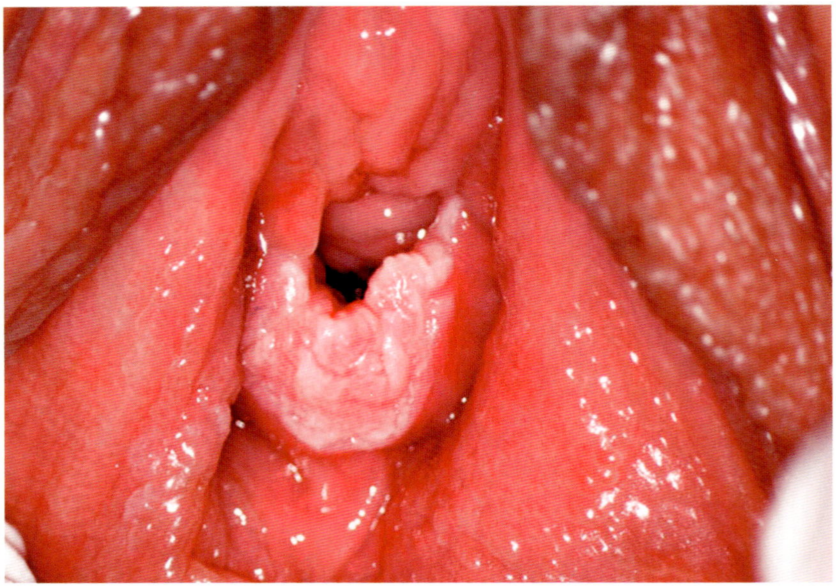

Figure 107 - Hymenal HPV flat condyloma.

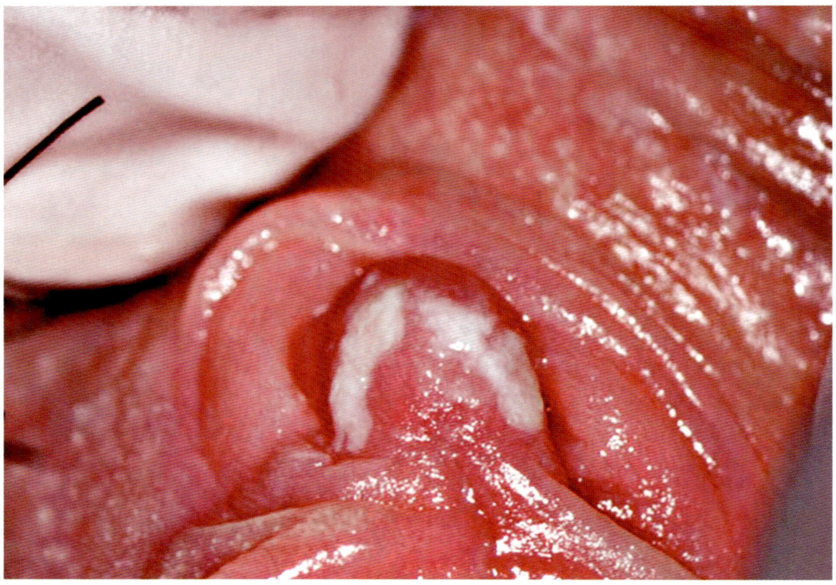

Figure 108 - Clitoral HPV flat condyloma.

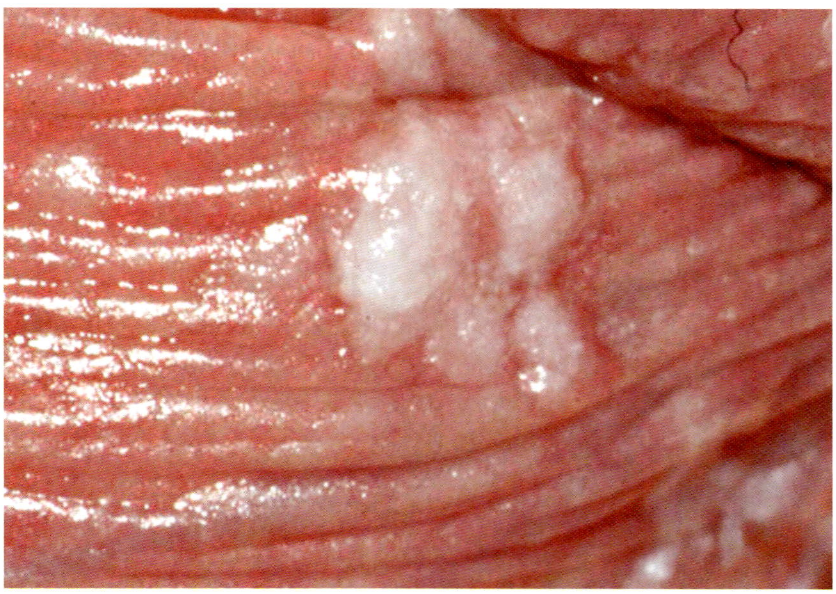

Figure 109 - Vaginal HPV flat condyloma.

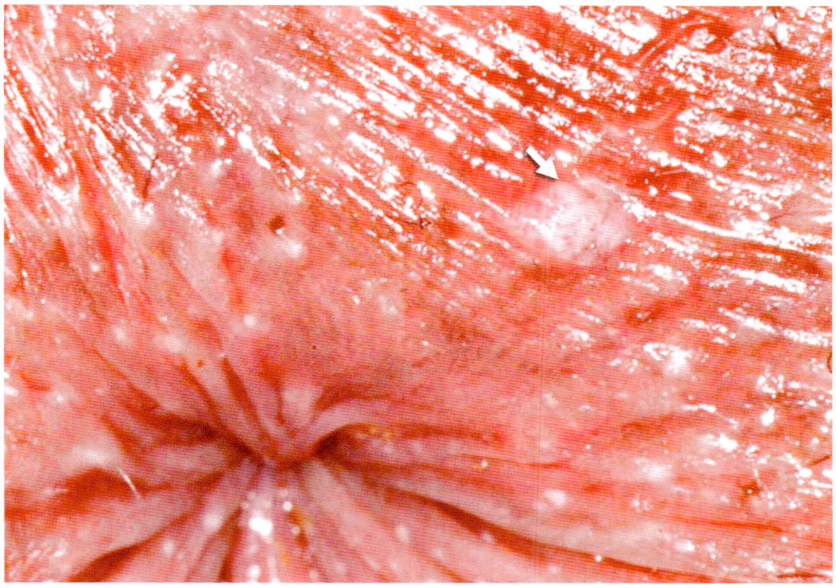

Figure 110 - Perianal HPV flat condyloma (arrow).

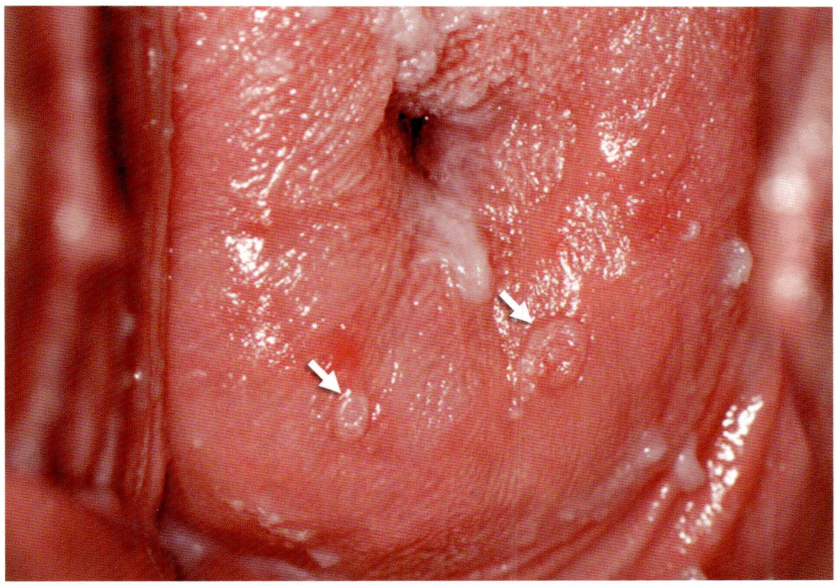

Figure 111 - Cervical HPV flat condylomas (arrows).

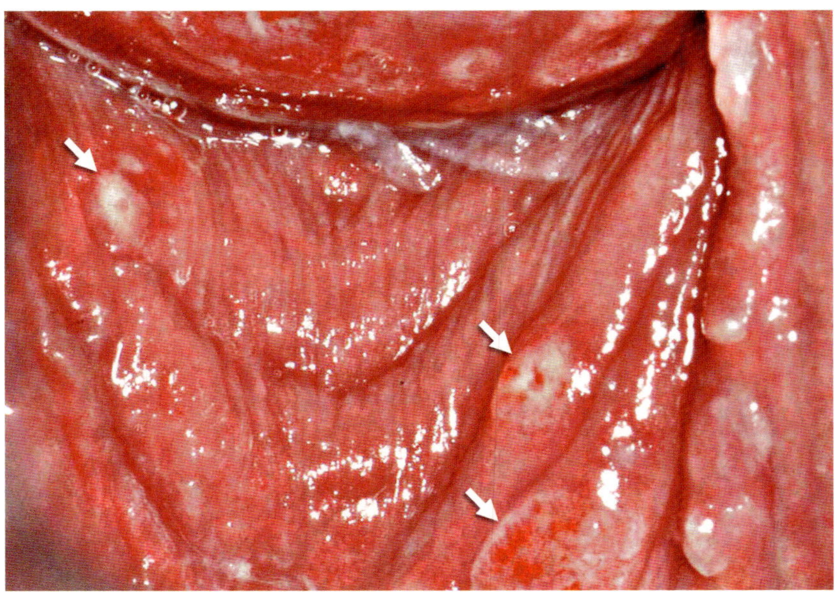

Figure 112 - Vaginal HPV flat condylomas (arrows).

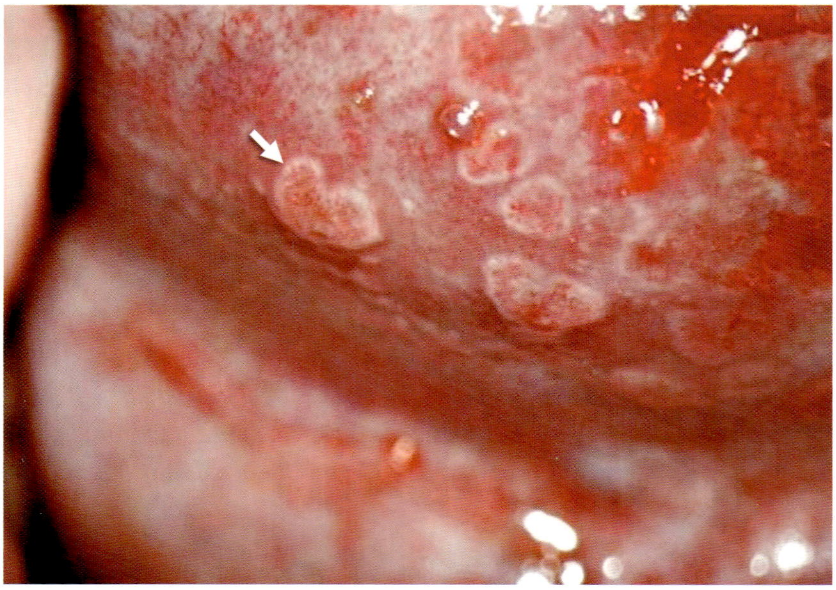

Figure 113 - Centrally depressed erythematous papules (arrow), caused by Candida infection.

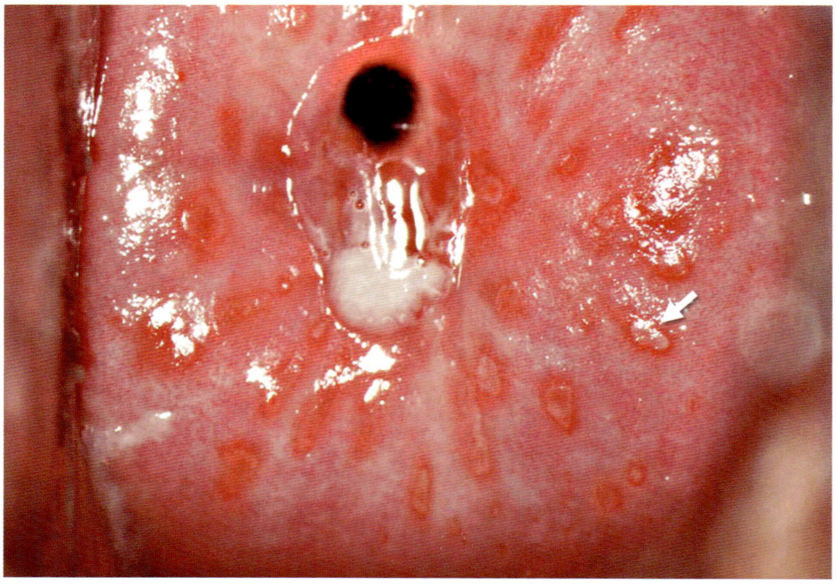

Figure 114 - After application of acetic acid, fungal papules induced by Candida infection remain reddish or appear faint white with a red contour (arrow).

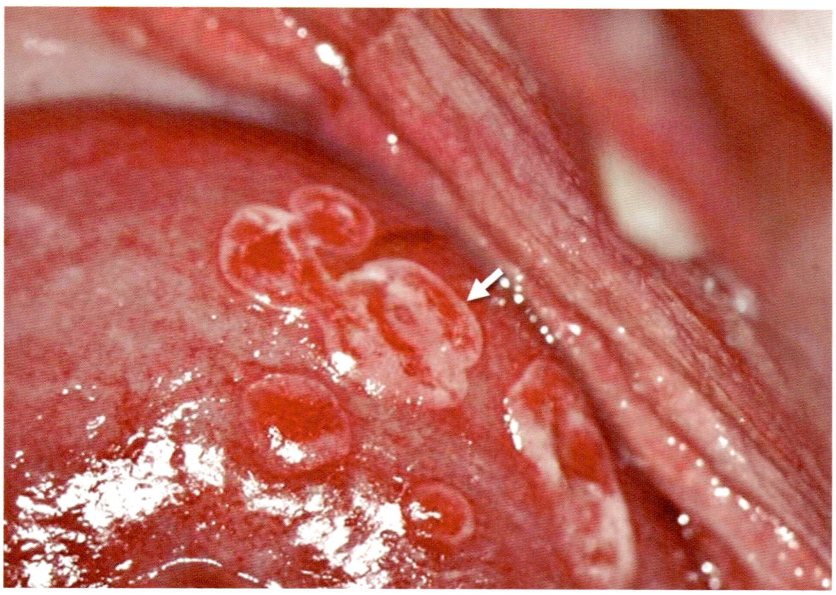

Figure 115 - Cervical decidual polyps (arrow) appear whitish before application of acetic acid.

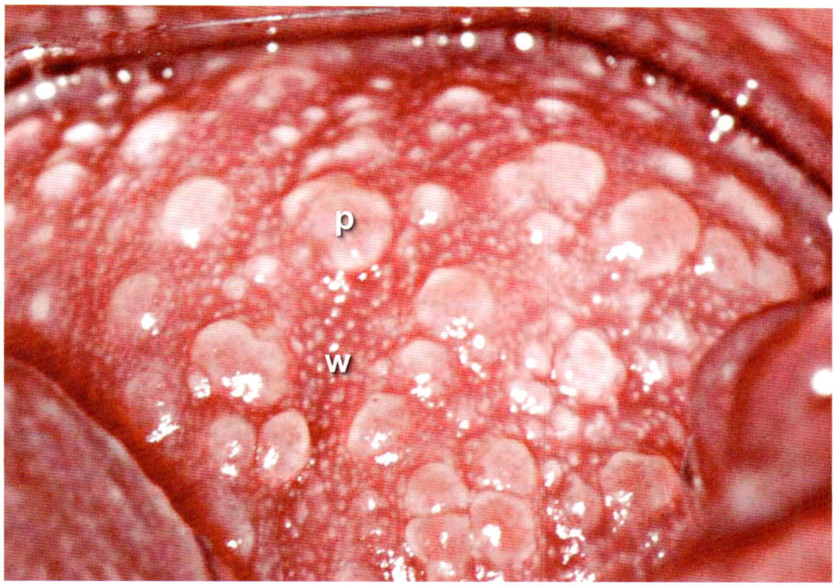

Figure 116 - Pregnant woman at 28th week of gestation. After application of acetic acid, vaginal decidual polyps (p) appear intensely white, and an interspersed white metaplastic punctation (w) can be observed.

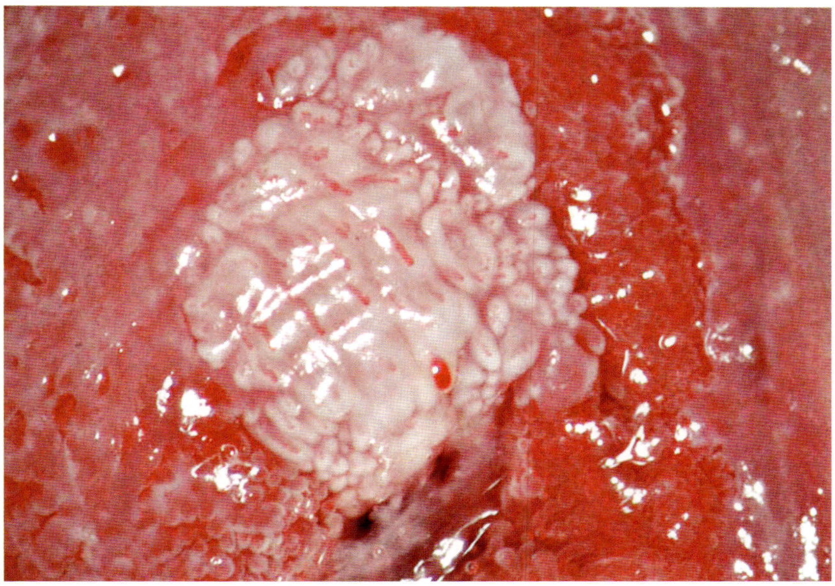

Figure 117 - Flat plaque of acetowhite epithelium without evident atypical vessels. The lesion was shown to be composed of HPV/CIN II epithelium.

for scattered flat condylomas. Decidual polyps appear whitish without application of acetic acid and show no epithelial covering. Decidual reaction takes place in the deeper cervical stroma.

Flat condylomas may seriously mislead the colposcopist because they can mask high-grade lesions particularly when present as a flat plaque of acetowhite epithelium without evident atypical vessels (Figures 117, 118). Although high-grade CIN and malignancy produce a coarser structure with a coarse vascular pattern, a biopsy is always necessary.

Vulvar visible sebaceous glands, known as Fordyce spots or granules (Figure 119) can mimic flat condylomas induced by HPV infection, but their uniform distribution and yellowish aspect provide helpful diagnostic hints. Fordyce spots appear as small, raised, pale, white or yellowish spots or bumps, 1 to 3 mm in diameter. They are completely normal, harmless and painless, and occur in 70 to 80 per cent of adults.

Care must be taken with perianal lesions because they may harbor intraepithelial lesions (Figure 120). Anal intraepithelial neoplasia (AIN) is a premalignant lesion of the anal mucosa that is a precursor to anal cancer. Because progression of AIN to anal cancer is known to occur in some individuals over several years, screening for AIN and early anal cancer, as well as, treatment of advanced AIN lesions, is reasonable in certain high-risk populations. Failure to examine the anal skin properly is often the reason for delays in diagnosis.

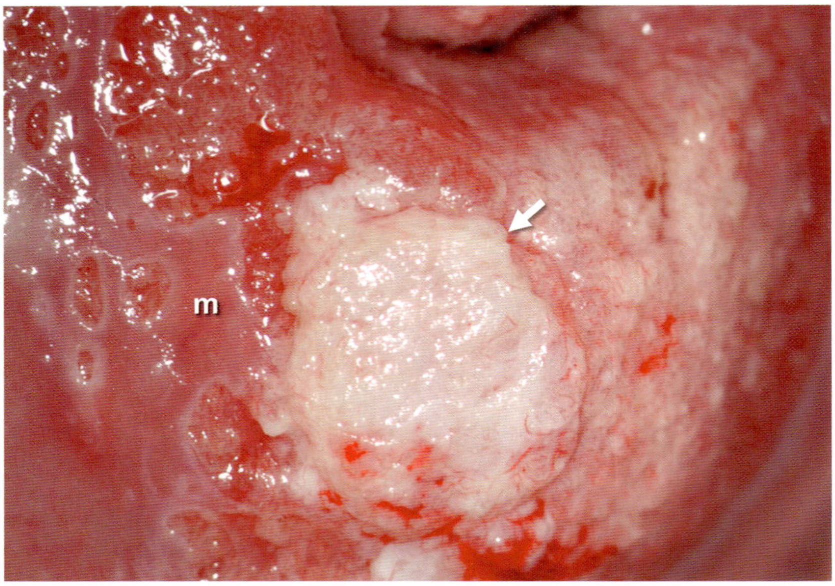

Figure 118 - No vascular pattern can be observed in this raised intense acetowhite lesion. Excision biopsy and resultant histology revealed adenocarcinoma.

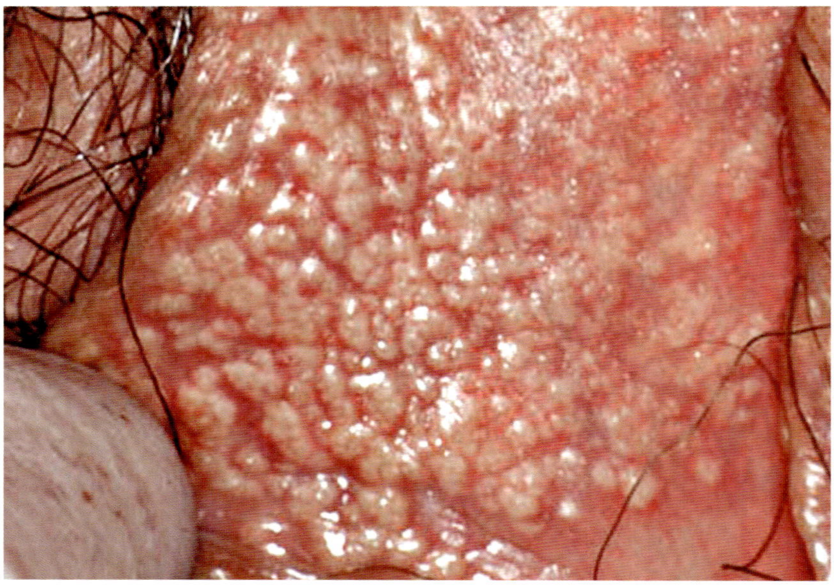

Figure 119 - Fordyce spots involve the inner surface of the left labium minus.

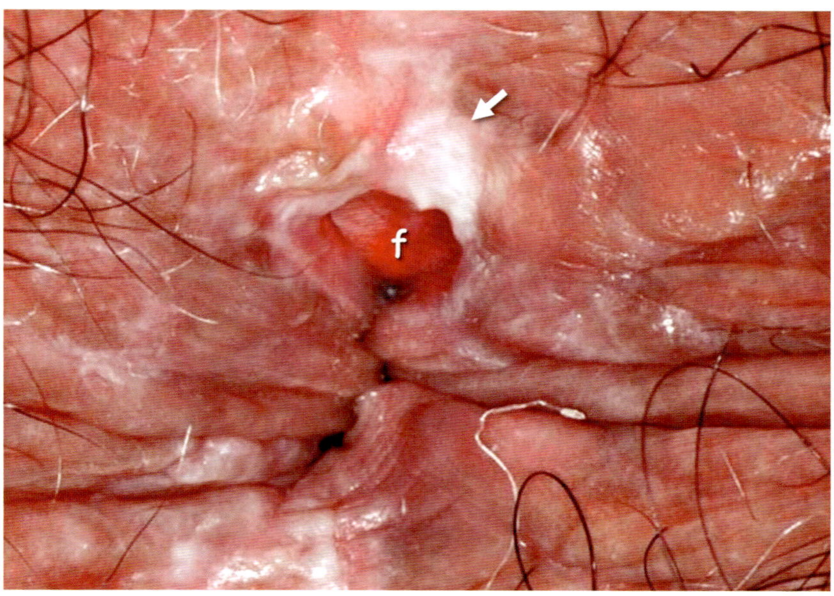

Figure 120 - The arrow indicates a shiny, dense acetowhite epithelium, in the form of a flat condyloma. Biopsy disclosed an anal high-grade SIL. Anal fissure (f).

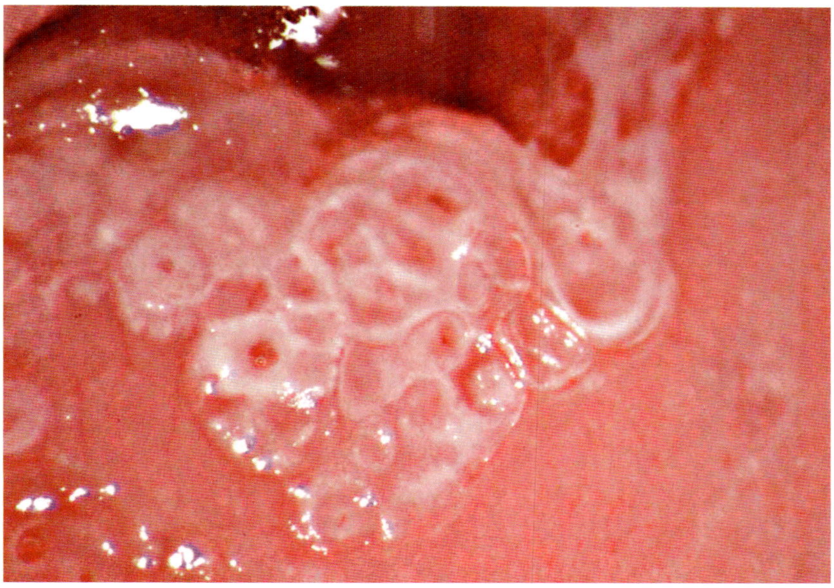

Figure 121 - This brain-like microconvoluted lesion is a variant of HPV flat condyloma.

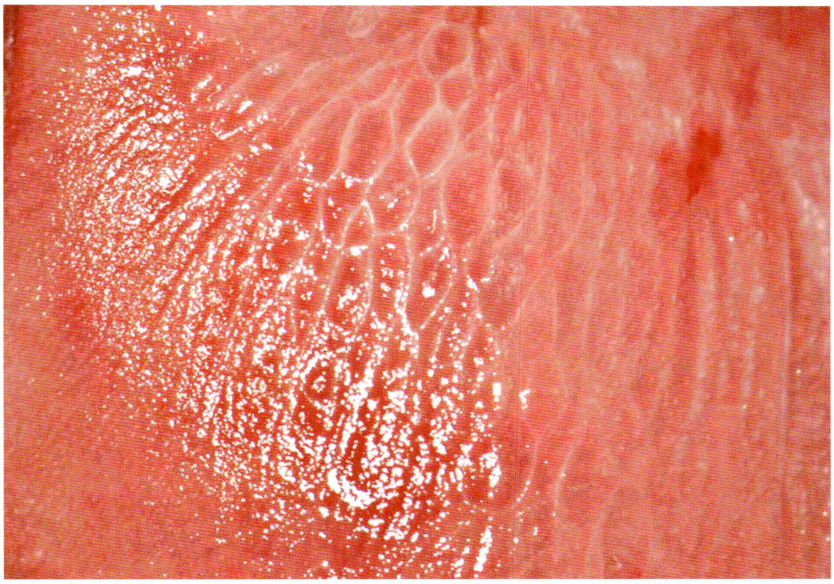

Figure 122 - Gyrated area of normal cervical mucosa, resulting from scarring at the site of surgical removal after LEEP.

A characteristic variant of flat condyloma is represented by brain-like microconvoluted epithelial changes where uniform-caliber capillaries are lying parallel to the surface, and delimitate micro convolutions with hyperkeratosis (Figure 121). Sometimes, this characteristic epithelial derangement induced by HPV may be difficult to distinguish from the encephaloid appearance seen in early verrucous carcinoma producing similar warty excrescences.

Brain-like microconvoluted flat condyloma must be differentiated from the gyrated areas of normal cervical mucosa, that result from scarring at the site of surgical removal after conization or LEEP (Loop Electrosurgical Excision Procedure) (Figure 122). In the presence of mucosal wrinkling, hyperkeratosis and vessel arrangement are absent.

Colposcopy may show three different types of **white punctation**: viral white punctation, fungal white punctation and metaplastic white punctation.

Viral white punctation, also called *condylomatous cervicitis* and *vaginitis* is a diffuse and poorly circumscribed lesion. Viral white punctation differs from fungal and metaplastic white punctation as the white dots appear coarse, irregular in size and slightly elevated (Figure 123). The cervix (Figure 124) and the vagina (Figure 125) are evenly studded with numerous white dots corresponding to the tall stromal papillae that lift the slightly altered epithelium. These poorly keratinized papillary spikes produce a colposcopic appearance of white stippling.

Viral white punctation is distinguishable from the same colposcopic finding induced by Candida in-

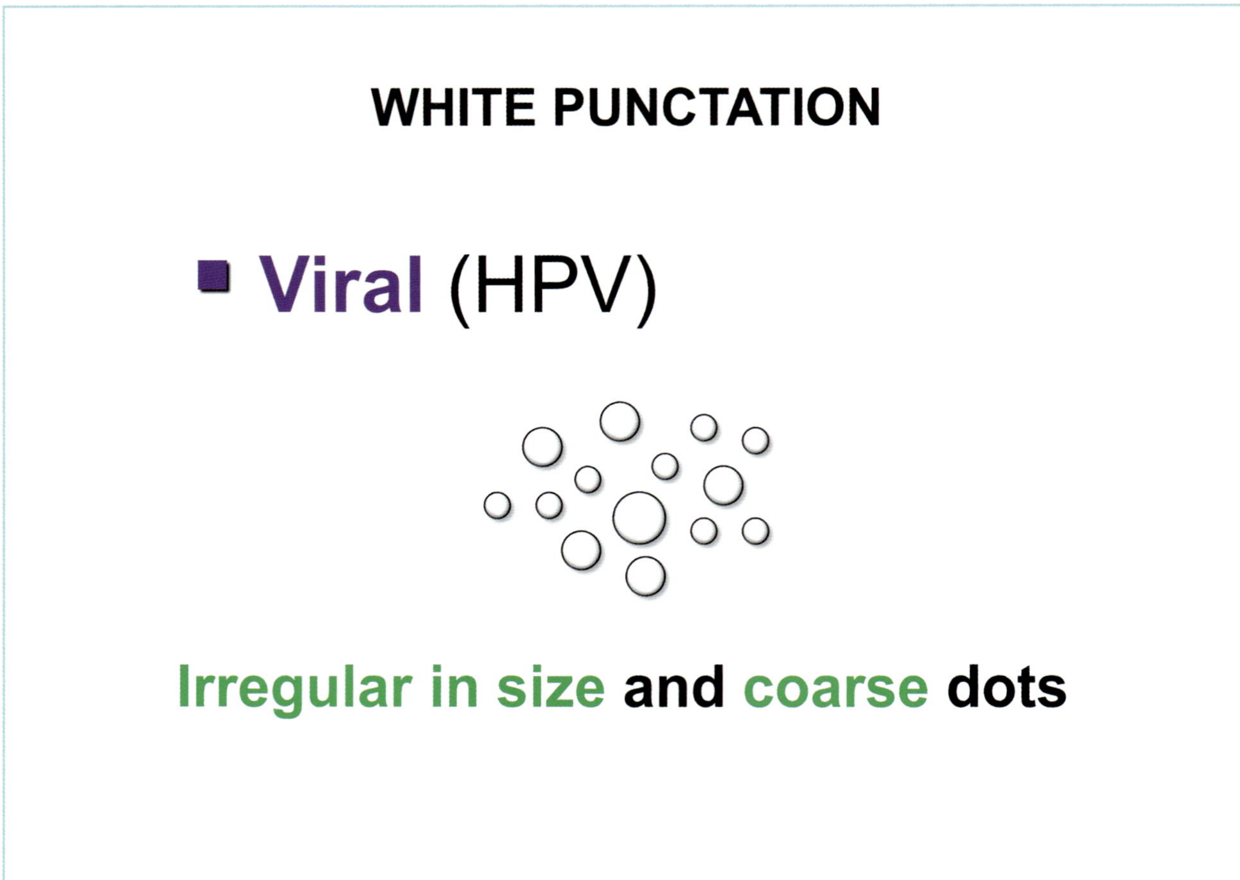

Figure 123 - Diagrammatic representation of viral white punctation.

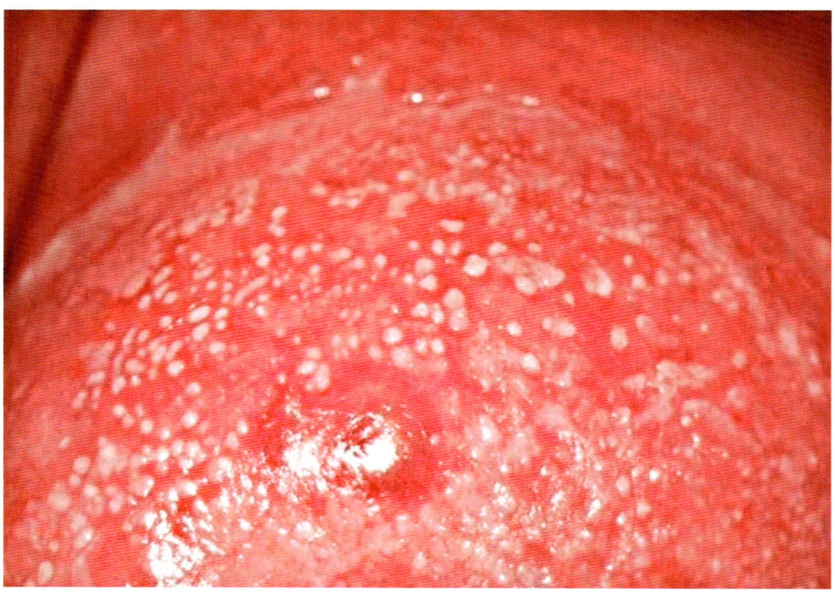

Figure 124 - Condylomatous cervicitis. After application of acetic acid, the white dots of viral punctation appear coarse, irregular in size and slightly elevated.

fection as fungal white punctation is often seen in association with centrally depressed erythematous papules (white dots colpitis) (Figures 126, 127).

Metaplastic white punctation is colposcopically distinguishable from the other white punctations (fungal and viral) due to it appearing fine and contiguous to the squamocolumnar junction (Figures 128, 129). Overspread small Nabothian follicles can mimic white punctation (Figure 130). Retention cysts look like shiny and tiny bumps on the surface of the cervix, in contrast with the opaque appearance of white punctation.

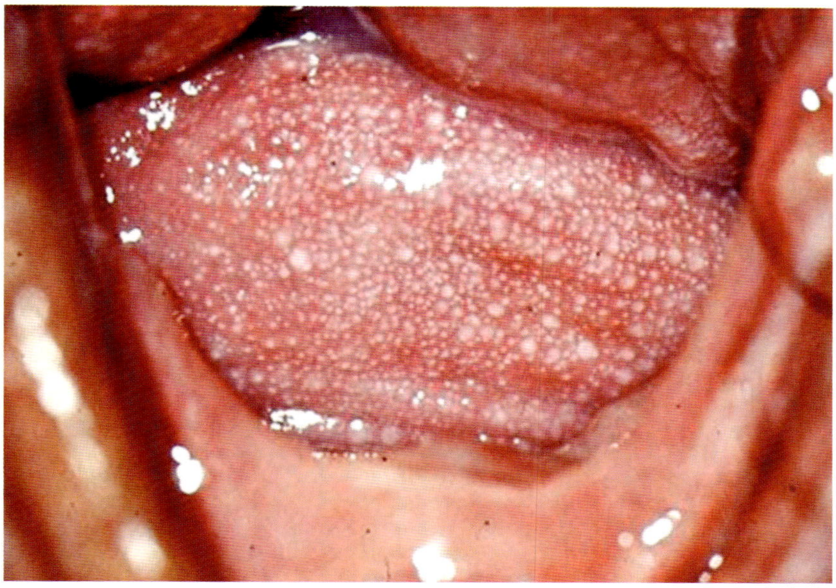

Figure 125 - Condylomatous vaginitis. Coarse, irregularly sized and raised white dots are scattered on the anterior vaginal wall.

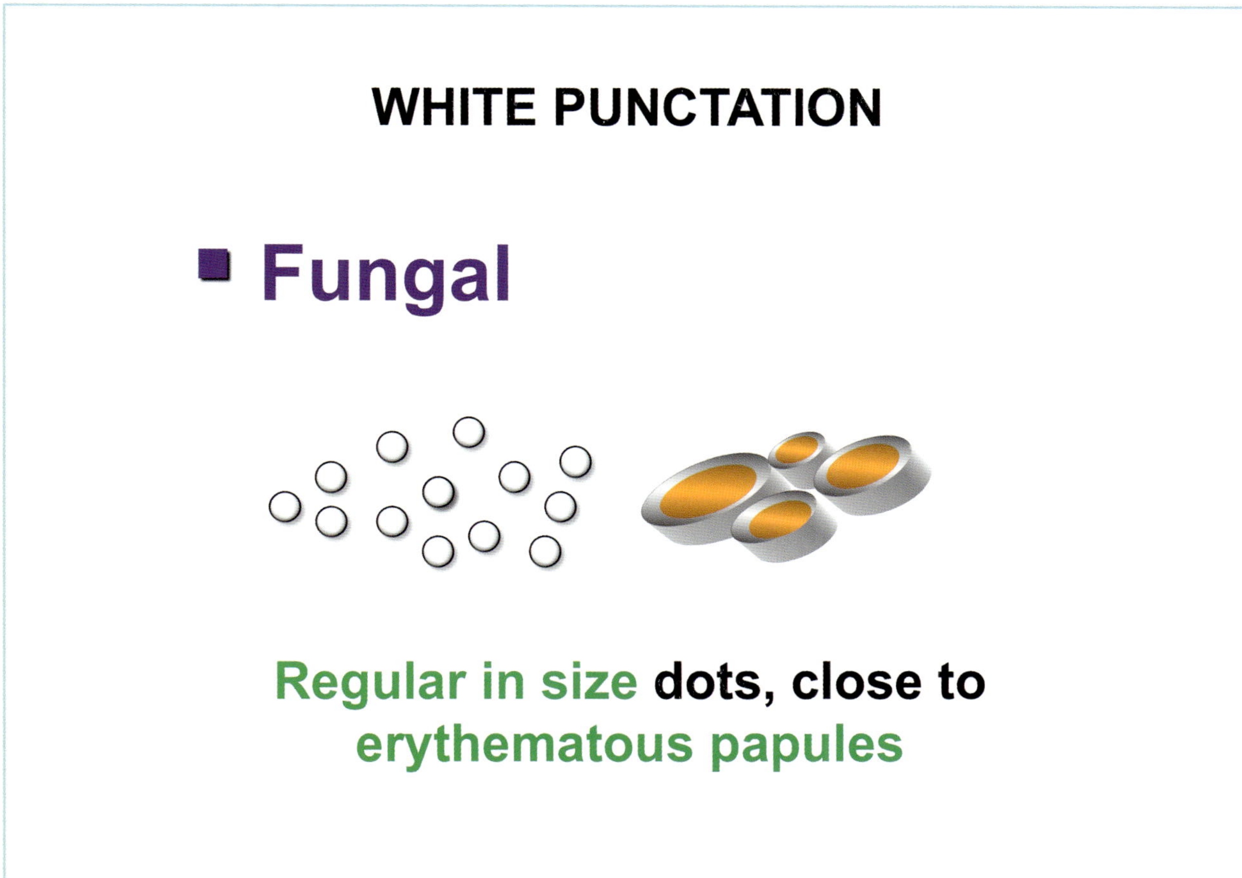

Figure 126 - Diagrammatic representation of fungal white punctation.

The cervix is composed of two regions: the ectocervix and the endocervix (Figure 131). The ectocervix is lined by a non-keratinized stratified squamous epithelium, whereas a single layer of columnar cells coats the endocervix. There is a sharp step-like white border between the ectocervix and the endocervix, called the squamocolumnar junction (SCJ) because it clearly separates squamous epithelium from columnar epithelium (Figure 132). The step between the columnar and the squamous epithelium is due to the difference in their thickness.

With advancing age, decreased hormonal levels af-

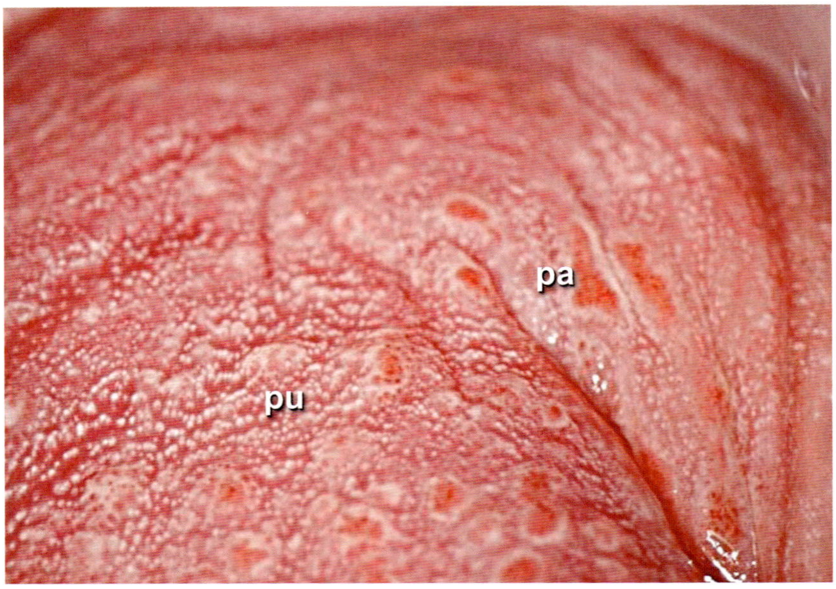

Figure 127 - Fungal white punctation (pu) is associated with erythematous papules (pa) (white dots colpitis).

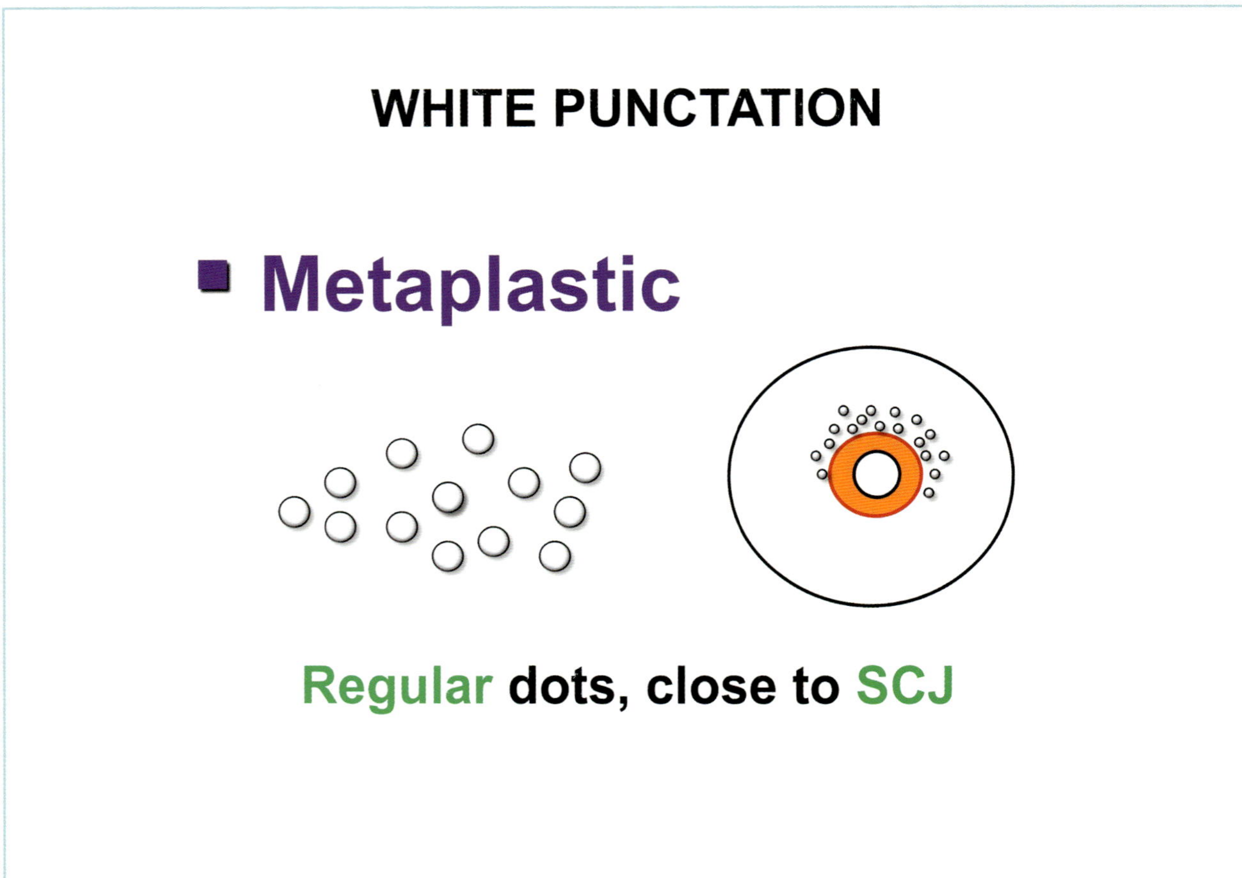

Figure 128 - Diagrammatic representation of metaplastic white punctation.

fect cervical stroma which becomes thinner along with a decrease in vascularity. Vessels become narrow and fragile, sub-epithelial hemorrhages may appear and the SCJ may be scarcely identifiable (Figure 133).

After the onset of menopause, the SC junction moves towards the external os and lastly recedes higher inside the endocervical canal so, it is mostly not visible (Figure 134).

When the squamo columnar junction cannot be identified, a cotton swab may be useful in exposing the endocervical canal. Should this procedure not

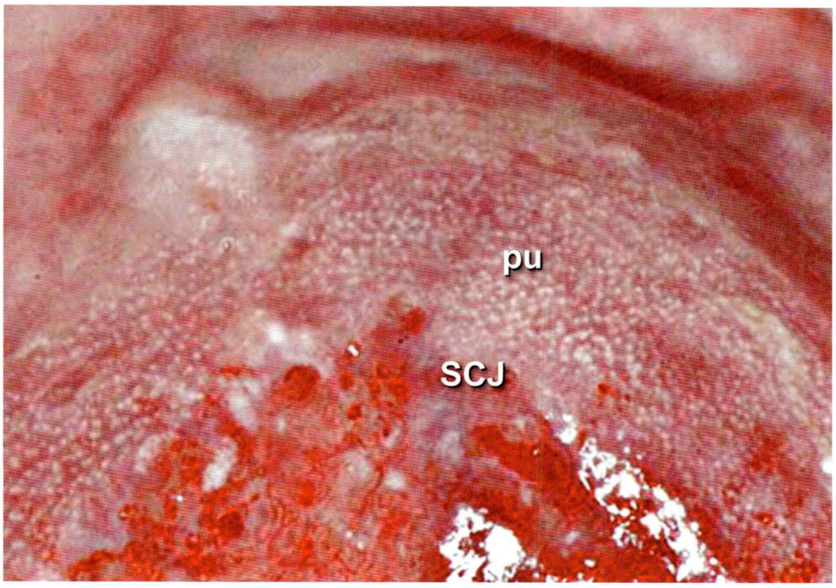

Figure 129 - Fine dots of metaplastic white punctation (pu) are seen contiguous to the squamocolumnar junction (SCJ).

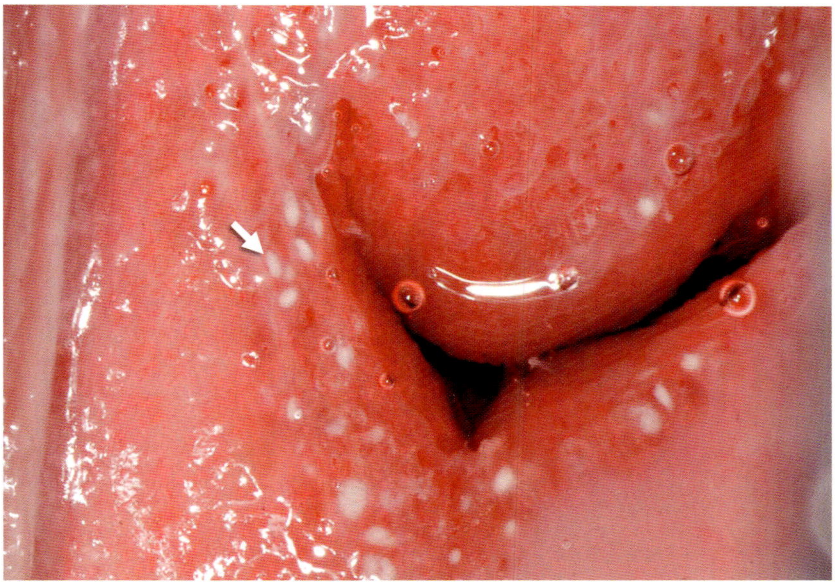

Figure 130 - Overspread small Nabothian follicles (arrow) can be misinterpreted as white punctation.

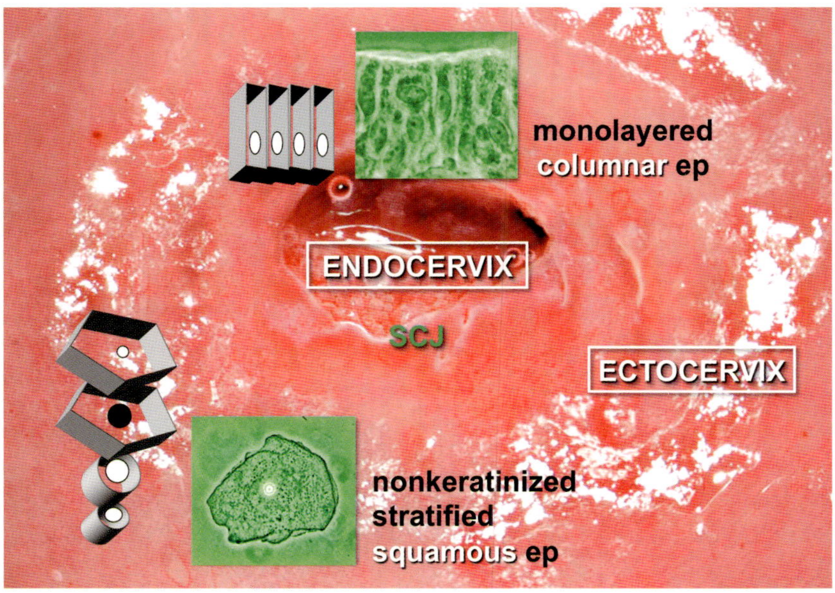

Figure 131 - Diagrammatic representation and microphotographs of the regions of the cervix and lining epithelia.

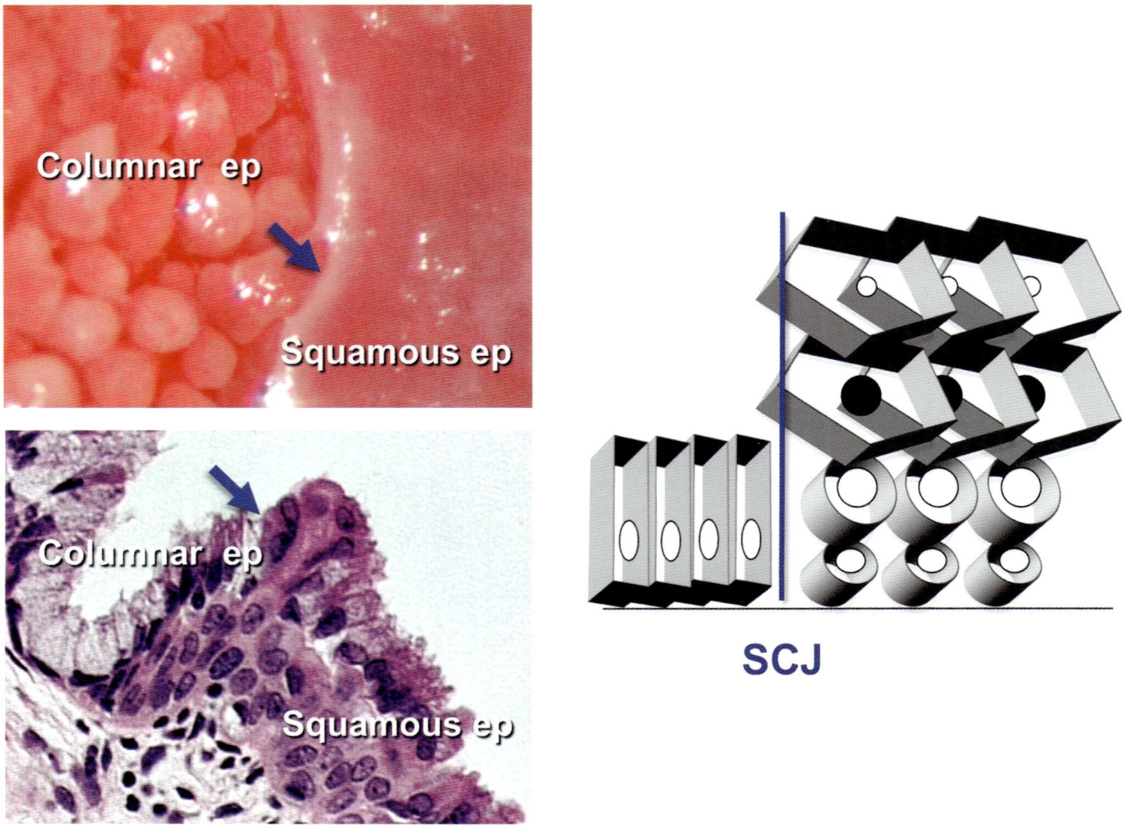

Figure 132 - Colpophotograph, histologic finding and diagrammatic representation of the squamocolumnar junction (arrows).

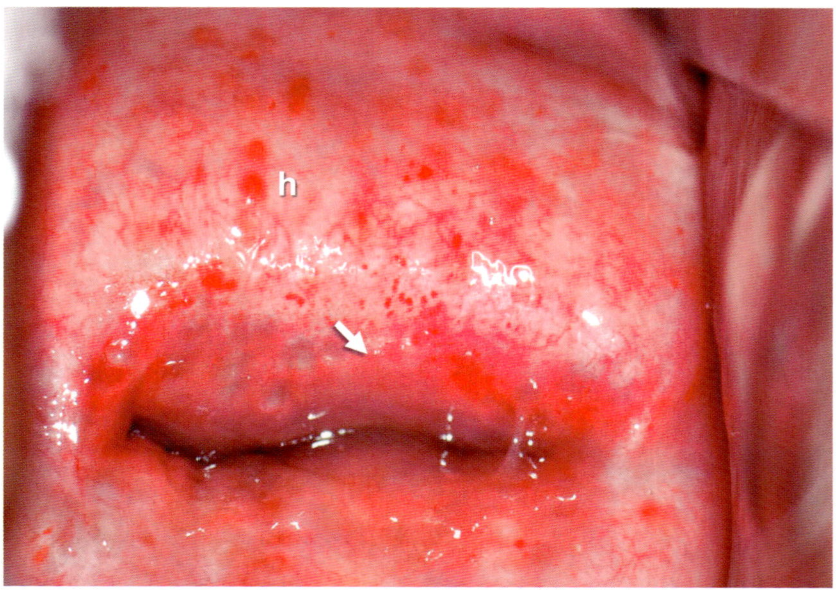

Figure 133 - The dystrophic cervix in menopause exhibits sub-epithelial hemorrhages (h) and a scarcely identifiable squamocolumnar junction (arrow).

sufficiently localize the SCJ or locate the upper margin of a lesion extending into the endocervical canal, Kogan's endocervical speculum can be used. Based on their visibility, colposcopic lesions can be graded in three groups:

- Group 1: lesion is fully visible on the ectocervix
- Group 2: lesion extends into canal, but upper limit is visible
- Group 3: lesion extends into canal and upper limit is not visible.

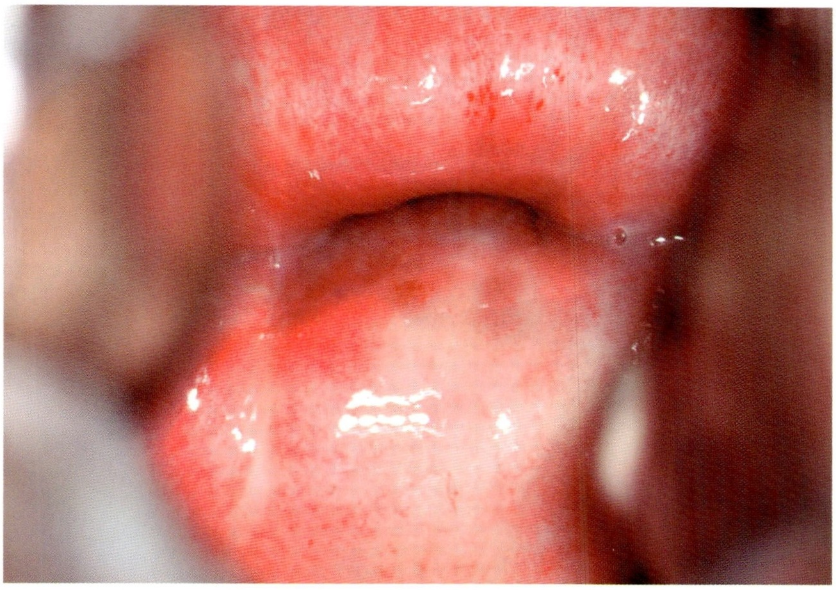

Figure 134 - Cervix after the onset of menopause. The squamocolumnar junction is not visible as it receded higher inside the endocervical canal.

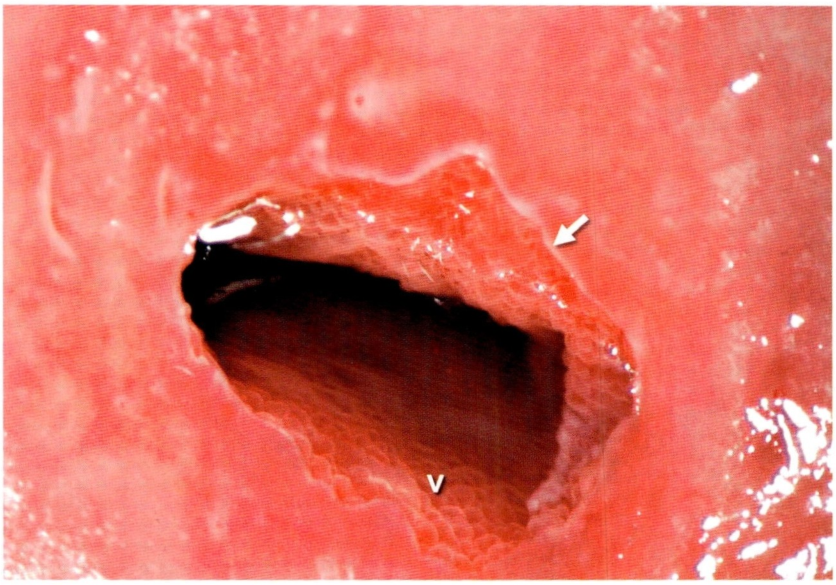

Figure 135 - Acetic acid causes swelling and whitening of the individual villi (v). The arrow indicates the SCJ.

After application of acetic acid (3% to 5%) with either soaked cotton balls, gauze pads or a sprayer, columnar epithelium assumes a grape-like appearance because acetic acid causes swelling and whitening of individual villi (Figure 135) that may raise the surrounding squamous epithelium. Within the endocervix itself, the villi are broader and less grape-like in appearance (Figure 136). The stratified squamous epithelium lines both the cervix and the vagina.
Proceeding from the basement membrane towards the surface, vaginal and cervical epithelia are composed of four cell types (Figure 137):

- *basal* cells
- *parabasal* cells
- *intermediate* cells
- *superficial* cells

With the maturation of cells towards the surface, the cellular elements progressively enlarge whereas the nuclei become smaller.
If we consider a fully mature squamous epithelium, it is predominantly composed of squamous cells (intermediate and superficial cells) and a thin layer of immature cells (basal and parabasal cells). Due to its low density and poor nuclear content, direct light passes through the entire mature squamous epithelium like a lens, reaches the stroma (Figure 138) and is reflected, giving the cervix a pink, translucent appearance (Figure 139).
Basal and parabasal cells have a predominant nucleus, rich in proteins (Figure 140). Acetic acid causes reversible coagulation of nucleoproteins. Although these proteins coagulate or precipitate after

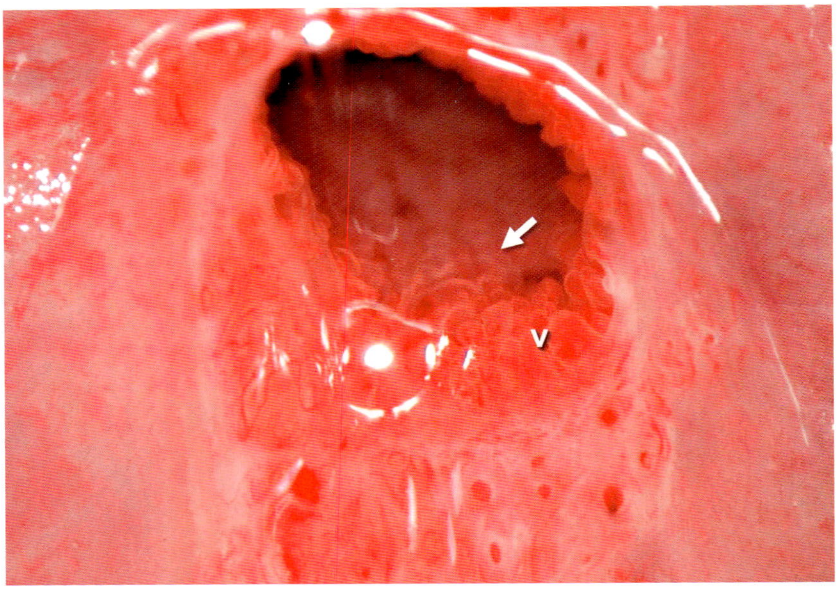

Figure 136 - Proceeding from the external os towards the endocervical canal, the villi (v) are broader and less grape-like in appearance (arrow).

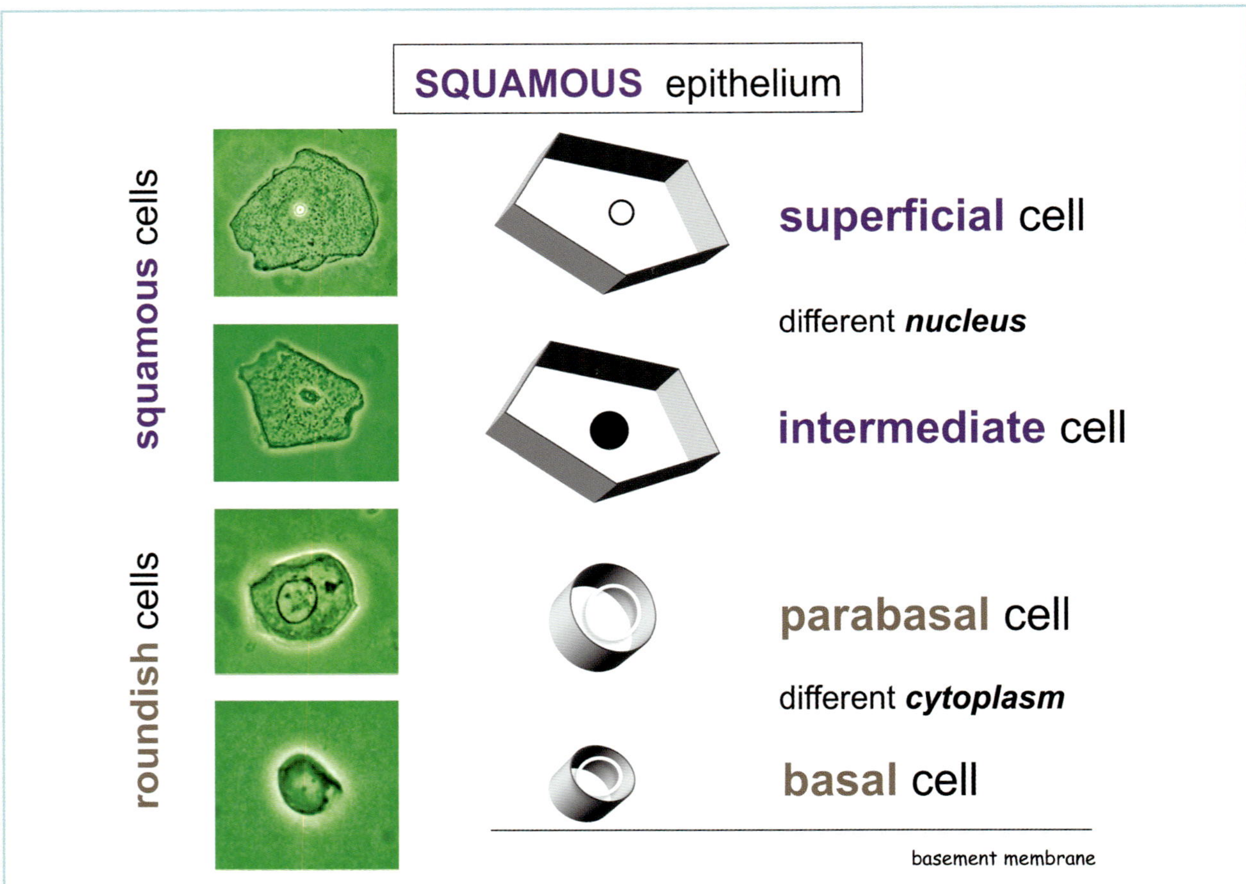

Figure 137 - Diagrammatic representation and microphotographs of the cervico-vaginal epithelium.

acetic acid application, producing **acetowhiteness**, the acetic acid may not penetrate sufficiently through the deeper cells, and the resulting scant protein coagulation is not sufficient to interfere with the light pathway. Acetic acid does not affect glycogen producing epithelium; thus, the direct light still reaches the stroma, reflects its tinge and the appearance of the epithelium does not change (Figure 141).

Both in original squamous epithelium and mature metaplastic epithelium, large squamous cells are rich in glycogen, responsible for iodine uptake (Figure 142). After application of Lugol's iodine solution

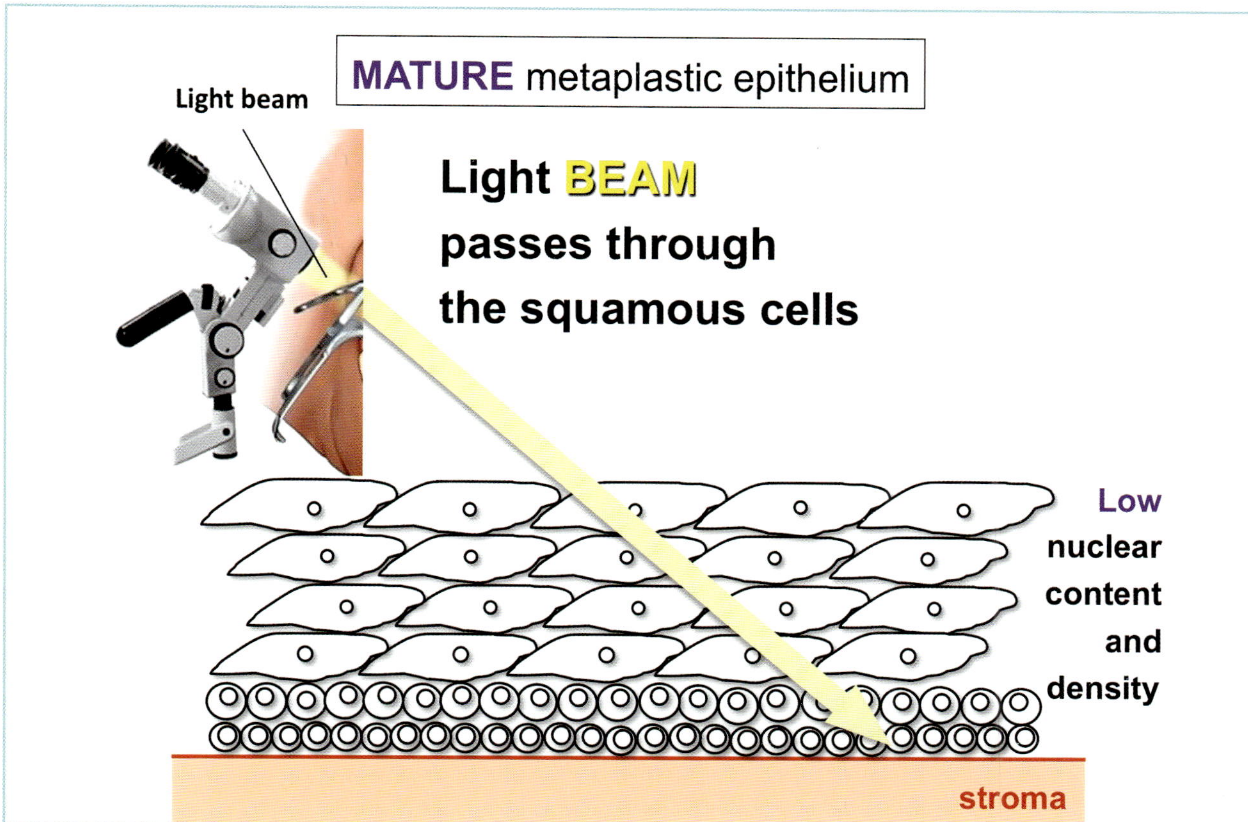

Figure 138 - Diagrammatic representation of the light pathway, through a mature squamous epithelium.

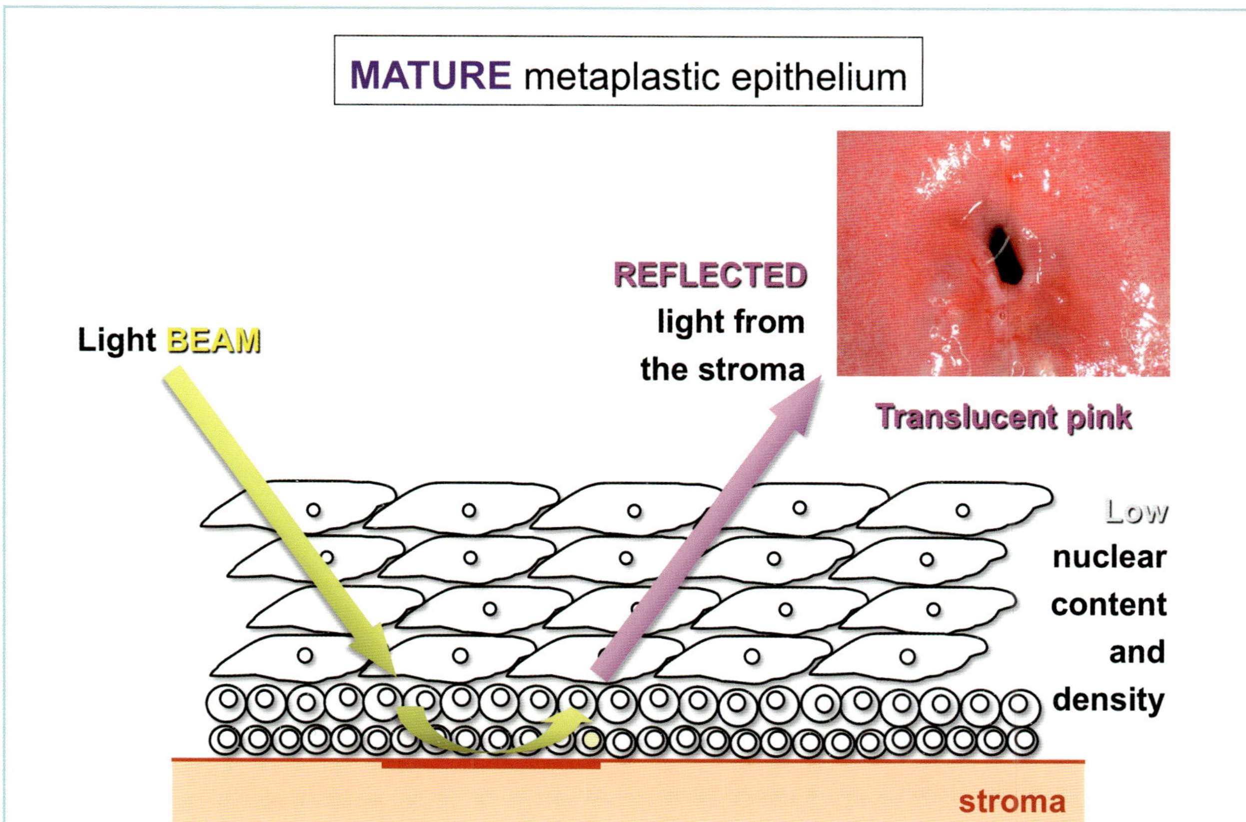

Figure 139 - Diagrammatic representation of the light pathway, through a mature squamous epithelium, and the colposcopic appearance of the cervix which appears translucent pink.

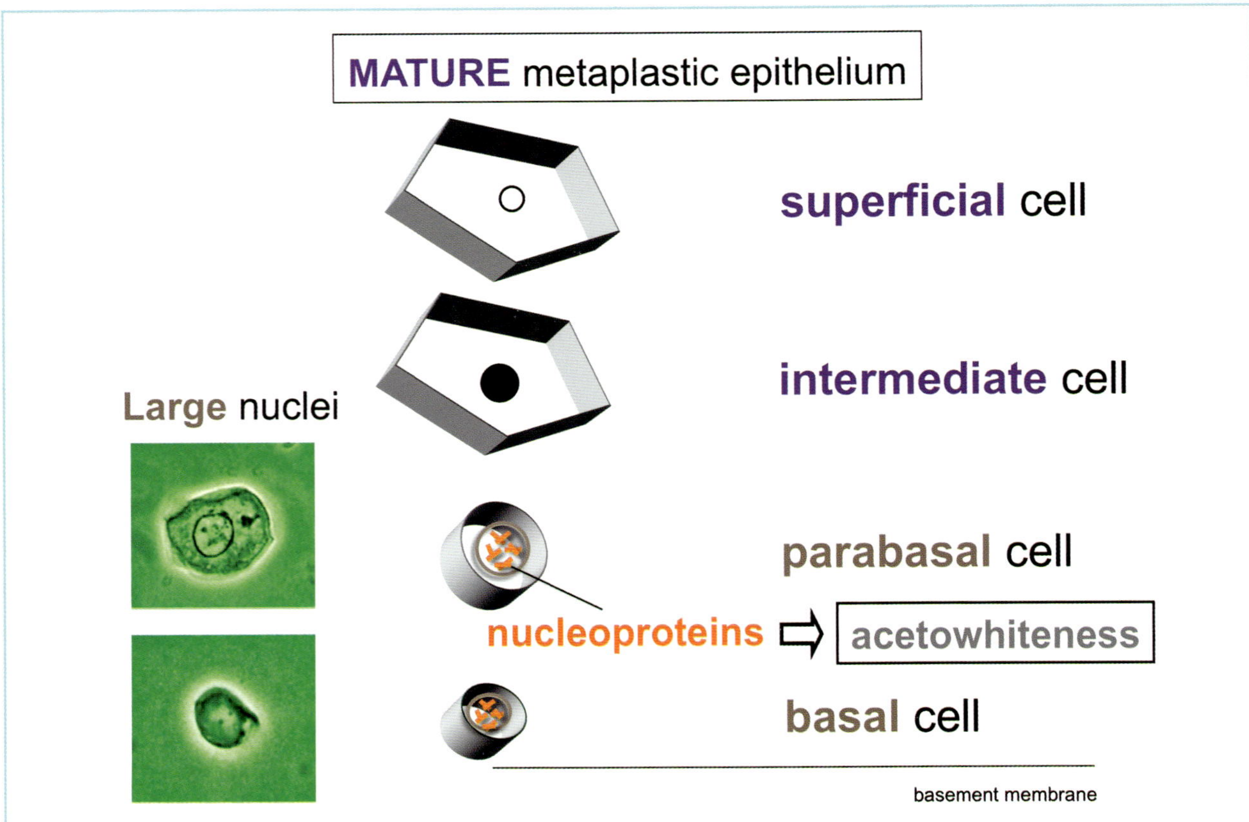

Figure 140 - Diagrammatic representation and microphotographs of the squamous epithelium which indicates the high content of nucleoproteins in immature nuclei, responsible for acetowhite reaction.

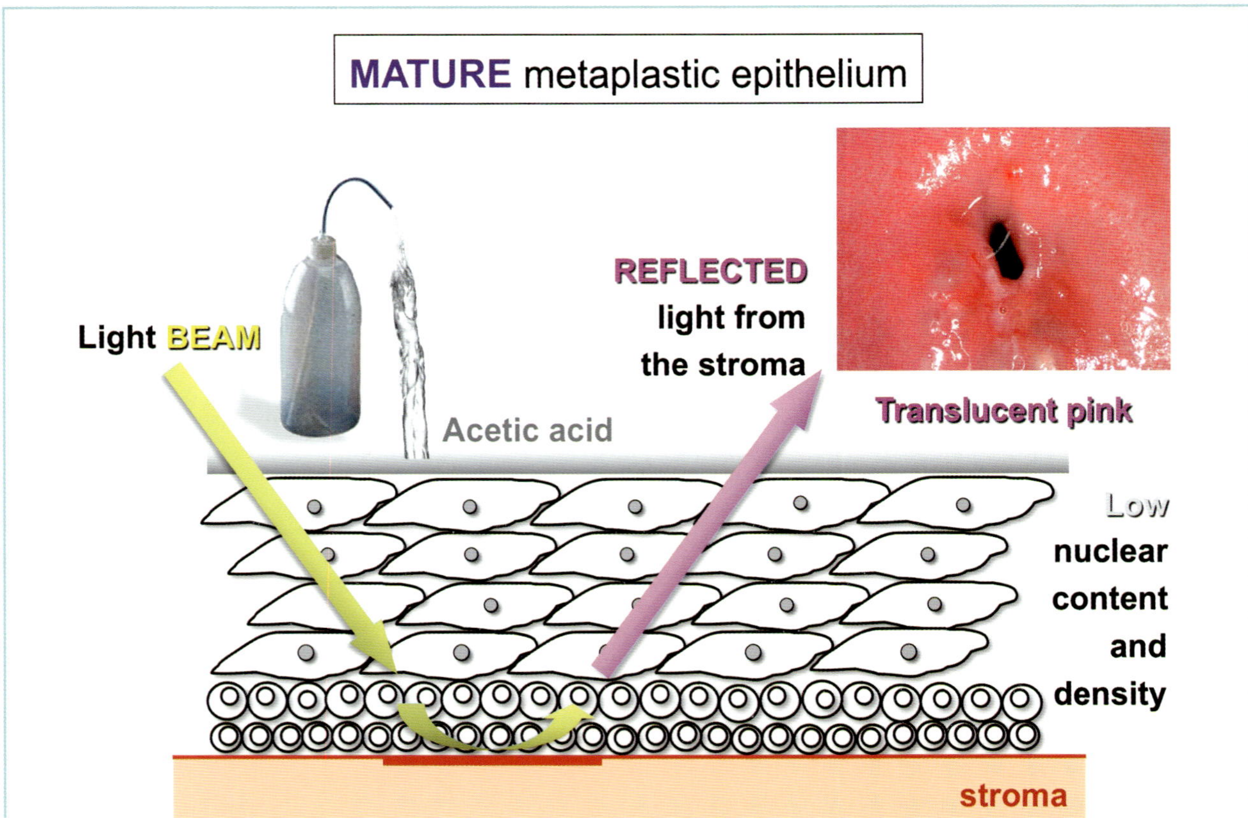

Figure 141 - Diagrammatic representation and microphotographs of the light pathway, through a mature squamous epithelium, after application of acetic acid. The colpophotograph shows that the cervix keeps its translucent pink appearance.

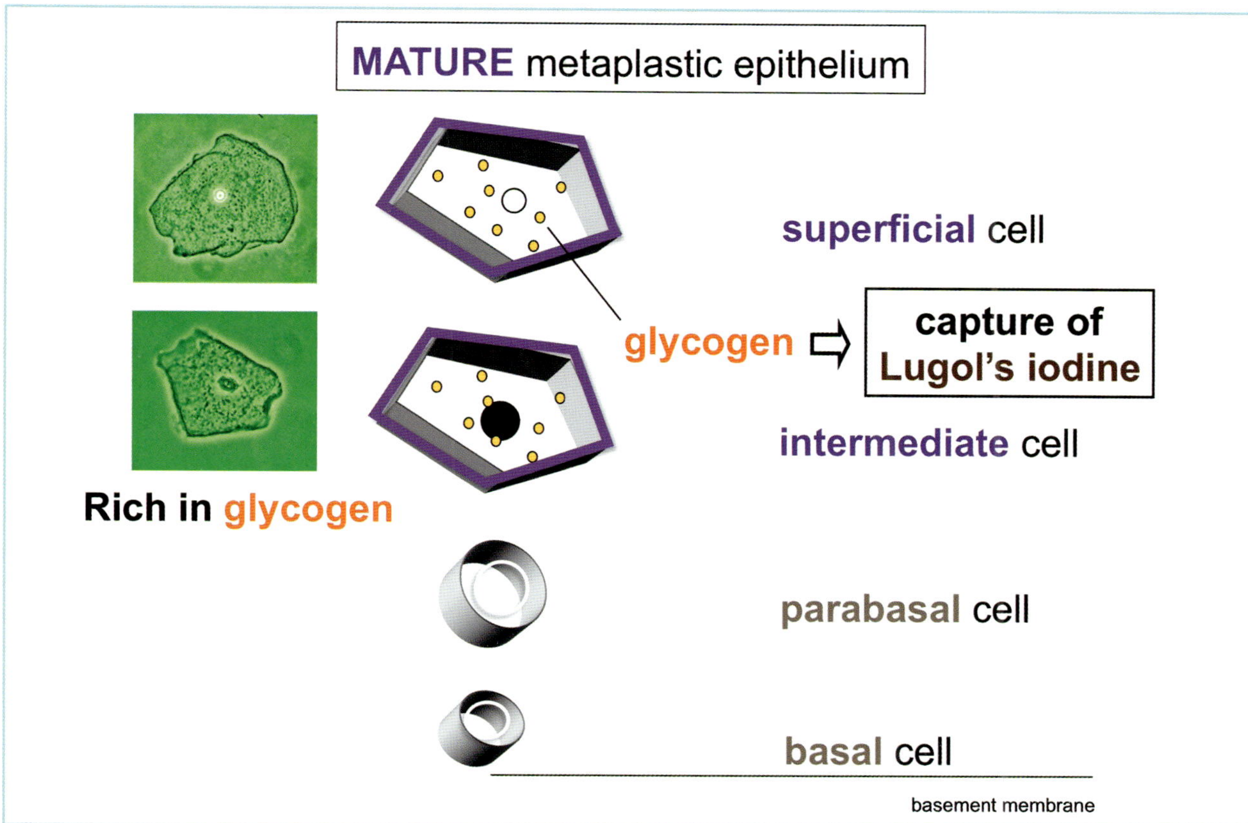

Figure 142 - Diagrammatic representation and microphotographs of the squamous epithelium which points out the high content of cytoplasmic glycogen in squamous cells, responsible for Lugol's iodine staining.

(Schiller's test), superficial and intermediate cells stain from mahogany brown to nearly black (Figure 143). Glycogenated epithelium is referred to as negative Schiller's test or iodine positive area. Columnar epithelium does not contain glycogen; therefore, it does not take up iodine and remains unstained. Sometimes, it is merely discolored by a thin film of iodine covering it. Erosions of the cervix or areas where shedding of squamous cells takes place do not stain with iodine and remain distinctly colorless in contrast with the surrounding mahogany brown background.

The squamo-columnar junction is not static but may come on to the cervix when high levels of estrogens cause the eversion of external os (Figure 144). Estrogen stimulation may be observed during intrauterine life, menarche, first pregnancy and luteal insufficiency. *Ectropion* is a marked eversion of the endocervical mucosa which often appears strikingly reddish and with raised margins. (Figure 145). Exposed columnar epithelium associated with Chlamydia infection appears hypertrophic, congested and reddened (Figure 146).

The low pH of the vagina causes the shedding of fragile columnar cells on exposed villi and, in a variable time, the columnar epithelium is replaced by newly developed tissue, which is initially called *immature metaplastic epithelium*. The upper limit of the transformation zone is the new squamocolumnar junction between the immature metaplastic epithelium and the columnar epithelium (Figure 147).

The metaplastic process begins at the tip of the columnar villi which are first exposed to an acidic vaginal environment (Figure 148a). When this multilayered but still undifferentiated immature squamous epithelium caps the villi (Figure 148b), this results in some opaqueness on their tip, after application of acetic acid (Figures 149, 150). This loss of translucency represents the earliest metaplastic change. As the metaplastic process continues, the immature metaplastic epithelium extends into the clefts of adjacent villi (Figures 148c, 151), until a smooth surface is produced within the original columnar epithelium (Figures 148d, 152).

Metaplastic epithelium forms patches and long projections which ramify and grow in a tongue-shaped manner (Figure 153), spreading towards the center in an irregular manner. Gradually, they fuse together to form a membrane-like area (Figure 154).

The wedge-shaped offshoots, often having a more

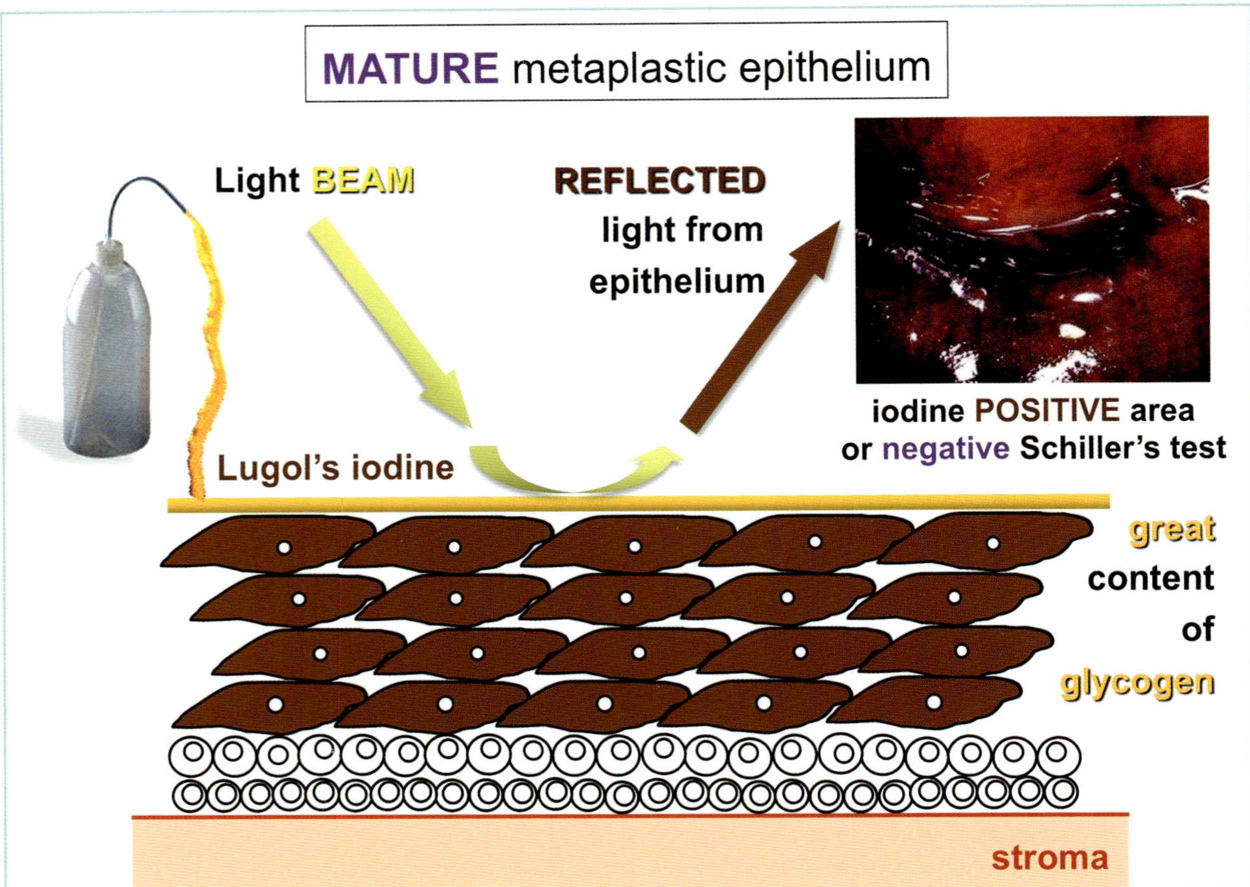

Figure 143 - Diagrammatic representation and colpophotograph of the effect of Lugol's iodine on mature squamous epithelium, which stains from mahogany brown to nearly black.

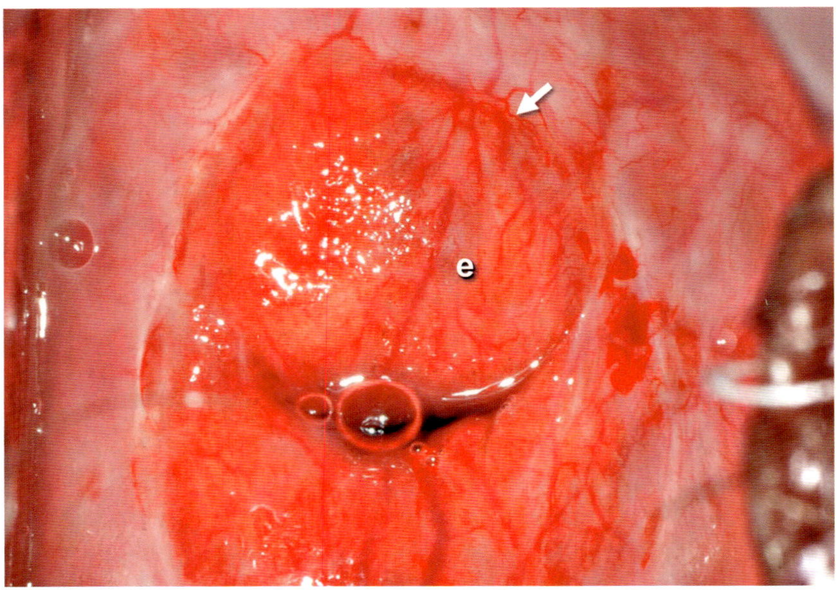

Figure 144 - Extensive reddish area of everted columnar epithelium (e). The original squamocolumnar junction (arrow) is located on the ectocervix, far away from the external os.

defined margin that originate from the original squamocolumnar junction, proceed towards the external os and eventually join to intra-junctional metaplastic patches, are termed by some authors as epithelialization (Figure 155).

When the metaplastic replacement is almost completed, the acetowhite metaplastic epithelium over the villi may exceed the height of the smooth surface. According to the protrusion of metaplastic epithelium over the villi, acetowhite dots or small humps

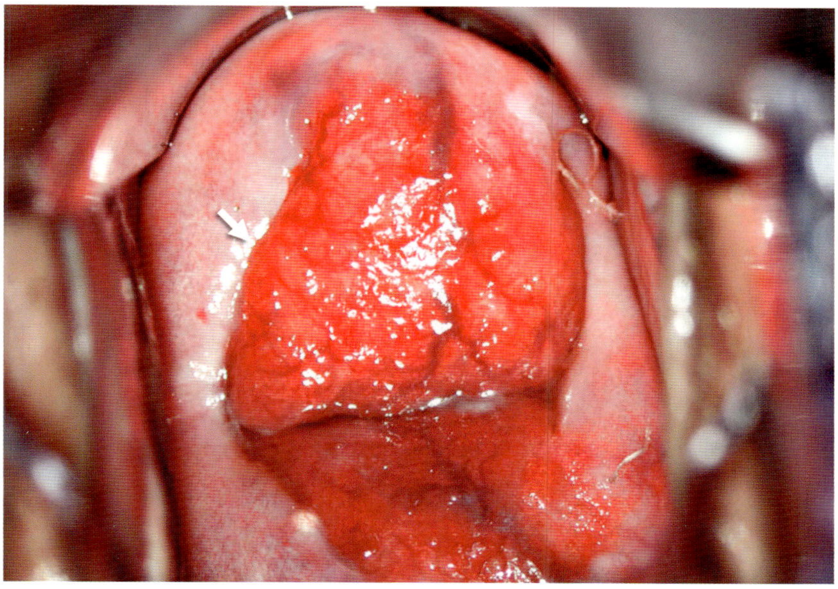

Figure 145 - Ectropion displays a strikingly reddish and marked eversion of the endocervical mucosa with raised margins (arrow).

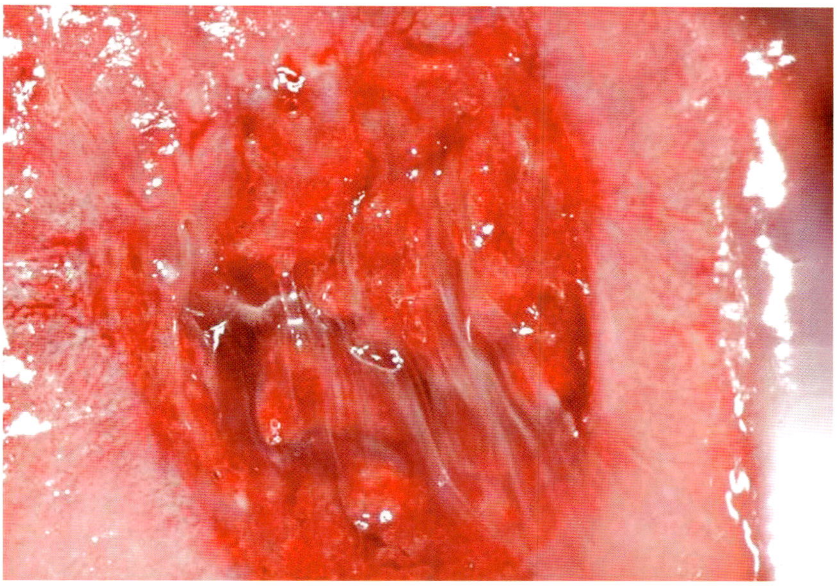

Figure 146 - Reddish "angry looking", inflamed columnar epithelium with loss of villous structure, in Chlamydia trachomatis infection.

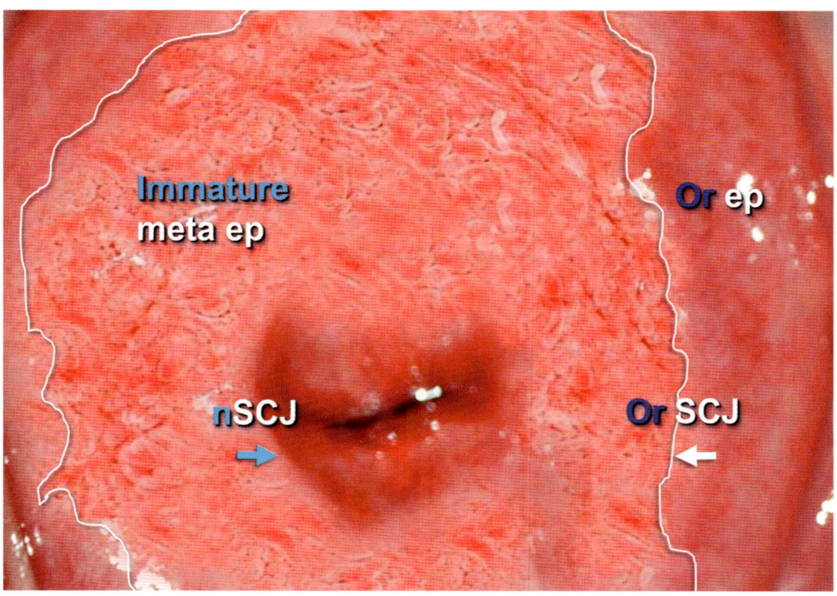

Figure 147 - The exposed columnar epithelium has been substituted by a faint acetowhite immature metaplastic epithelium. The original SCJ (white arrow) separates the transformation zone from the translucent darker pink original squamous epithelium (Or ep).
The light blue arrow indicates the new squamocolumnar epithelium (nSCJ).

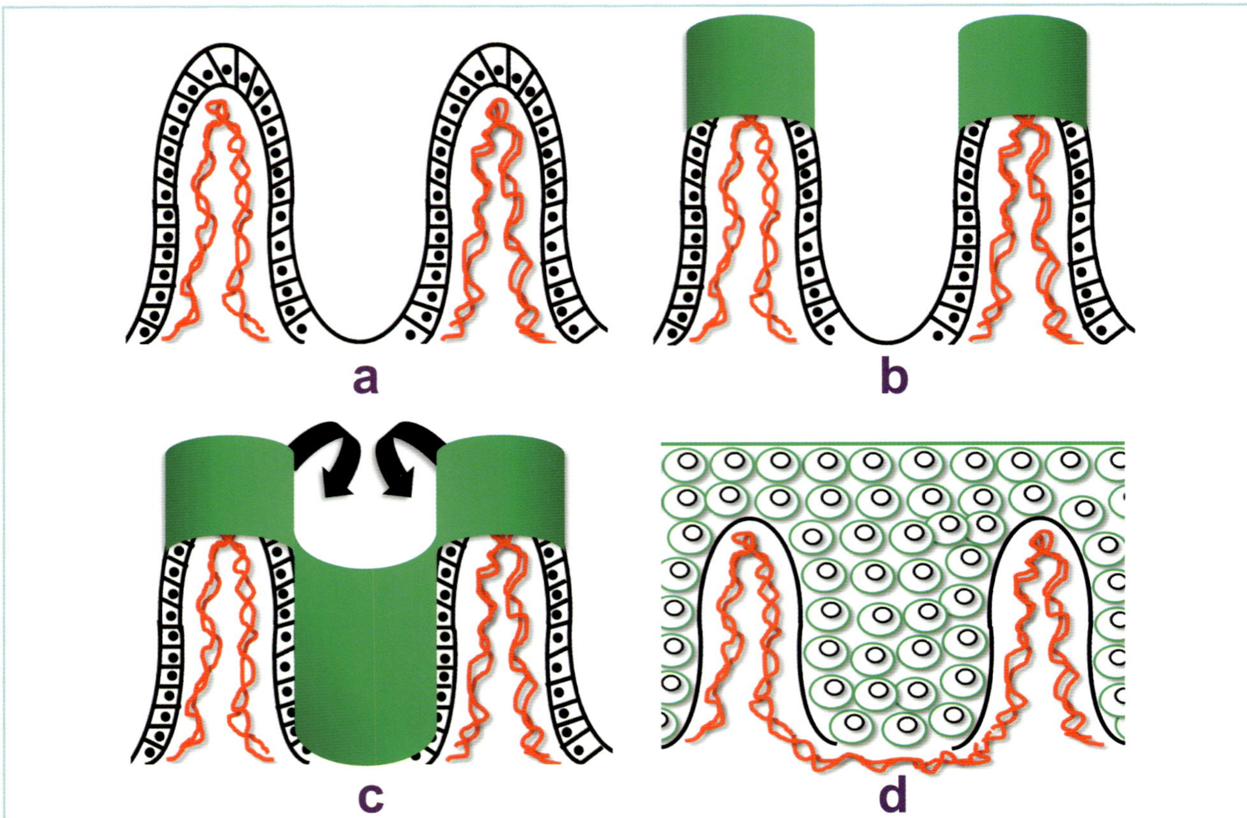

Figure 148 - Diagrammatic representation of squamous metaplasia: a) columnar villi; b) the immature metaplastic epithelium caps the villi; c) the immature metaplastic tissue extends into the clefts of adjacent villi; d) a smooth surface is produced within the original columnar epithelium.

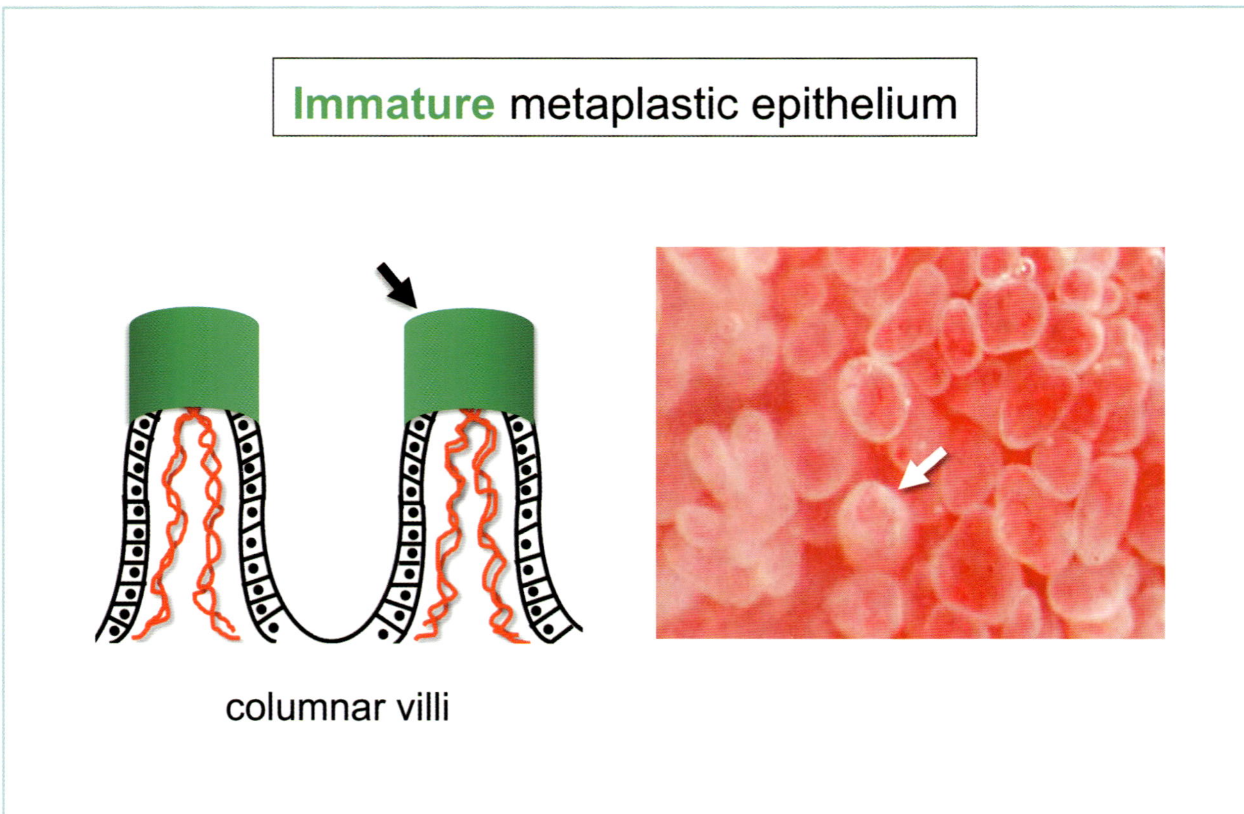

Figure 149 - Diagrammatic representation and colpophotograph of the effect of acetic acid on the tip of columnar villi (arrows).

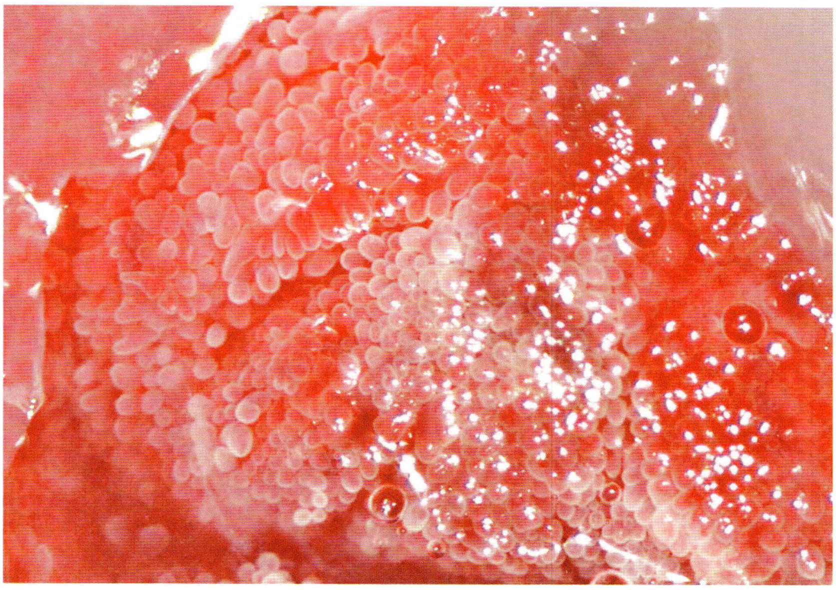

Figure 150 - Application of acetic acid causes some opaqueness on tip of columnar villi.

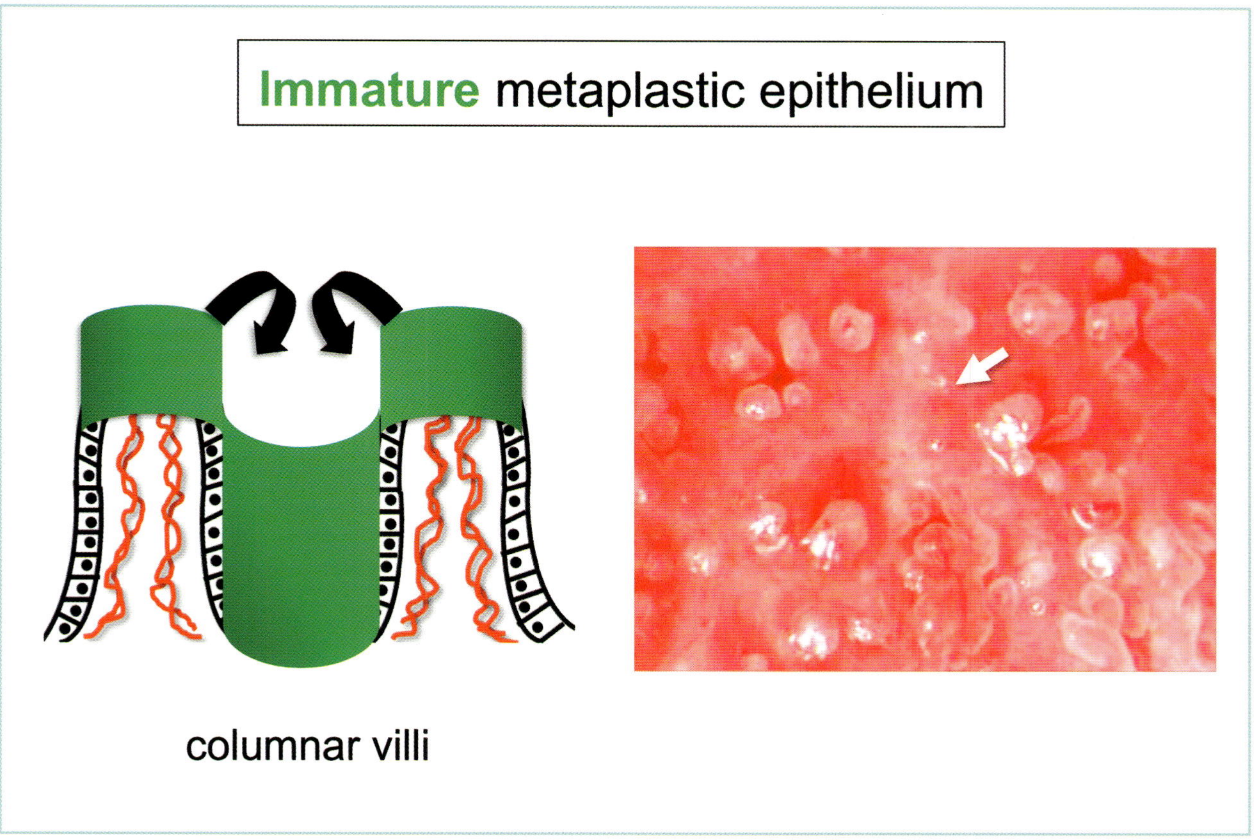

Figure 151 - The immature metaplastic tissue extends into the clefts of adjacent villi, as shown in the colpophotograph (arrow) and in the diagrammatic representation.

can be produced (Figure 156). Scattered acetowhite dots characterize metaplastic white punctation, colposcopically distinguishable from the other white punctations (fungal and viral) due to it appearing fine and contiguous to the squamocolumnar junction (Figure 157).

Metaplastic changes can also involve the distal portion of a cervical polyp protruding in the acidic vaginal environment (Figure 158). This immature metaplastic tissue may undergo the same dysplastic noxae seen on the cervical epithelium (Figure 159). When a typical metaplastic change occurs, after the

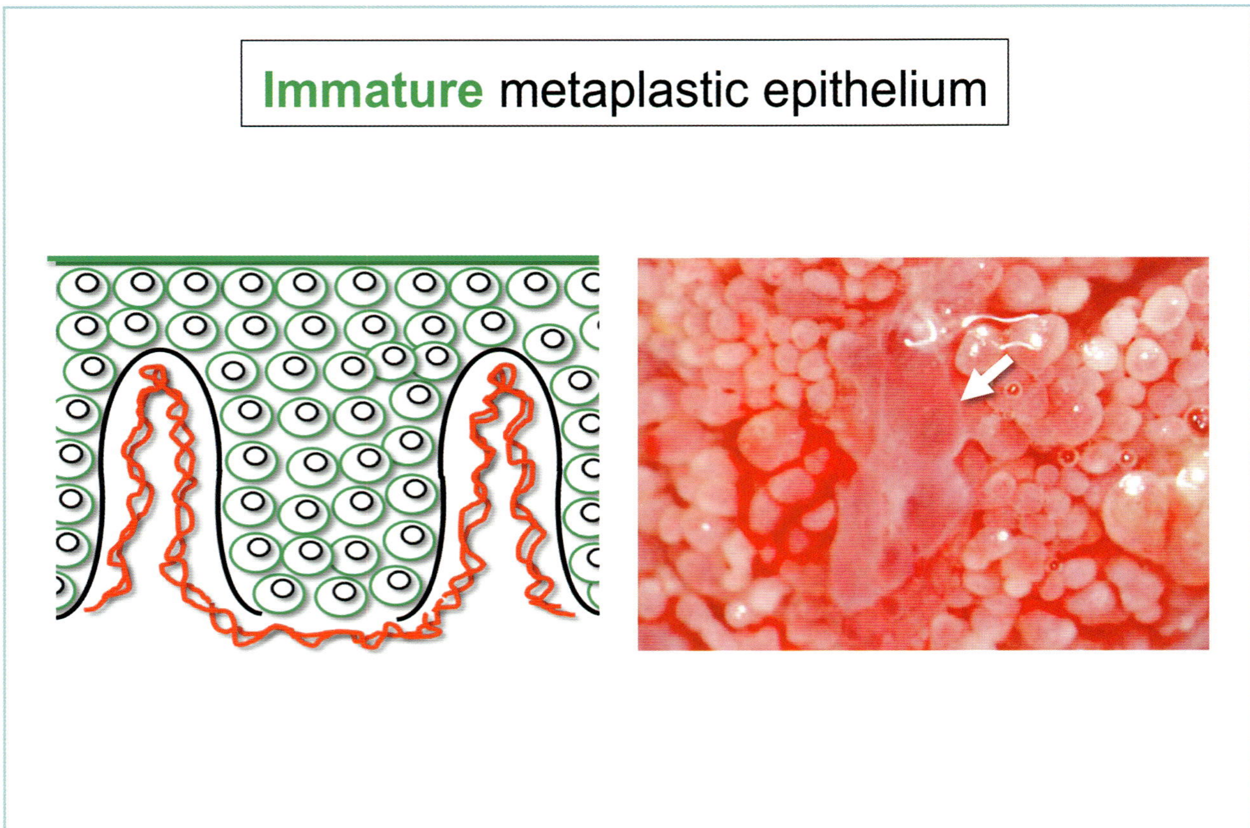

Figure 152 - The colposcopic feature shows a faint acetowhite, immature metaplastic epithelium, characterized by a smooth and translucent surface (arrow).

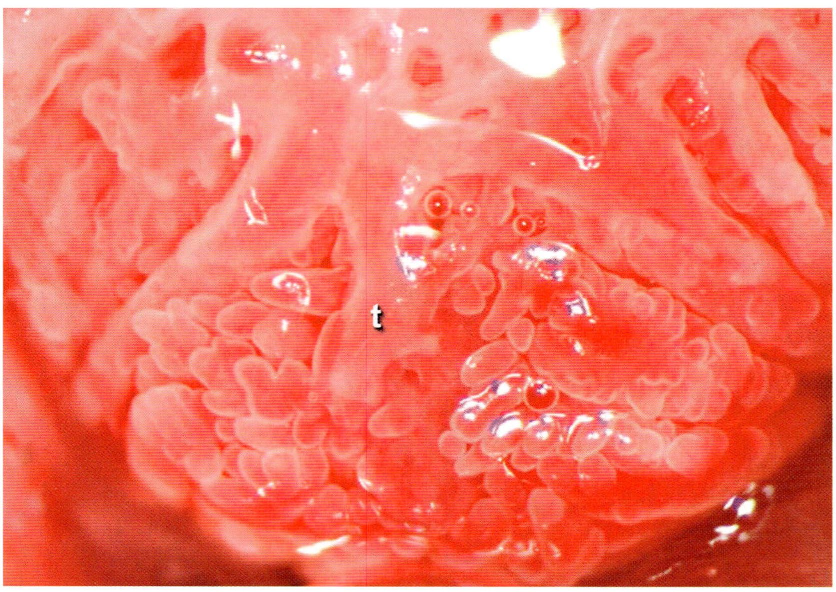

Figure 153 - The immature metaplastic epithelium appears faint acetowhite and produces well-defined tongue-like projections (t).

immature metaplastic epithelium has extended into the clefts of adjacent villi, until a smooth surface is produced (Figure 160a), individual stromal papillae become progressively flattened (Figure 160b) and the capillary structures in the villi are compressed and reduced in height. Lastly, capillaries form a fine network below the basement membrane and are not incorporated into the newly formed squamous epithelium (Figures 160c, 161).

How may this single layer of columnar cells turn into a thick stratified squamous tissue? The irritation of everted columnar epithelium by the acidic vaginal

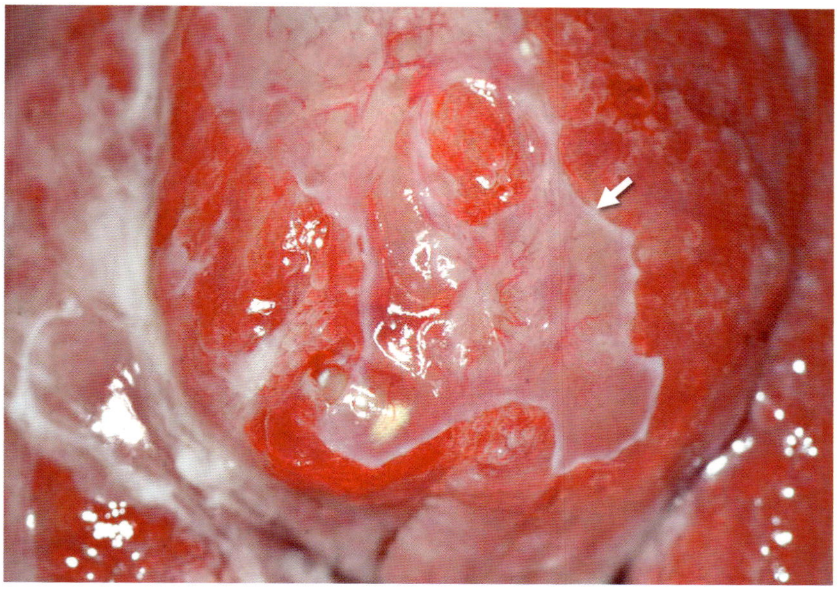

Figure 154 - The membrane-like area of immature metaplastic epithelium shows a smooth and translucent surface (arrow).

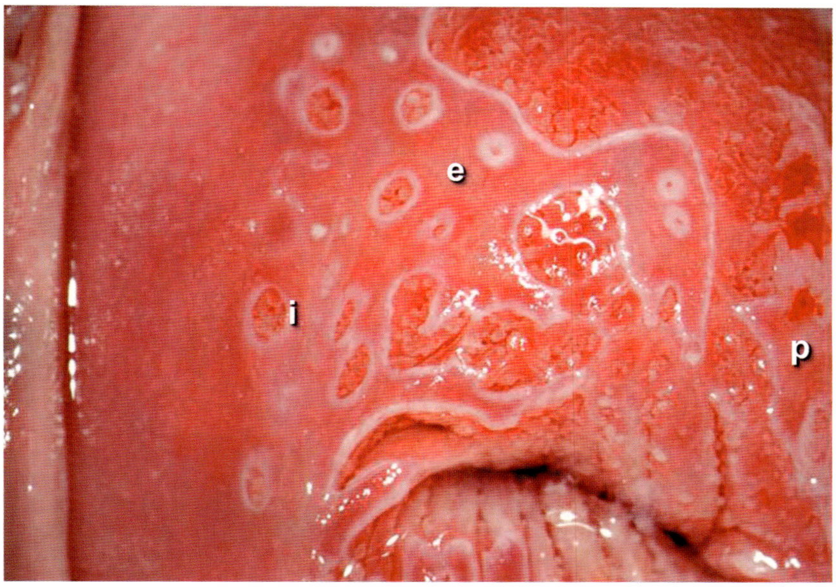

Figure 155 - The wedge-shaped offshoots originating from the original squamocolumnar junction (epithelialization) (e), proceed towards the intra-junctional metaplastic patch (p). Islands of the original columnar epithelium (i) are scattered in the new developed metaplastic epithelium.

environment results in the progressive shedding and destruction of columnar cells. Simultaneously, in response to irritation caused by vaginal acidity, small staminal cells known as sub-columnar *reserve cells* appear between columnar cells and the basement membrane (Figure 162a). In a variable time, reserve cells multiply (reserve cell hyperplasia) (Figure 162b) and the original columnar epithelium, that sometimes remains atop these new elements, is shed.
The metaplastic squamous epithelium is produced from the multiplication of reserve cells which turn into different maturative stages of metaplastic cells. These changes lead to the formation of a multilayered but still undifferentiated epithelium, referred to as *immature metaplastic epithelium* (Figure 163).
Immature metaplastic epithelium differs from mature squamous epithelium in that it is more cellular and most of its cells contain a large and immature nucleus, rich in proteins. The great amount of these nucleoproteins is responsible for acetowhiteness. At this time, after application of acetic acid, the direct light will be reflected from the epithelium and no longer from the stroma, giving the epithelium an opaque white appearance (Figure 164).
Once acetic acid has been applied, the speed of the appearance and disappearance of whiteness, as well as, its intensity and duration of stay, are related to different cytologic conditions such as increased cellularity, increased nucleo-cytoplasmic ratio, increased nuclear density, and thus relate to the degree of underlying histologic changes or abnormality.
Changes induced by acetic acid may be minor or

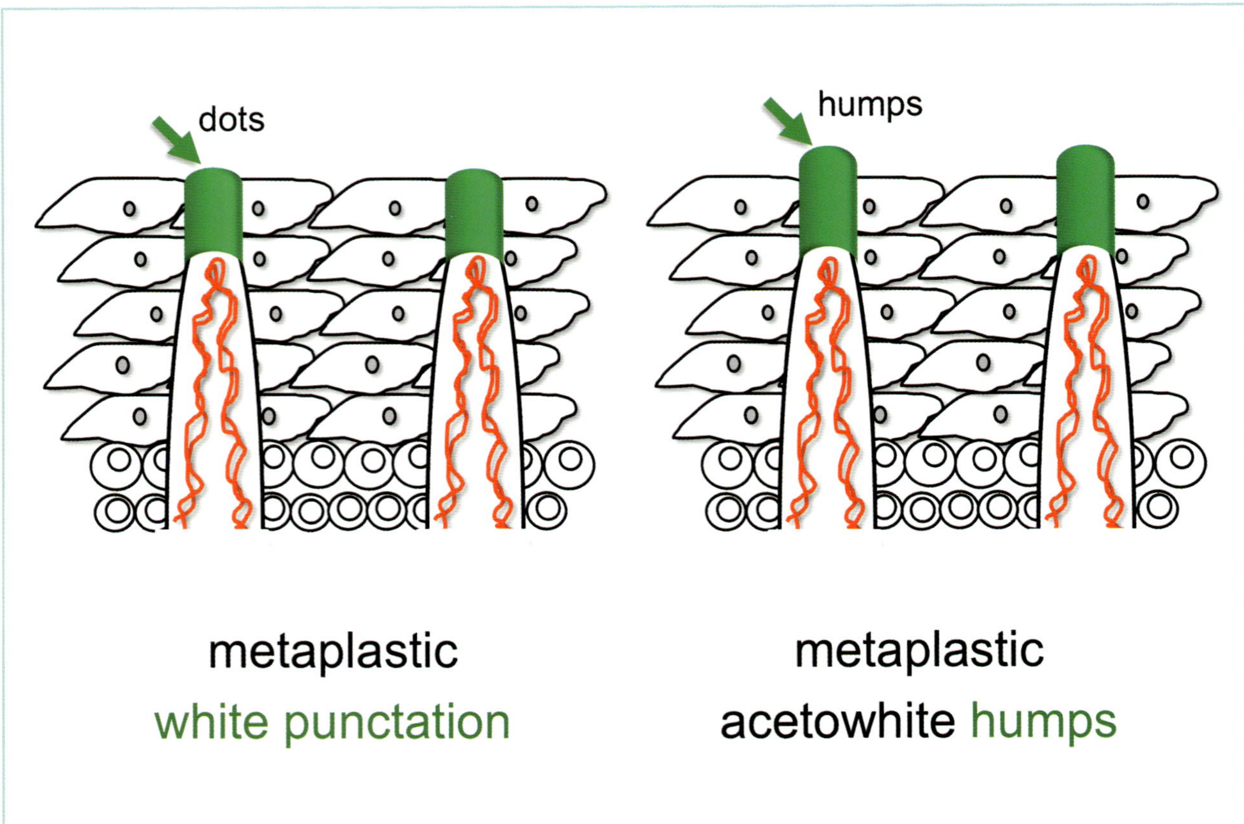

Figure 156 - Diagrammatic representation of metaplastic acetowhite dots (metaplastic white punctation) and small humps.

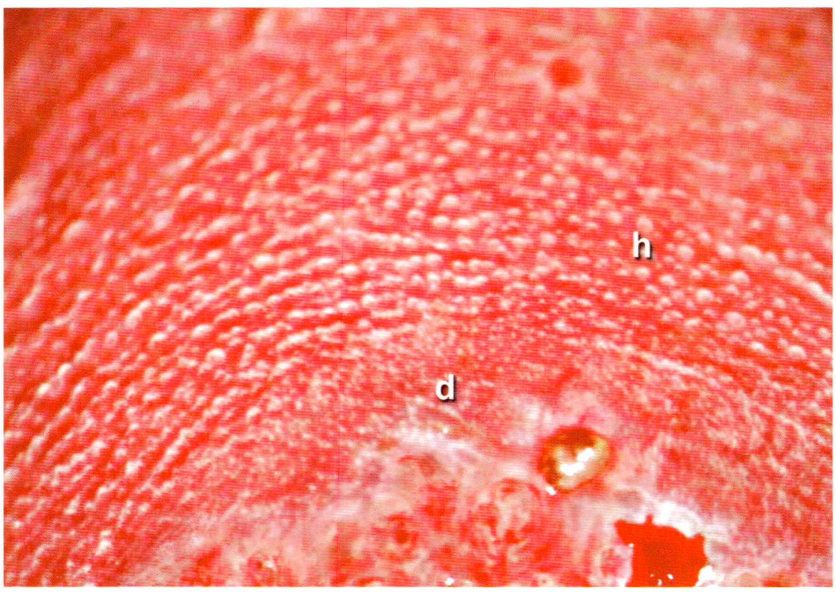

Figure 157 - Metaplastic acetowhite small humps (h) progressively turn into white dots (d) (metaplastic white punctation), close to the squamocolumnar junction.

major (2011 IFCPC Nomenclature). In the former case, acetowhite epithelium is *thin* with irregular, feathery, geographic or angular margins (Grade 1) (Figure 165). The appearance of whitening is delayed because the most nuclear density is located in the lower third of the epithelium and quickly disappears. Minor changes have a diffused margin and can merge almost imperceptibly with the surrounding normal epithelium. When dysplastic areas are too thin, they may escape colposcopic detection. Immature metaplastic epithelium may appear thickened and white after application of acetic acid (*dense* ace-

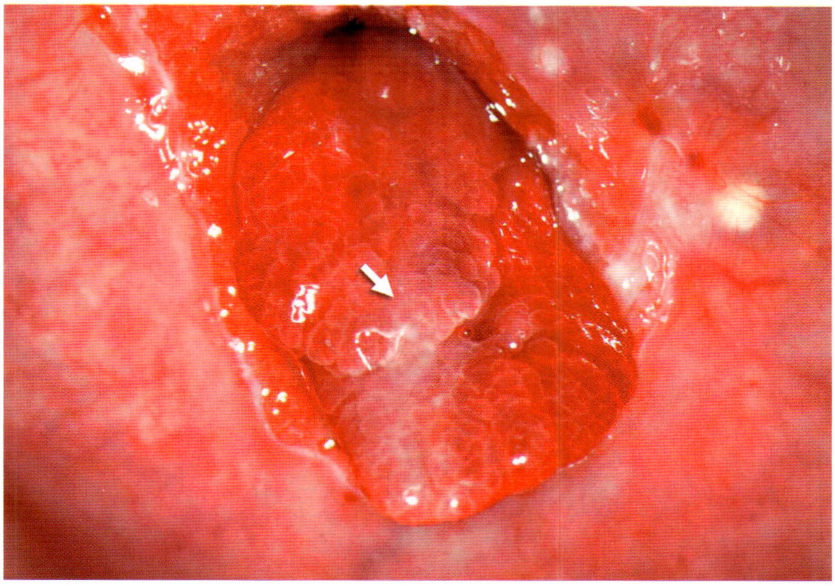

Figure 158 - The tip of the polyp protruding from the endocervical canal is coated with faint acetowhite immature metaplastic epithelium (arrow).

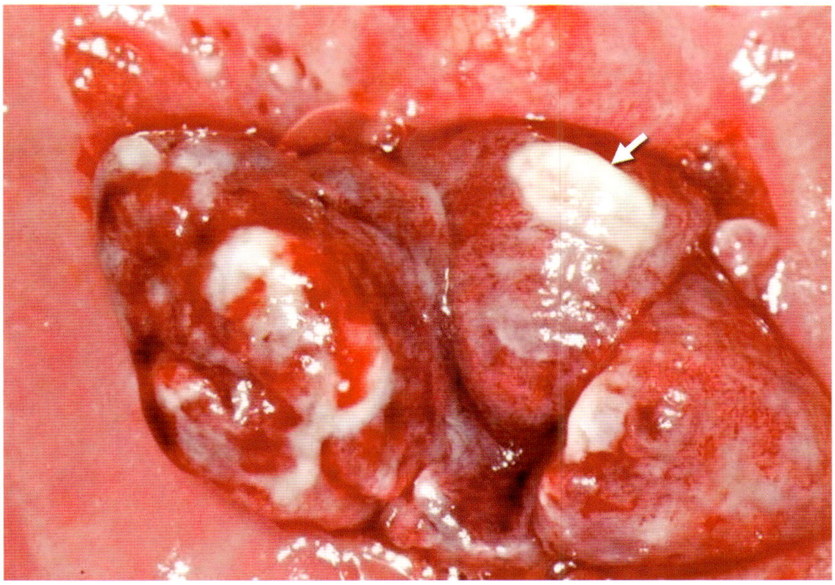

Figure 159 - The tip of the arrowed endocervical polyp displays a thick and intense acetowhite epithelium. Histology of the polyp disclosed a focal CIN III.

towhite epithelium) when its content in nuclear proteins is particularly high, although histology does not reveal any cytologic abnormality (Figures 166, 167).

Inflammation may produce a faint acetowhitening, which is ill-defined and widely distributed in the cervix, not restricted to the transformation zone (Figure 168). Diffuse acetowhitening or scattered white and sometimes raised dots may be observed on the vulva in the presence of poorly glycogenated epithelium (Figure 169) or inflammation (Figure 170). These acetowhite changes may present the colposcopist with a problem in diagnosis versus flat condyloma and the white punctation induced by HPV. The low content of glycogen in immature metaplastic epithelium is responsible for the partial capture of iodine after Lugol's iodine solution application, depending on the various stages of development of the metaplastic process. This focal glycogen retention gives a speckled appearance of epithelium (iodine partial positive area) (Figure 171).

Iodine staining is a must before performing biopsy or ablative procedures, to ensure free margins of the healthy mucosa. It should be pointed out that Schiller's test is extremely useful in the evaluation of all the vaginal folds and above all in the presence of iodine-negative areas that have shown faint acetowhitening.

Furthermore, iodine staining is helpful for novel colposcopists in order to localize abnormal areas and confirm the colposcopic suspicion. Nevertheless, many colposcopists have stopped Schiller's test, con-

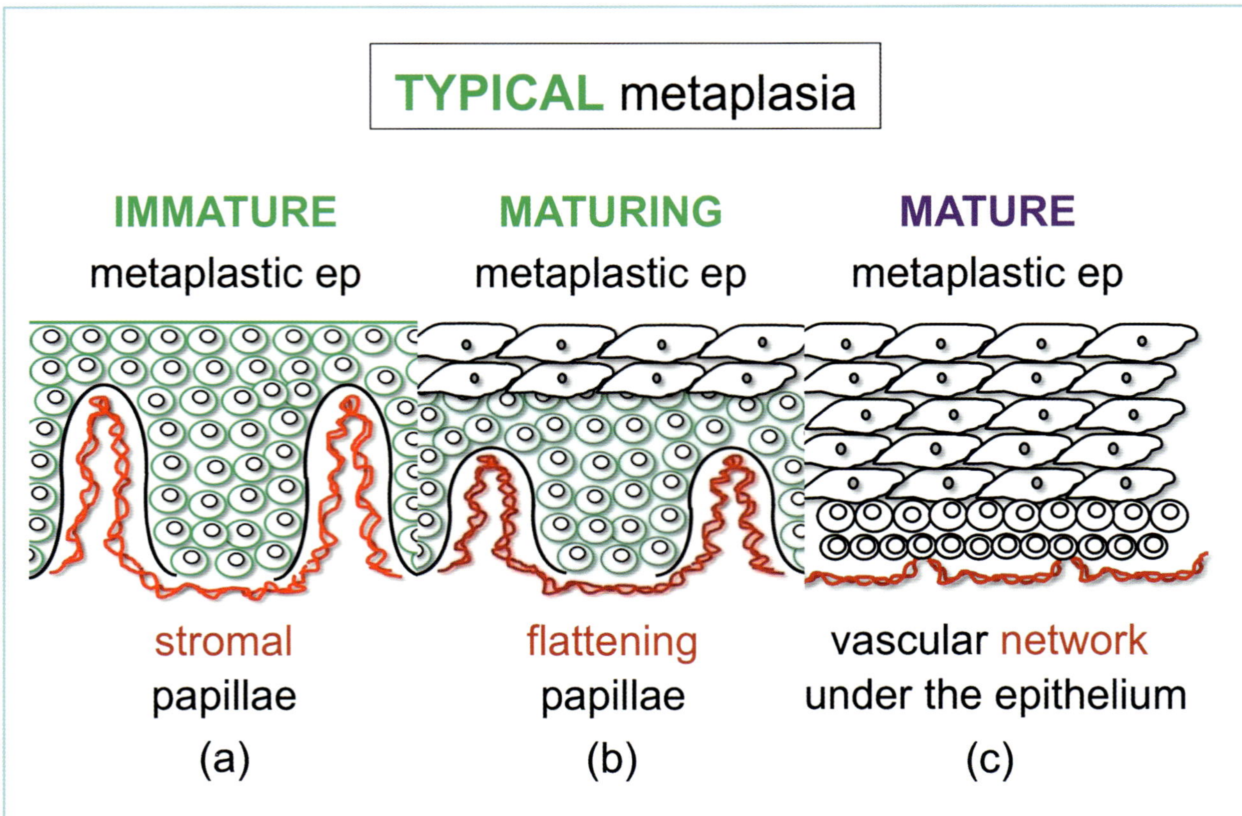

Figure 160 - Diagrammatic representation of stromal papillae in immature metaplastic epithelium (a) which progressively flatten (b), until a fine network below the basement membrane is formed (c), in the presence of a newly developed mature squamous epithelium.

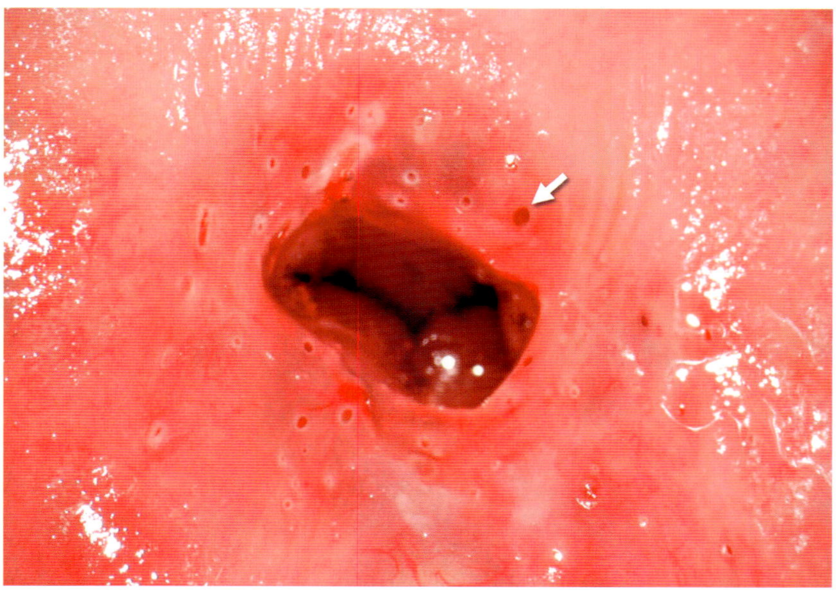

Figure 161 - Mature metaplastic epithelium with scattered gland openings (arrow).

sidering it a non-specific test that does not add further information to the colposcopic evaluation. Furthermore, iodine staining may obscure very minute vascular details and it is often difficult to differentiate between atrophic mucosa lacking in glycogen and iodine-negative dysplastic areas. Additionally, possible cervical trauma caused by insertion of the vaginal speculum may result in an iodine negative-area.

Finally, in normal conditions, immature metaplastic epithelium will produce a *mature squamous epithelium*. The fully mature metaplastic epithelium ap-

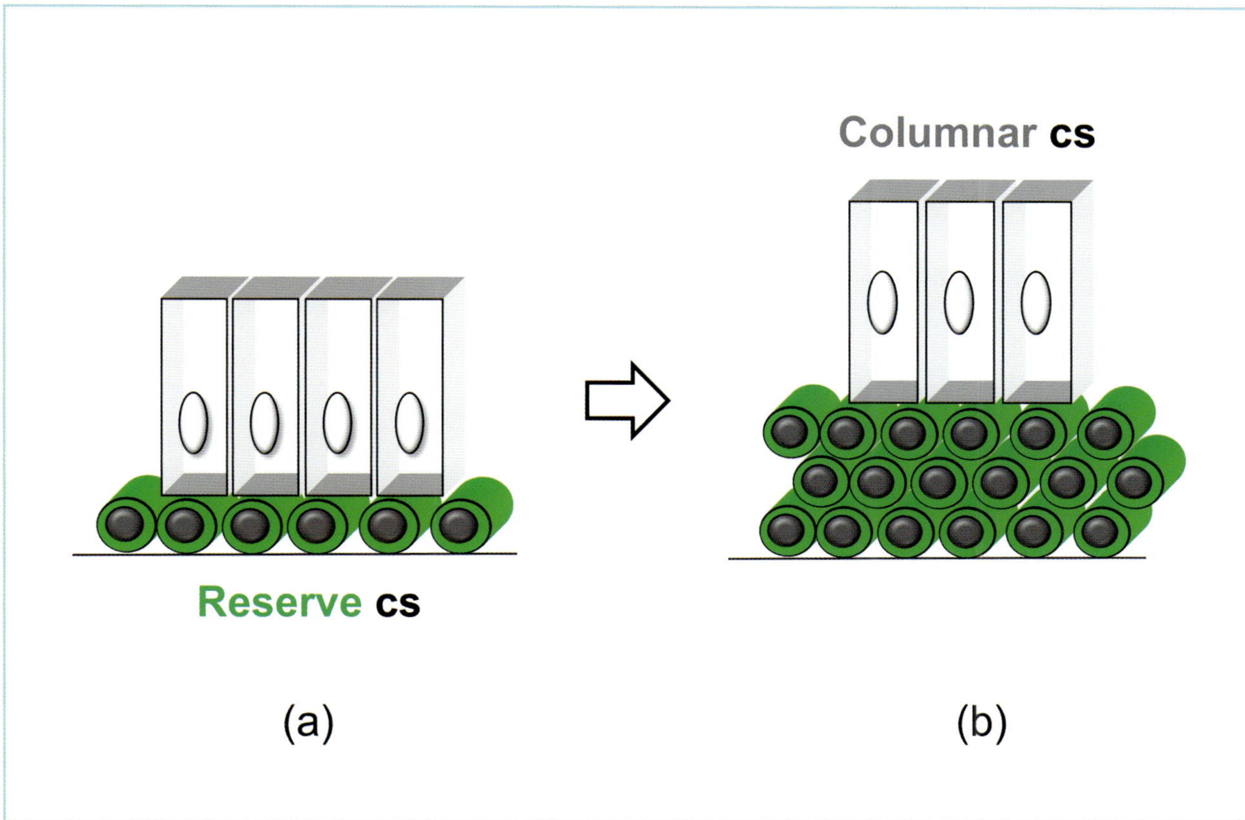

Figure 162 - Diagrammatic representation of reserve cells, located between the basement membrane and columnar cells.

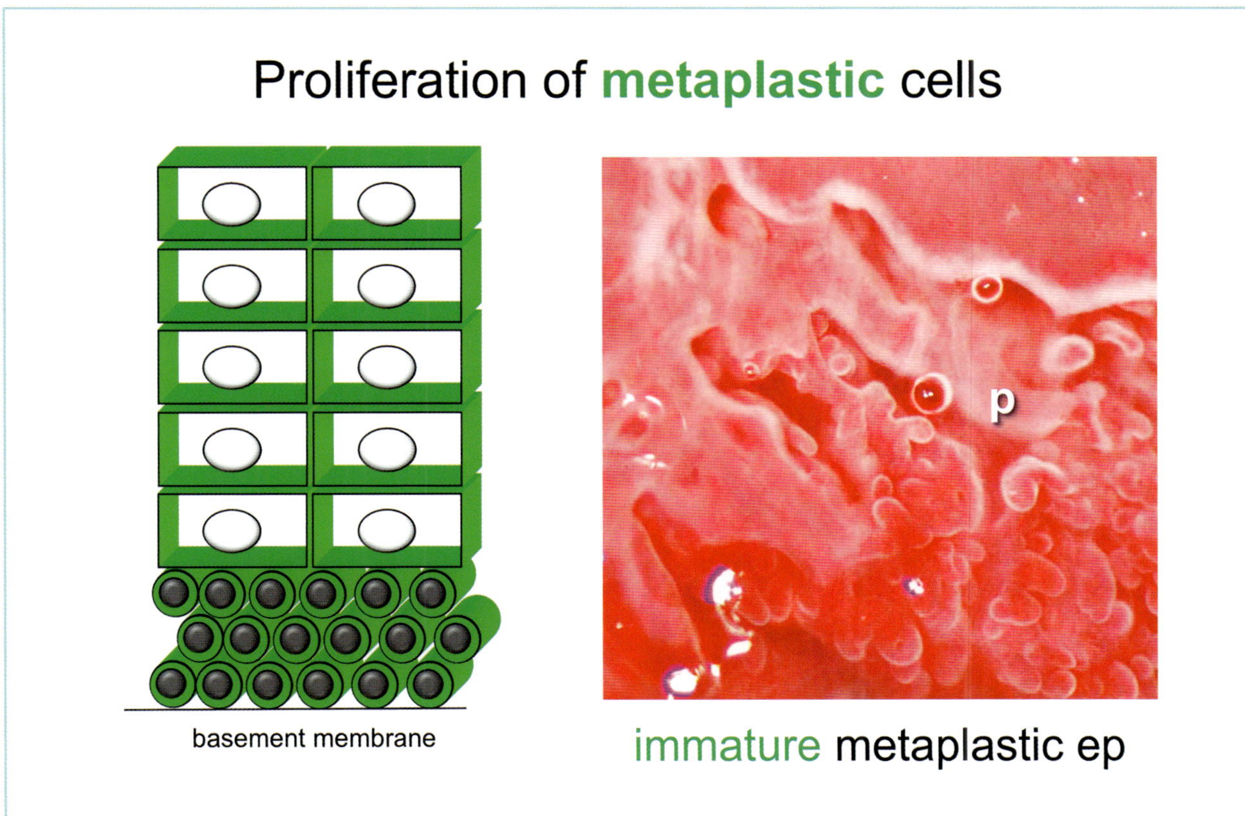

Figure 163 - The diagrammatic representation shows a stratified but not yet differentiated immature metaplastic epithelium. On colposcopy, the same epithelium appears faint acetowhite with tongue-like projections (p).

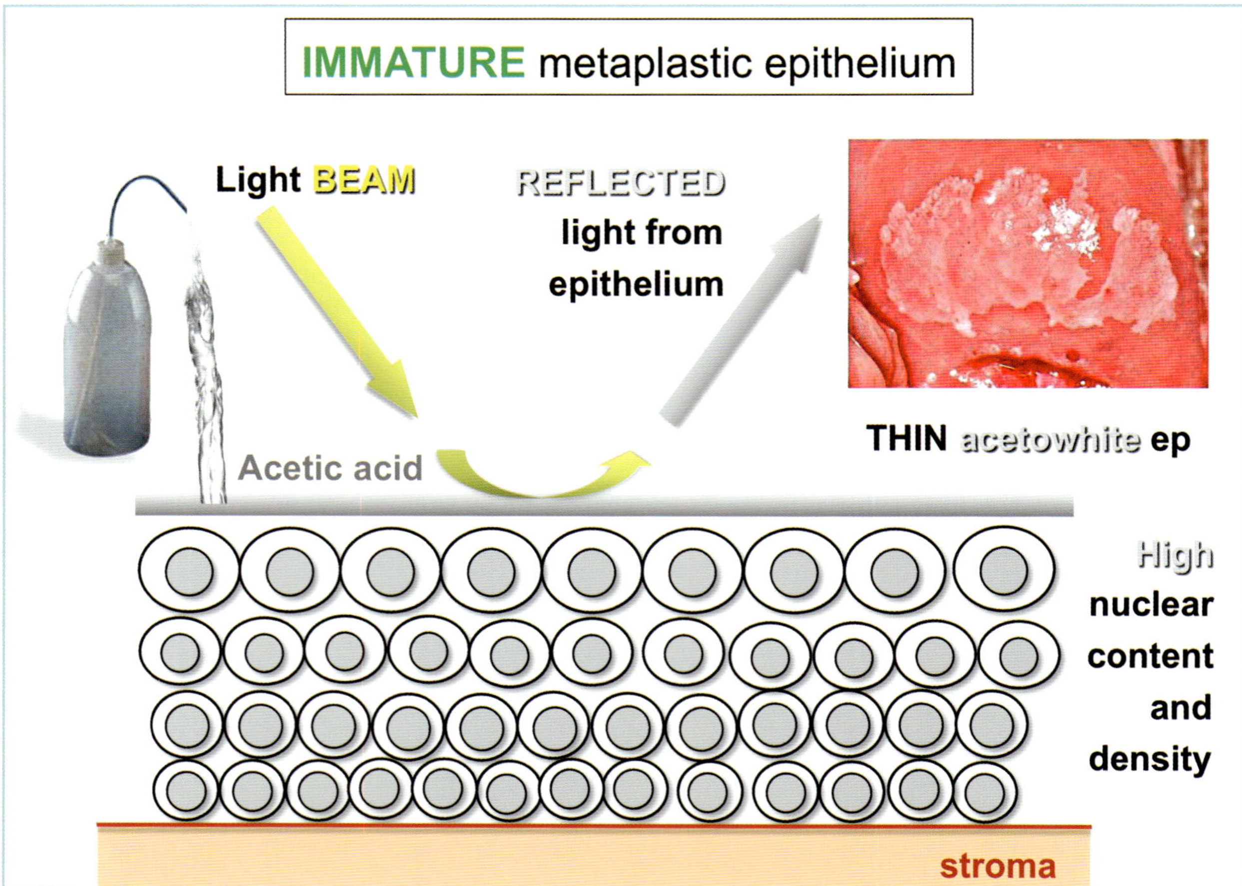

Figure 164 - Diagrammatic representation of the light pathway, through an immature metaplastic epithelium, after application of acetic acid. The colpophotograph exhibits a thin acetowhite area, with geographic margins.

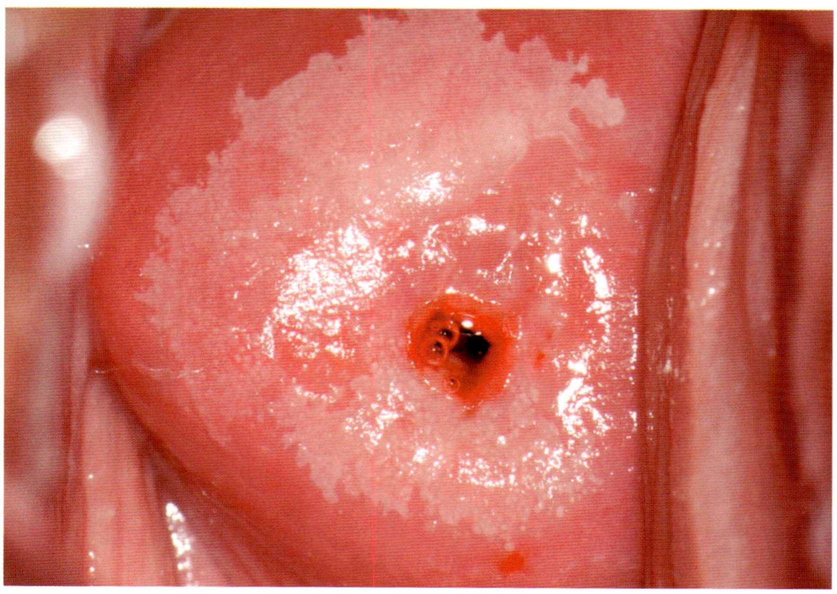

Figure 165 - Thin acetowhite epithelium with irregular, feathery, geographic or angular margins.

pears smooth like the original squamous epithelium, but it is distinguishable from the latter due to the following aspects:

- The mature squamous metaplastic epithelium appears light pink or whitish-pink, compared with the translucent darker pink original squamous epithelium (Figure 172). Sometimes a reddish border separates original squamous epithelium from fully developed metaplastic epithelium (Figure 173).

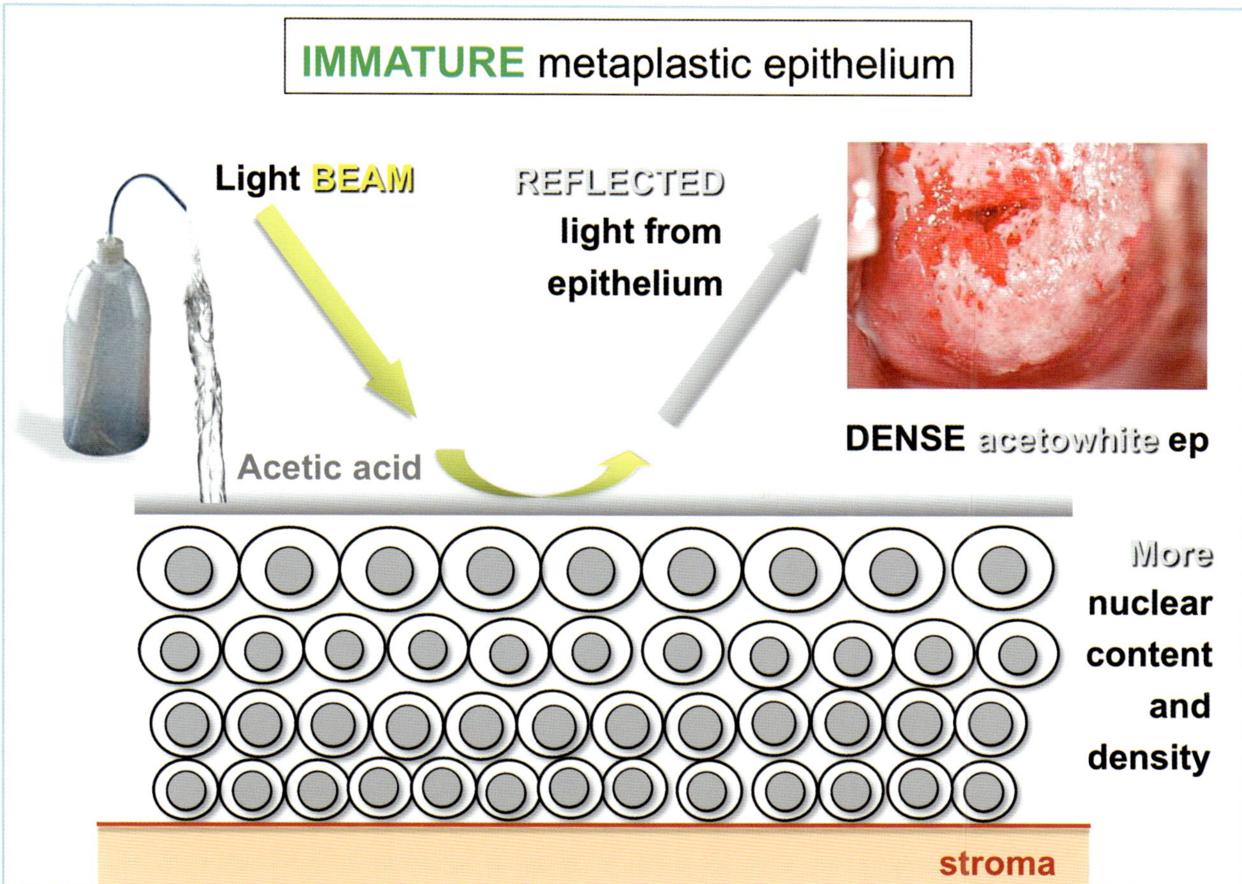

Figure 166 - Diagrammatic representation of the light pathway, through an immature metaplastic epithelium, after application of acetic acid. The colpophotograph exhibits a thick acetowhite area, with well-defined margins.

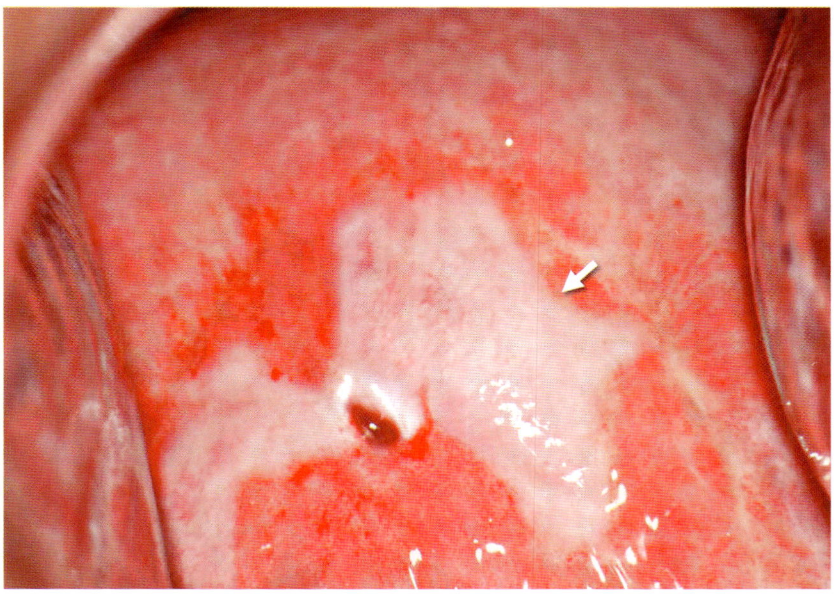

Figure 167 - Thick and raised acetowhite, immature metaplastic epithelium without any cytologic abnormality.

- Islands of the original columnar epithelium are scattered in the adjacent mature squamous epithelium (Figure 174). Sometimes, when the islands of columnar epithelium are completely covered by mature metaplastic epithelium, some dimples are observed on the cervical surface (Figure 175).
- The gland openings, that are not yet covered by metaplastic epithelium, indicate that transformation from the original columnar epithelium

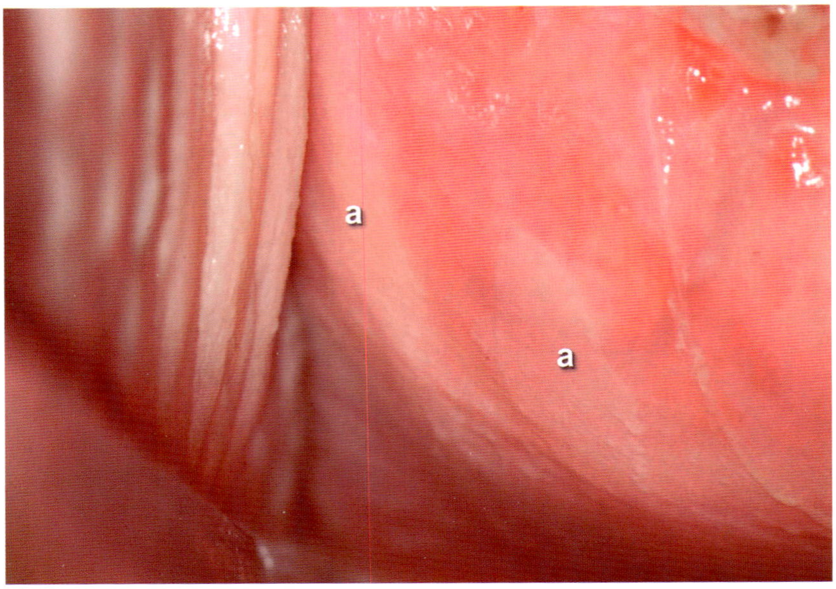

Figure 168 - Faint acetowhite areas (a) produced by inflammation.

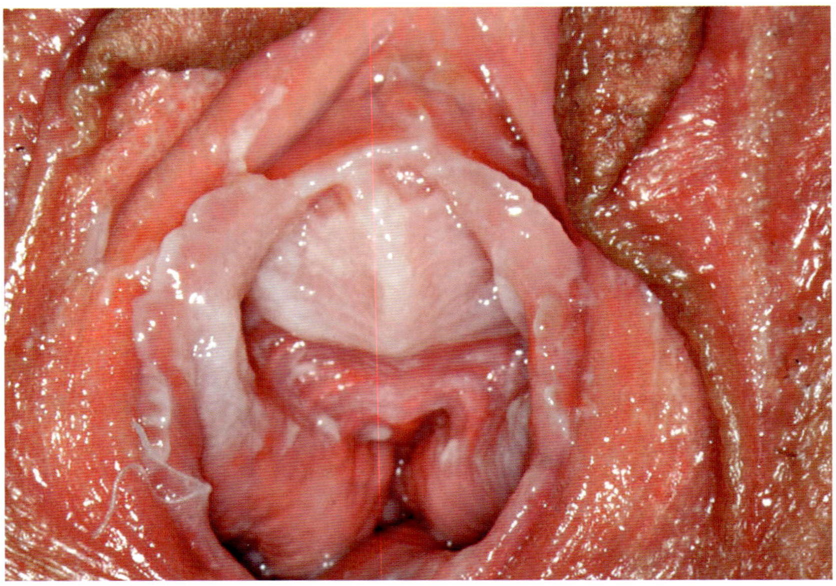

Figure 169 - Diffuse acetowhitening due to poorly glycogenated epithelium.

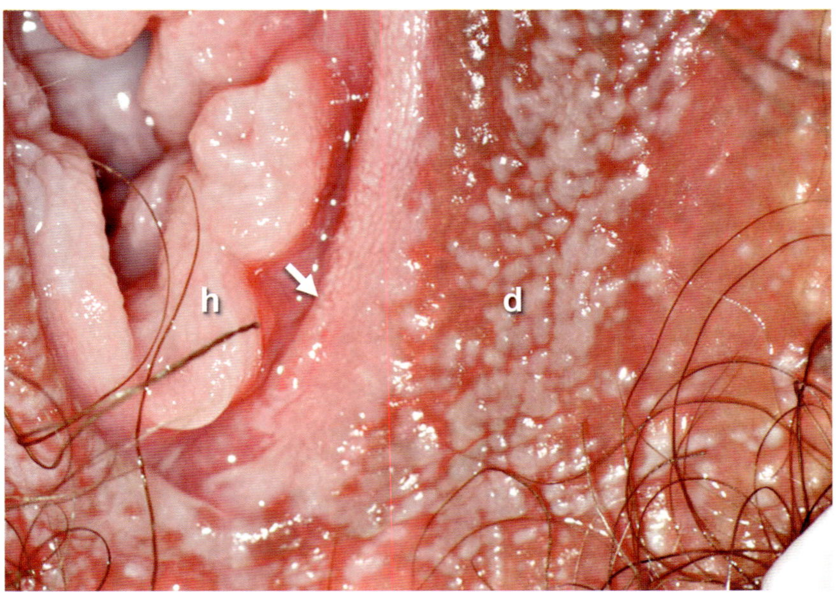

Figure 170 - Inflammation produces acetowhitening on the hymenal ring (h), extending to the fourchette (horse-shoe shape) (arrow) and to the vestibule in the form of raised white dots (d).

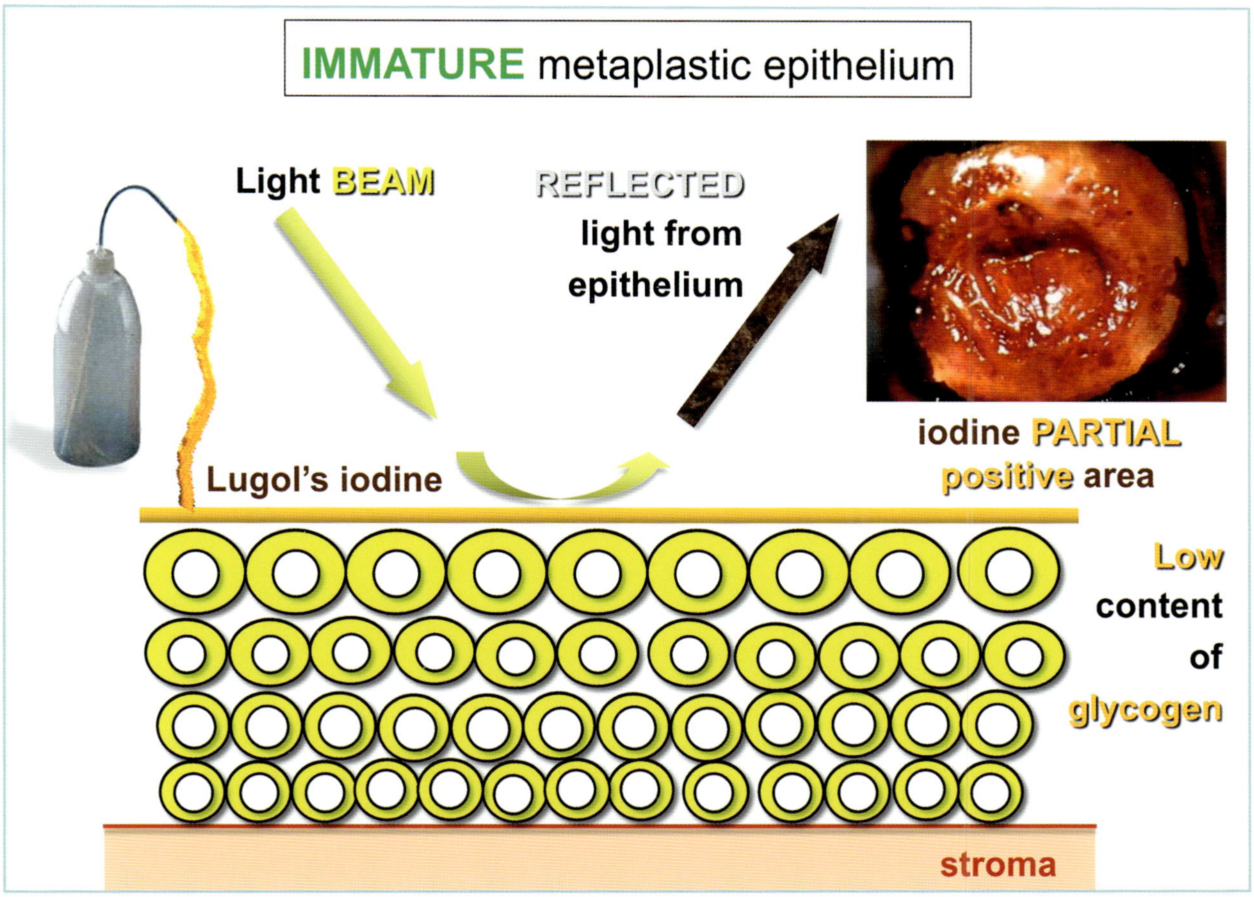

Figure 171 - Diagrammatic representation of the light pathway, through an immature metaplastic epithelium, after Lugol's iodine application. The colpophotograph reveals a focal glycogen retention, which gives a speckled appearance of epithelium.

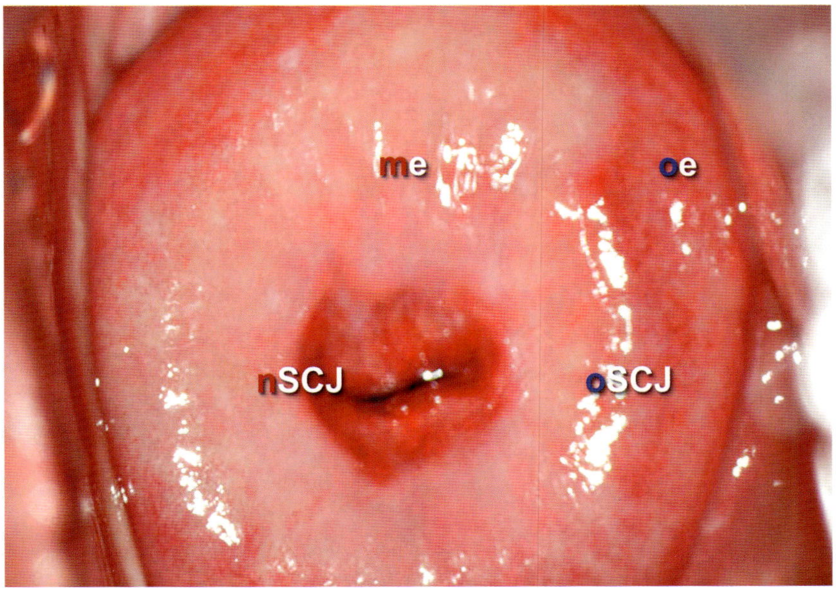

Figure 172 - The mature squamous metaplastic epithelium (me) appears light pink, compared with the darker pink original squamous epithelium (oe). Original squamocolumnar junction (oSCJ), new squamocolumnar junction (nSCJ).

occurred. The most distal crypt opening (Figure 176) or nabothian follicle (Figure 177) usually indicate the distal limit of the transformation zone. Gland openings may appear in different aspects, defining five grades which progressively reflect normal metaplastic changes and different degrees of atypical epithelium (Figure 178):

- Grade I. Gland openings without a surrounding ring, colposcopically seen as red craters only (Figure 179). Sometimes the crypt outlets

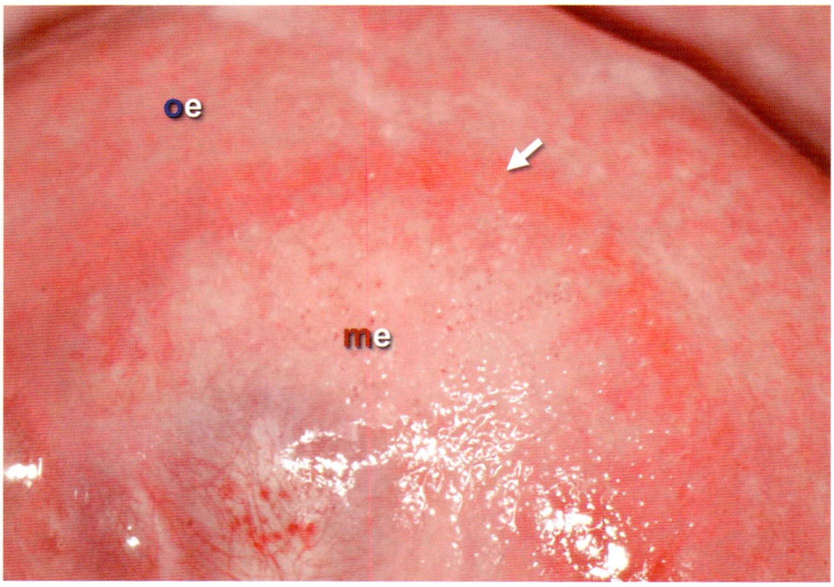

Figure 173 - A reddish border (arrow) separates the whitish-pink mature squamous metaplastic epithelium (me) from the original squamous epithelium (oe).

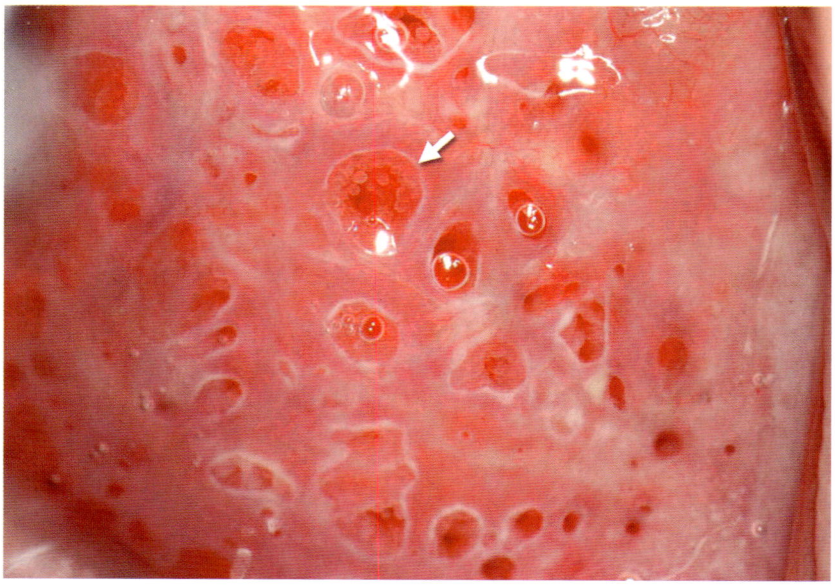

Figure 174 - Multiple islands of original columnar epithelium (arrow) are disseminated in the adjacent almost mature squamous epithelium.

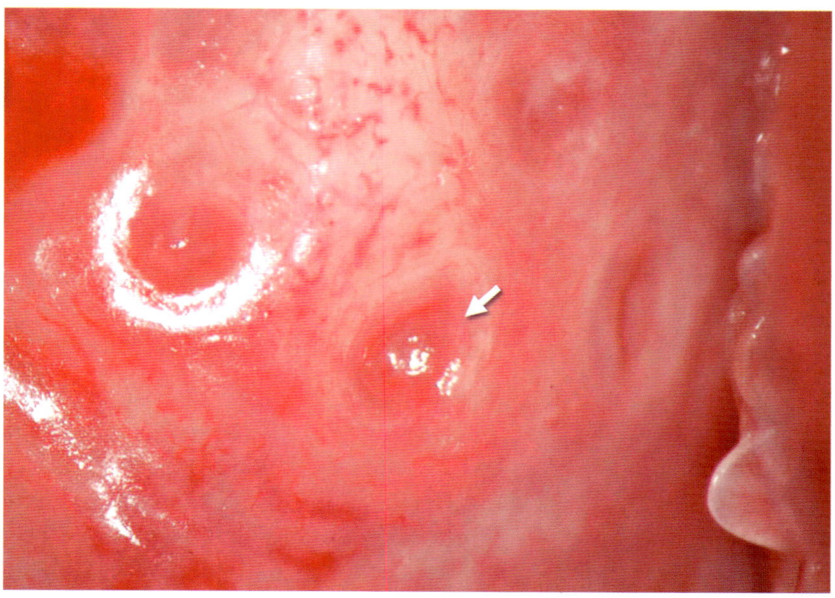

Figure 175 - The arrowed dimple indicates an island of columnar epithelium completely covered by mature metaplastic epithelium.

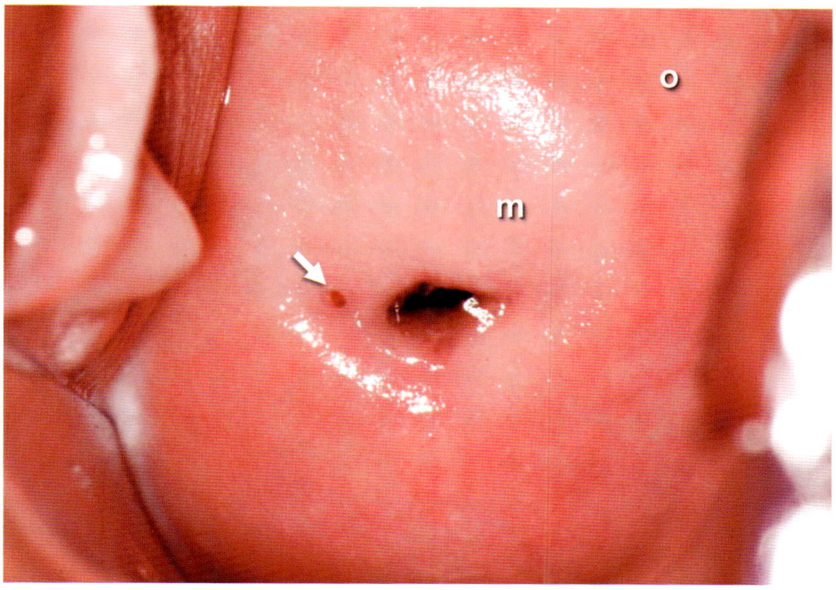

Figure 176 - The most distal crypt opening (arrow) from the external os usually indicates the outer limit of the transformation zone. The colposcopic feature shows the difference between the light pink mature metaplastic epithelium (m) and darker pink original squamous epithelium (o).

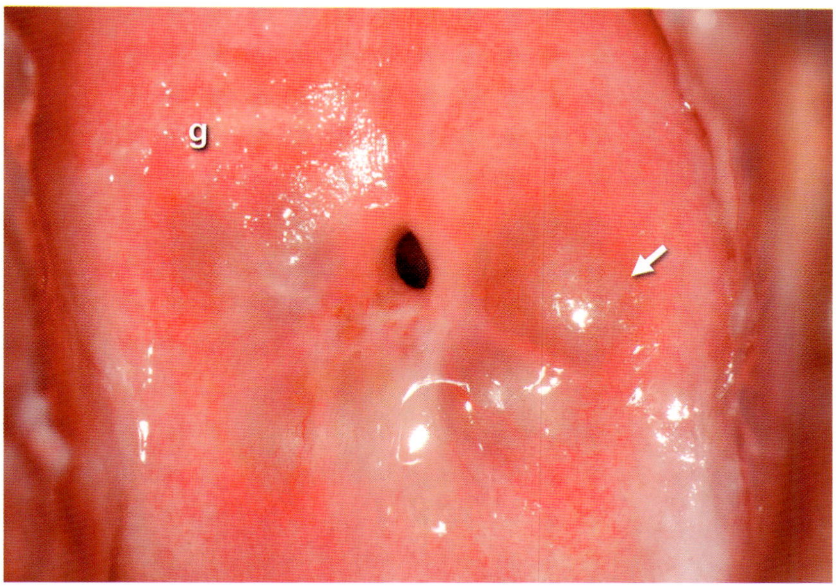

Figure 177 - The arrowed nabothian follicle indicates the outer limit of the transformation zone. Keratotic granules (g).

may be observed while secreting abundant mucus (Figure 180).

- Grade II. Gland openings with a narrow, indistinct white ring (Figure 181).
- Grade III. Gland openings with a distinct but non-raised white ring (Figure 182).
- Grade IV. Gland openings with a dense acetowhite rim, raised from the surface like a doughnut (cuffed gland openings) (Figure 183).
- Grade V. Solid gland openings (Figure 184).

- Nabothian follicles or cysts develop as a result of the occlusion of crypt outlets by the overlying metaplastic squamous epithelium. Regular branching vessels with gradual decreasing caliber and a regular vascular network or flattened capillaries may be seen more prominently over nabothian follicles. When new, nabothian cysts appear transparent (Figure 185) or bluish in color (Figure 186). In the latter case, it is not always easy to distinguish them from endometrial cysts which are usually single, smaller than 1 cm and appear purplish (Figure 187). Histology establishes the diagnosis revealing endometrial glands, classically circular, with conspicuous mitotic figures. Nuclei appear hyperchromatic and cigar-shaped, endometrial stroma is classically cellular and hyperchromatic, and hemosiderin-laden macrophages may be granular.

Some operative procedures such as biopsy or detachment of the eschar following cautery can produce a breach of the cervical epithelium

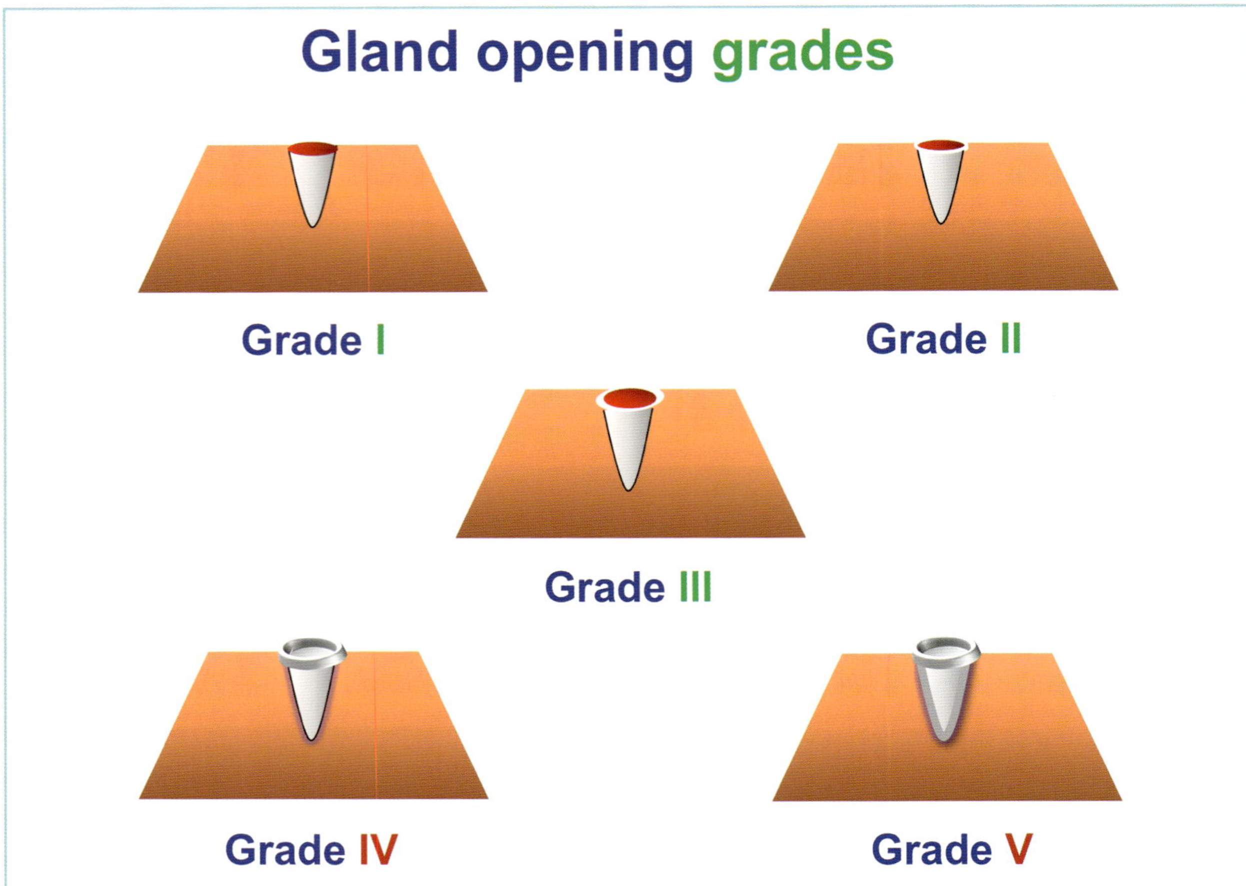

Figure 178 - Grade I to III gland openings reflect normal metaplastic changes whereas grade IV to V gland openings may indicate different degrees of atypical epithelium.

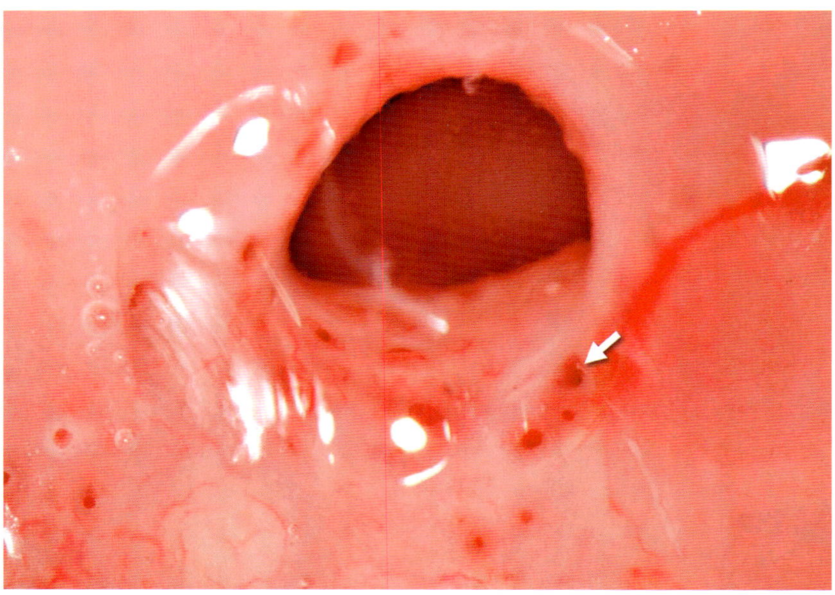

Figure 179 - The arrowed grade I gland opening shows no surrounding acetowhite ring and is seen as a red crater.

which allows the implantation of endometrial tissue. This condition, known as cervical endometriosis, may produce endometrial foci, cysts or ulcers. Endometrial foci are detectable when cervical endometriosis lies deep in the cervical stroma, showing a circumscribed bluish stippling beneath squamous epithelium (Figure 188). Bluish new nabothian cysts must be histologically differentiated from the rare cervical blue nevus (Figure 189).

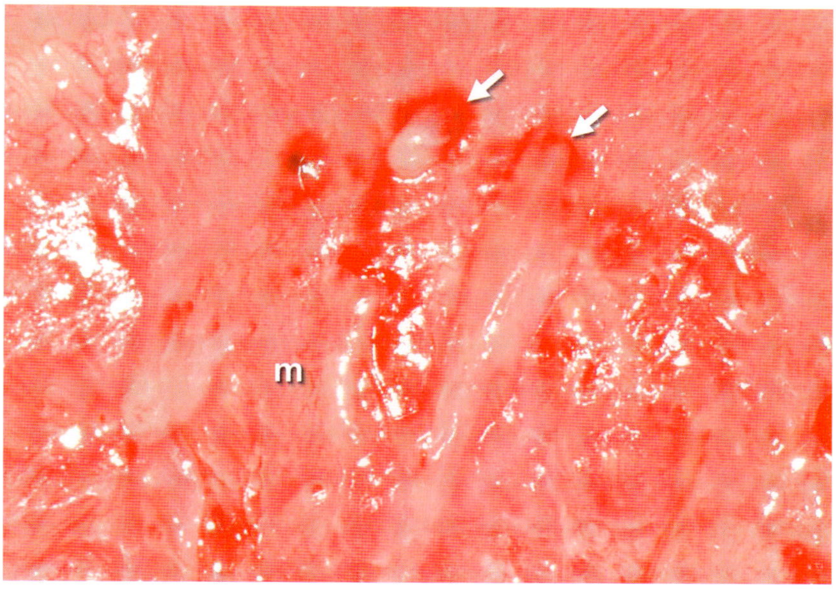

Figure 180 - The arrowed grade I gland openings show no surrounding acetowhite ring and are seen while secreting abundant mucus. Mature metaplastic tissue (m).

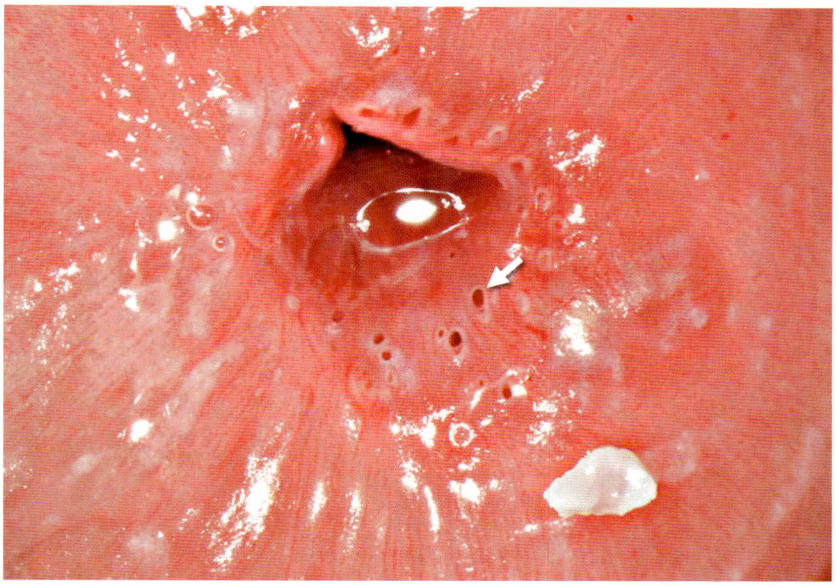

Figure 181 - After application of acetic acid, the grade II gland opening (arrow) shows a narrow, indistinct white ring.

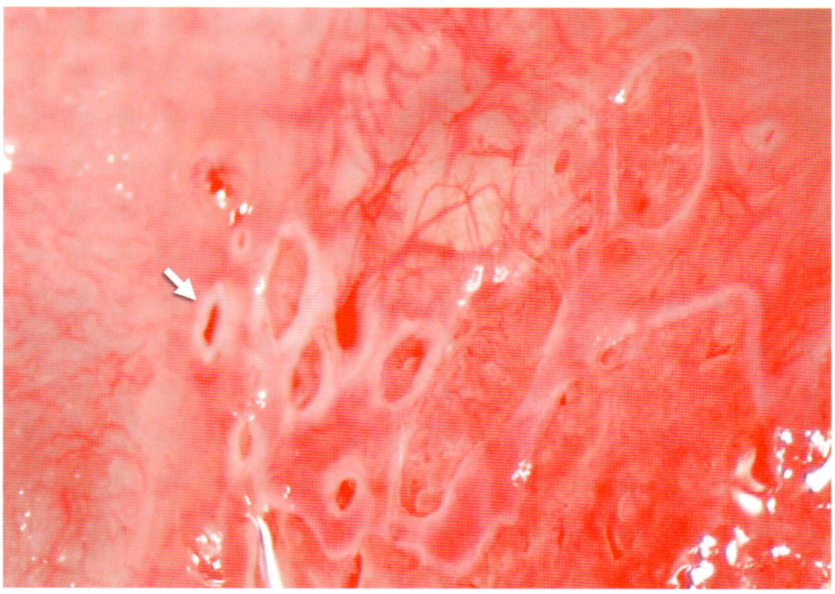

Figure 182 - The arrowed grade III crypt opening is surrounded by a distinct but non-raised white ring.

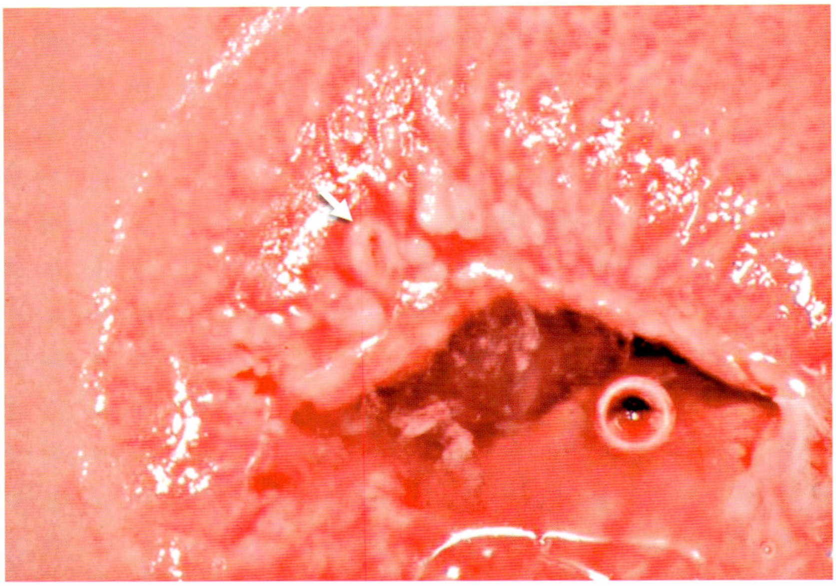

Figure 183 - The arrow indicates a grade IV gland opening, characterized by a distinct and elevated white ring (cuffed gland openings). Histology showed CIN III.

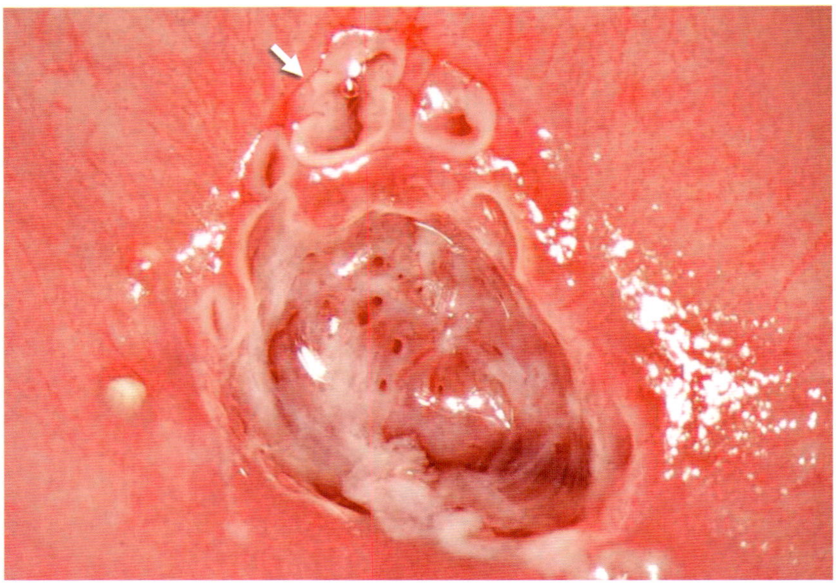

Figure 184 - Solid crypt opening (arrow). On histology, carcinoma in situ was reported.

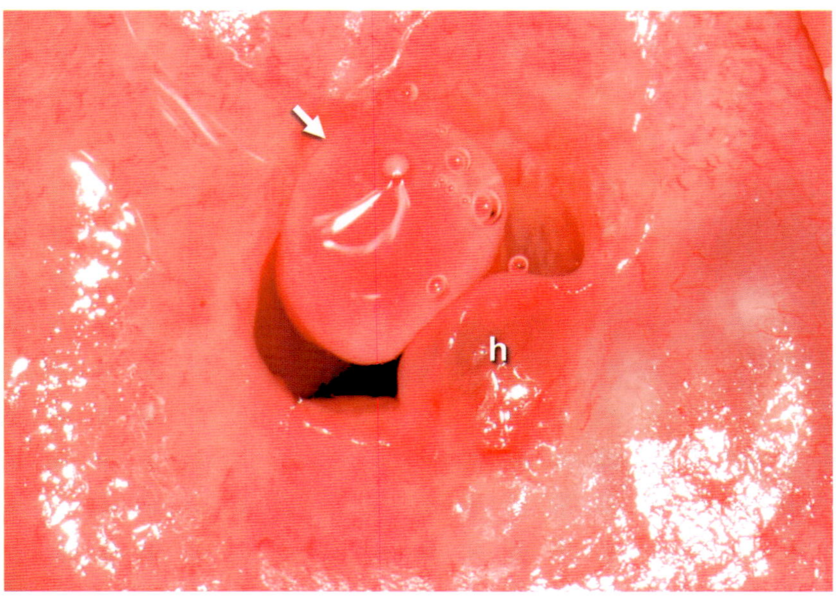

Figure 185 - The arrowed new nabothian cyst appears transparent. Focal hypertrophy of the posterior cervical lip (h).

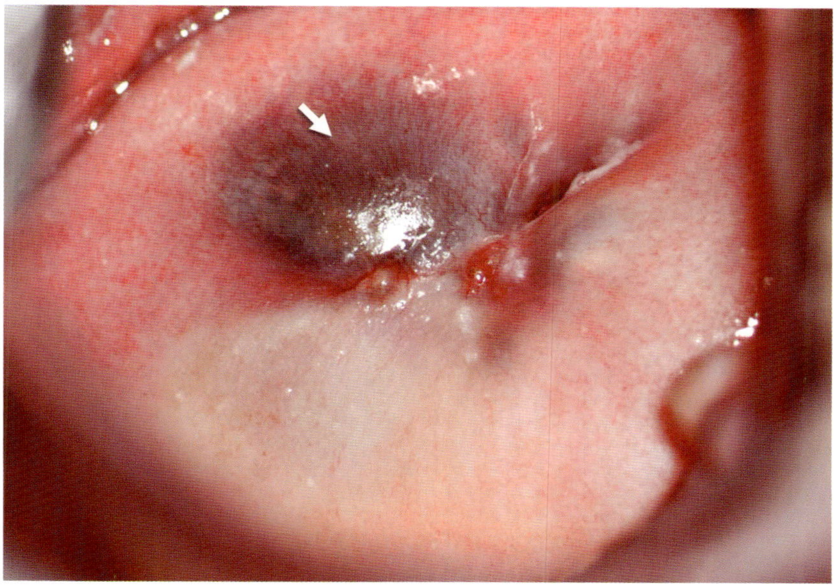

Figure 186 - When new, nabothian cysts may appear bluish in color (arrow).

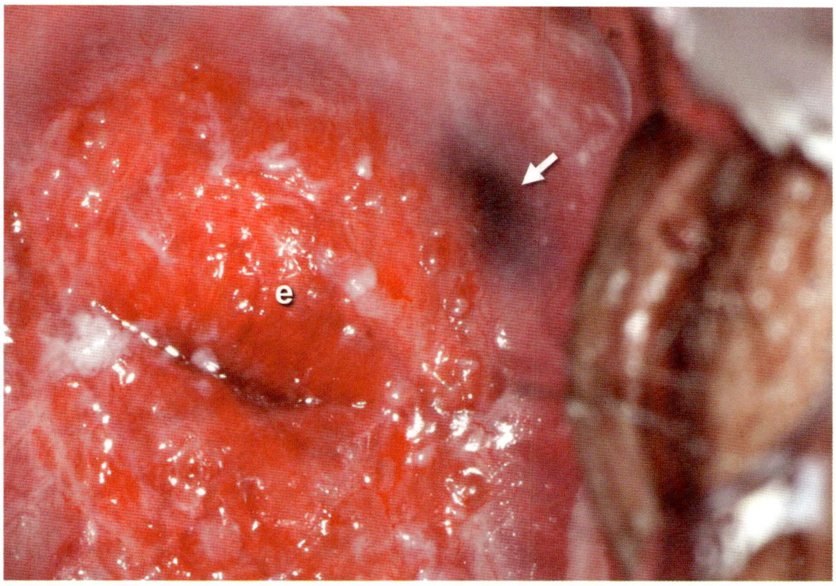

Figure 187 - The arrowed deep endometrial cyst appears purplish. Exposed columnar epithelium (e).

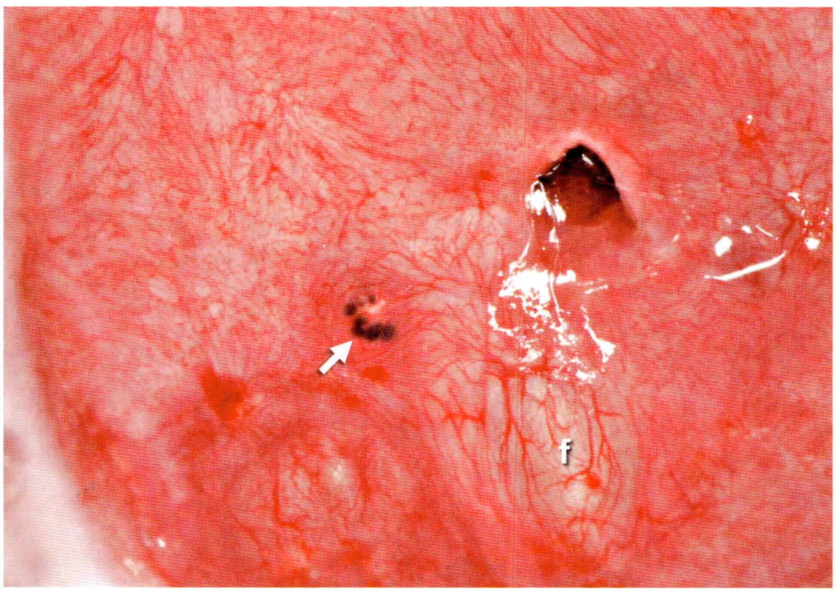

Figure 188 - Focus of endometriosis appears as a circumscribed bluish stippling, beneath the squamous epithelium (arrow). Branching vessels with decrease in caliber are seen over the surface of a deep nabothian follicle (f).

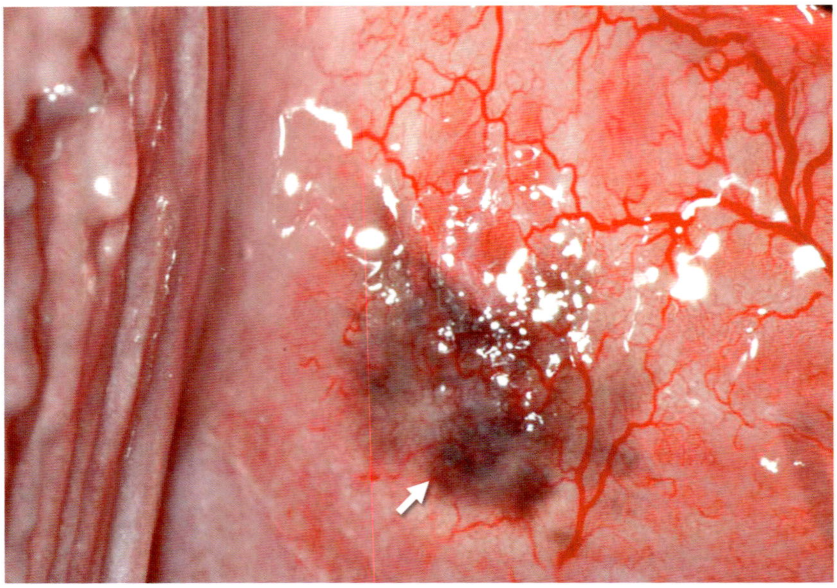

Figure 189 - Cervical blue nevus (arrow).

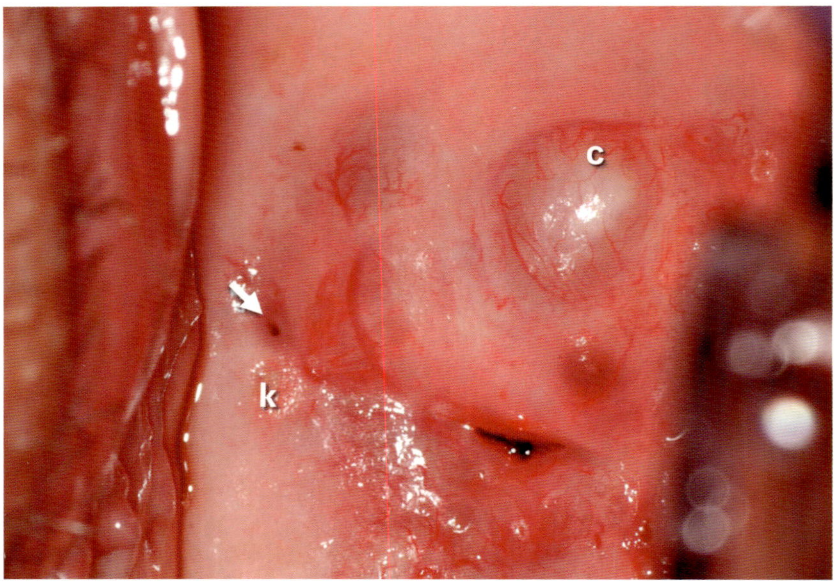

Figure 190 - Whitish nabothian cyst (c). The arrow indicates the most distal crypt opening. Keratotic granules (k).

On becoming old, bluish nabothian cysts turn ivory-white (Figure 190) or yellowish (Figure 191). Several cysts of different formation age may appear chambered (Figure 192). Glandular cysts may be seen also on the surface of endocervical polyps (Figure 193).

Sometimes, large vessels over nabothian cysts may mimic an abnormal vascular pattern, showing completely irregular and haphazard distribution with abrupt angular change (Figures 194, 195).

- Capillary vessels are more numerous than beneath original squamous epithelium (Figures 196, 197).
- During metaplastic maturation or in neovascularization occurring after ablative procedures, the tip of hairpin capillaries which extend high-up into stromal papillae that are not yet flattened, may be seen as fine punctation arranged in radiating lines from the external os (healing lines) (Figures 198, 199). Later, these punctate lines disappear and are eventually replaced by subepithelial fibrosis, seen as white areas before the application of acetic acid (Figure 200). Subepithelial fibrosis differs from dense immature metaplastic epithelium in that the latter appears translucent (see Figure 167).

Mature metaplasia is a permanent condition, but immature metaplastic changes make epithelium prone to potential neoplastic noxae. In fact, the transformation zone, the area in the columnar epithelium where a new squamous metaplastic epithelium forms, is the site where cervical intraepithelial neoplasia (CIN) originates.

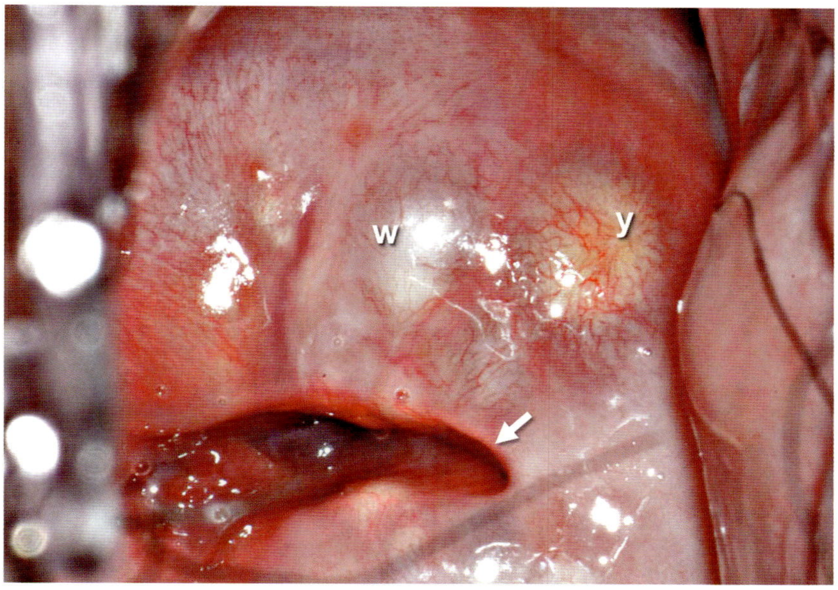

Figure 191 - The whitish nabothian follicle (w) and yellowish cyst (y) have not been recently produced. The arrow indicates the new squamocolumnar junction.

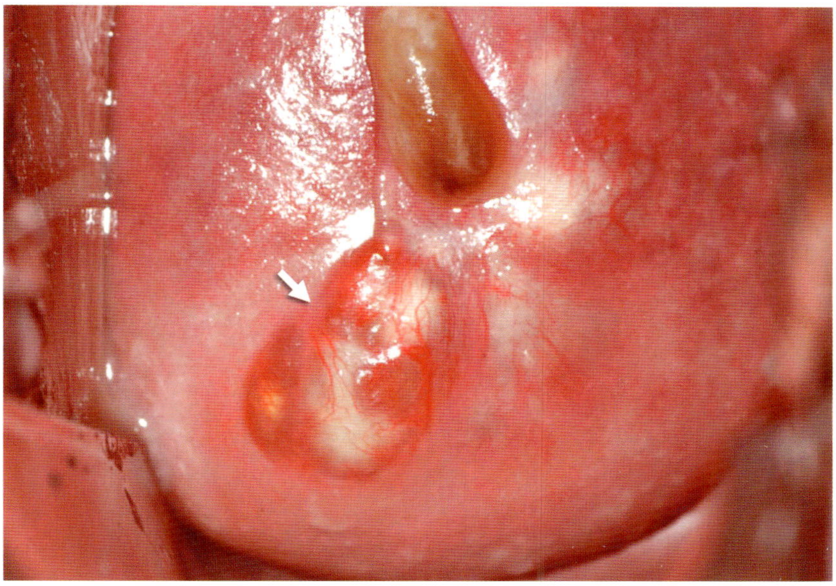

Figure 192 - Chambered cysts (arrow) indicate different formation age.

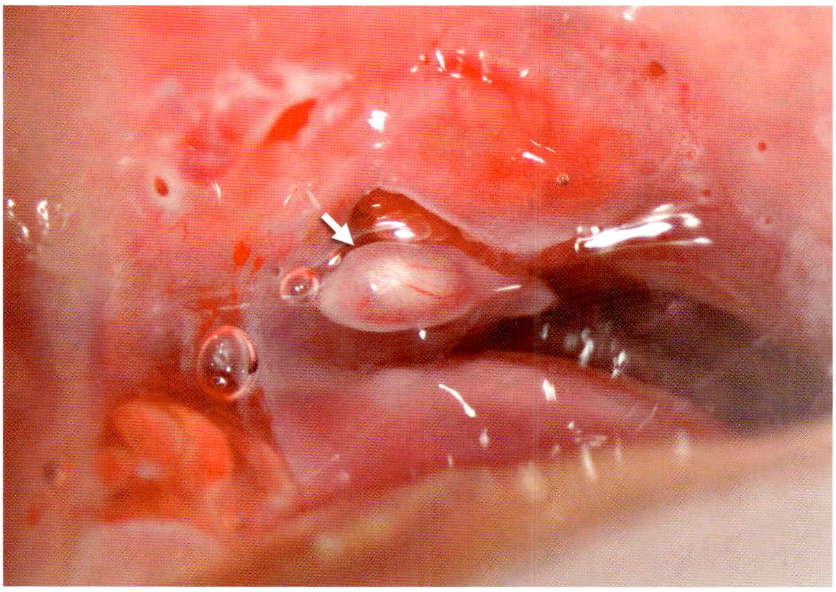

Figure 193 - A glandular cyst is contained in cervical polyp (arrow).

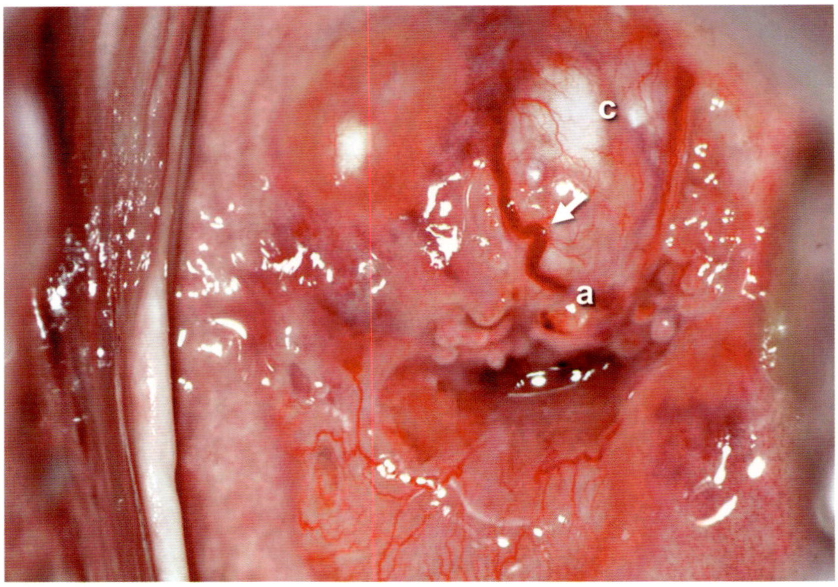

Figure 194 - The arrowed capillary over the nabothian cyst (c) shows an abrupt angular change (arrow) and appearance (a). Despite the abnormal vascular pattern, no atypia is present.

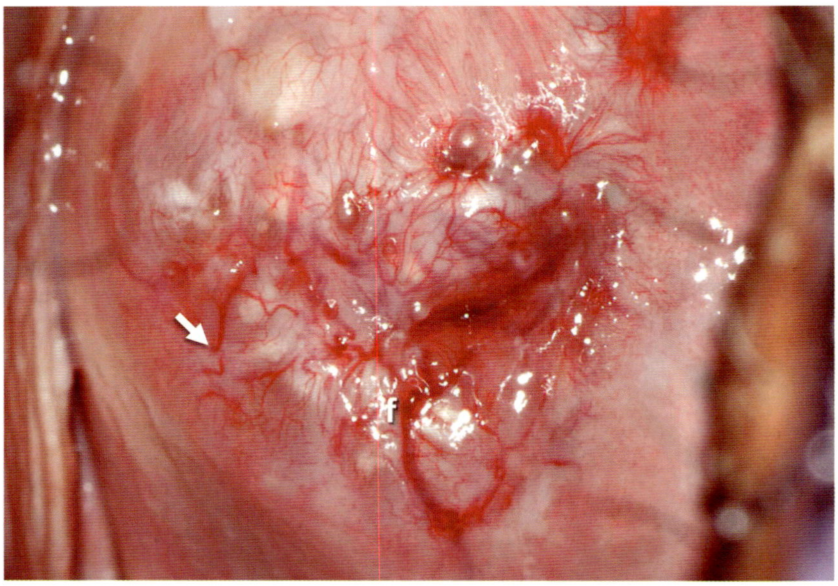

Figure 195 - Atypical vessels appear and disappear abruptly (arrow) and show gross fluctuations in width (f). No atypia is present.

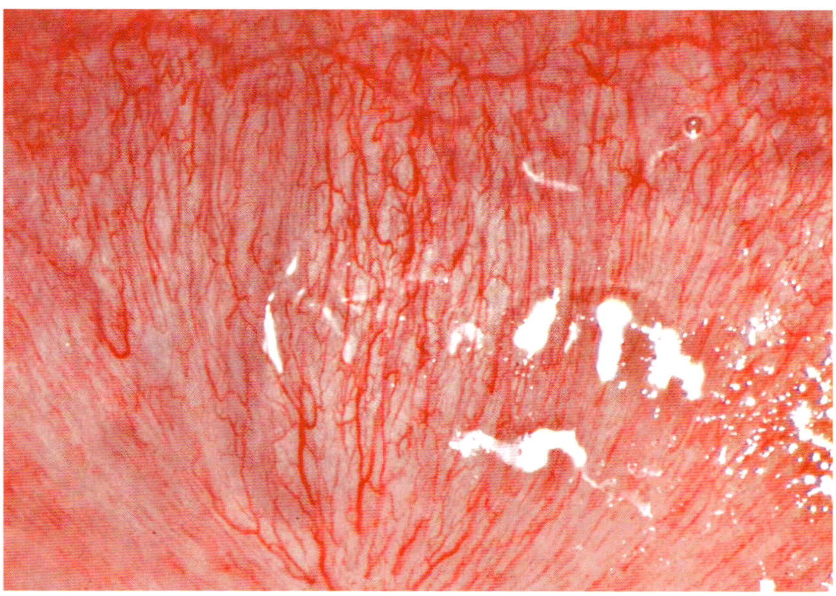

Figure 196 - Long parallel blood vessels with regular branching run over mature metaplastic epithelium.

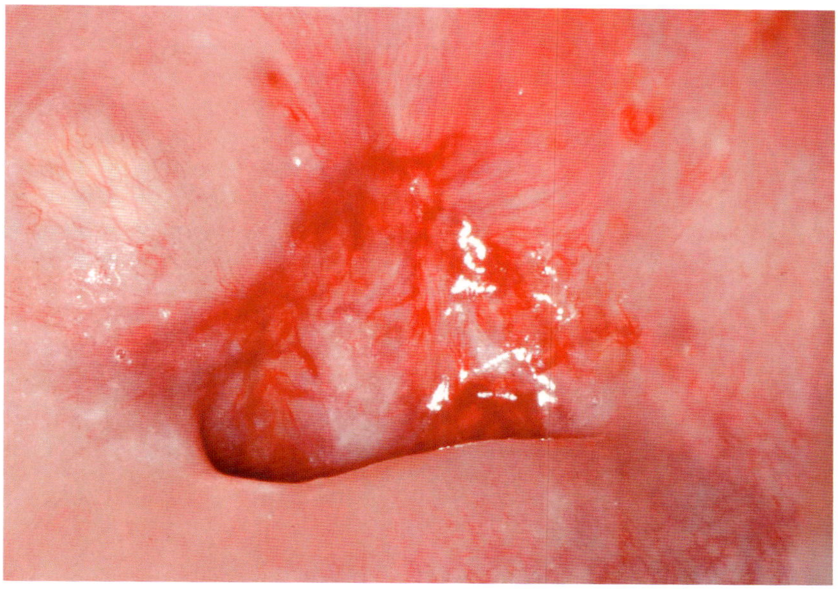

Figure 197 - Prominent vascular network over the mature metaplastic tissue, extending into the endocervical canal.

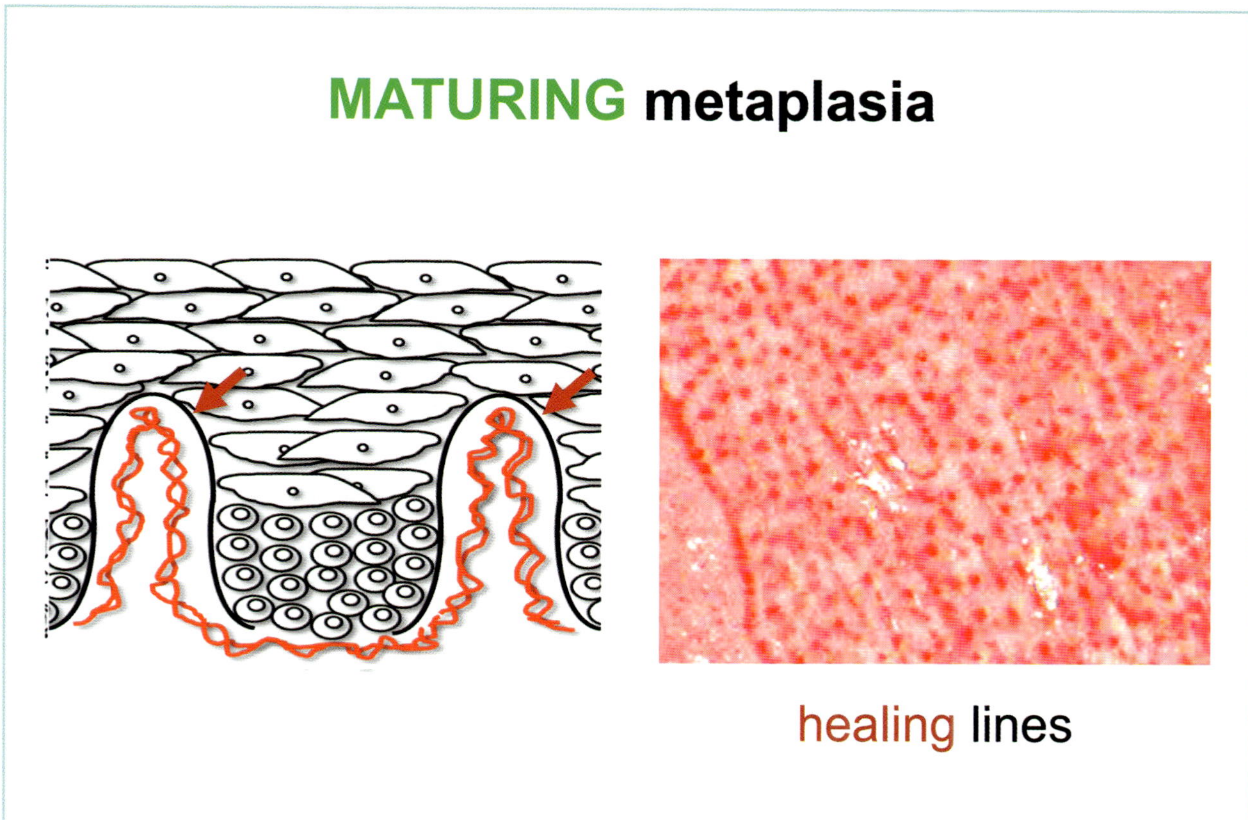

Figure 198 - Diagrammatic representation and colposcopic appearance of fine punctation arranged in radiating lines (healing lines).

Different conditions can induce metaplastic changes (Figure 201):

- exposed columnar epithelium
- biopsy or ablative procedures
- congenital transformation zone

In about 4% of women, the colposcopist may observe some zones of nonglycogenated epithelium that extend onto the anterior and posterior lips of the cervix and the vaginal fornices. For the comprehension of these unusually located areas, we must remember that during early embryonic life, the vaginal tube is lined by a cuboidal epithelium. Before birth, this epithelium is replaced by a stratified squamous epithelium, proceeding along the lateral walls and then the anterior and posterior walls, and upwards to reach the external os.

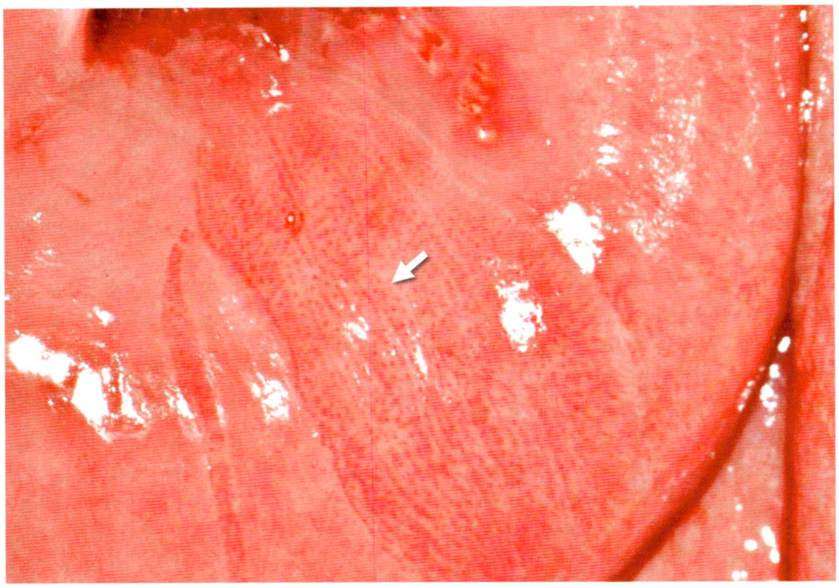

Figure 199 - Healing lines (arrow) after ablative procedure.

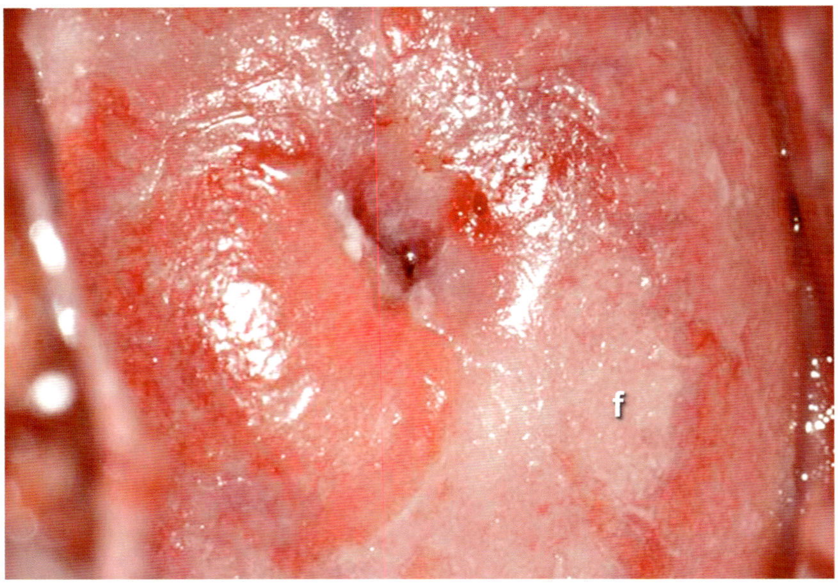

Figure 200 - Subepithelial fibrosis (f) appears as a white, opaque area, before application of acetic acid.

If this replacement is incomplete, the cuboidal epithelium remains distal to the external os, progressively involving the cervix, the anterior and posterior fornices and rarely the anterior and posterior vaginal walls. These areas where a late metaplastic conversion to squamous epithelium takes place, are termed *congenital transformation zone*.

Congenital metaplasia has many similarities with the squamous metaplasia found later in life and may undergo disorders of maturation such as thin or dense acetowhite areas, punctation or mosaic patterns and some solid white points detectable within the transformation zone. These solid epithelial pegs correspond to stratified and sometimes atypical epithelium in the glands (Figure 202). Although usually with the increasing severity of the lesion, the edge demarcation becomes sharper, the congenital transformation may exhibit very sharp borders, despite producing insignificant histologic changes (Figure 203).

Further development of the immature metaplastic epithelium may take two directions (Figure 204). In the vast majority of women, this newly formed tissue turns into a mature metaplastic epithelium and the area where the transformation occurs is termed as the normal transformation zone (NTZ). In a very small minority of women, the metaplastic epithelium may become atypical within an atypical transformation zone (ATZ).

During the immature metaplastic change, epithelium may attain exposure to a mutagenic agent and may become abnormal. Human Papillomavirus (HPV)

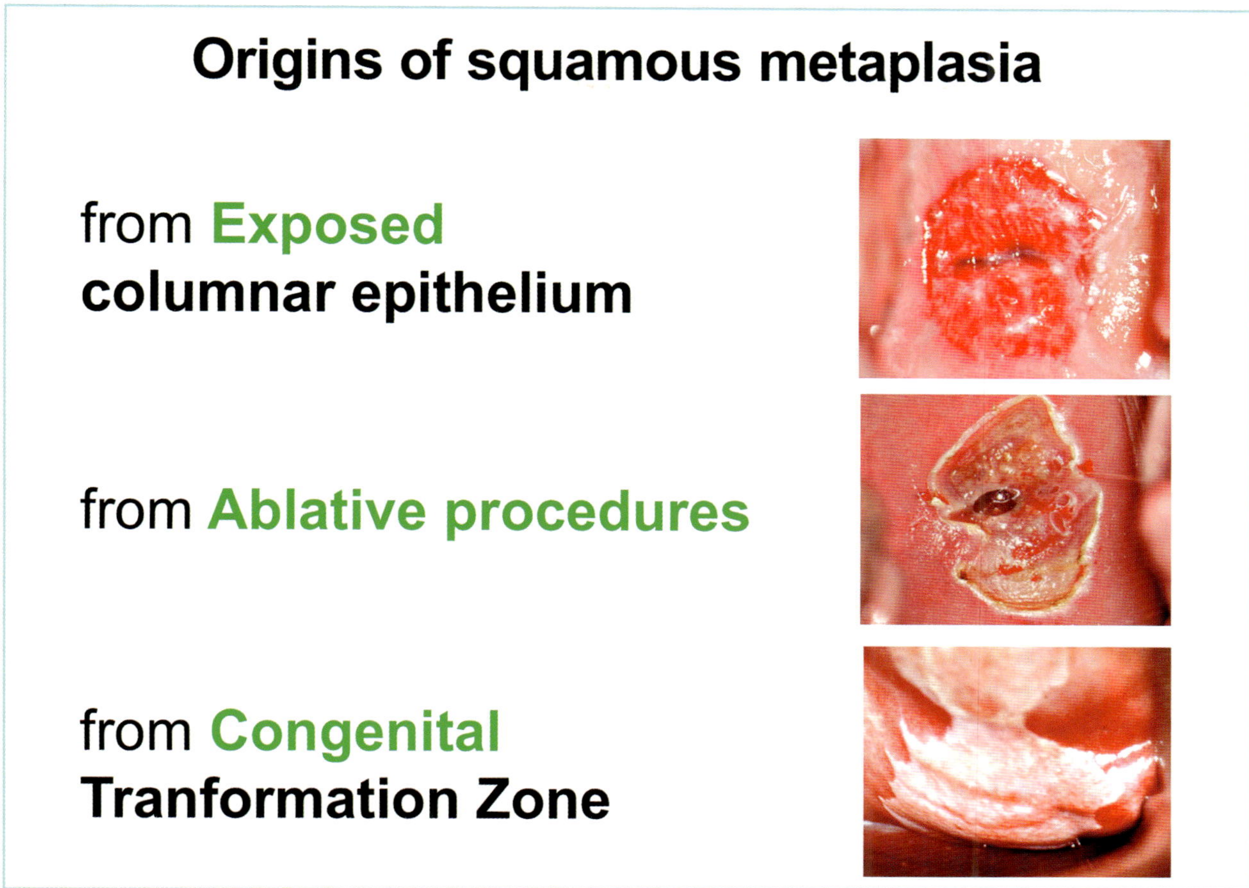

Figure 201 - Different origins of squamous metaplasia.

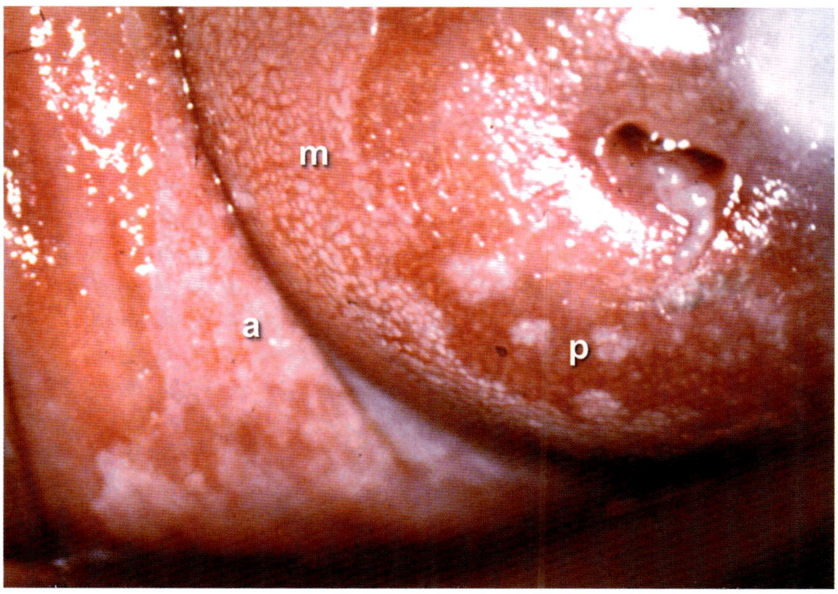

Figure 202 - Congenital metaplasia extends on to the posterior vaginal wall with an acetowhite area (a).
The cervix shows fine mosaic (m) and solid acetowhite epithelial pegs (p), corresponding to stratified epithelium in the glands.

is the major infectious etiological agent that is associated with the development of pre-cancerous lesions of the cervix.

Invasive cervical cancer is usually preceded by a long phase of cellular atypia, collectively referred to as cervical intraepithelial neoplasia (CIN). Pre-cancerous lesions of the cervix have different terminology (Figure 205): cervical intraepithelial neoplasia (CIN) (Richart CIN grading), cervical dysplasia (Reagan WHO) or squamous intraepithelial lesions (SIL) (Bethesda System). CIN is further categorized into grades 1, 2 and 3 whereas dysplasia is divided

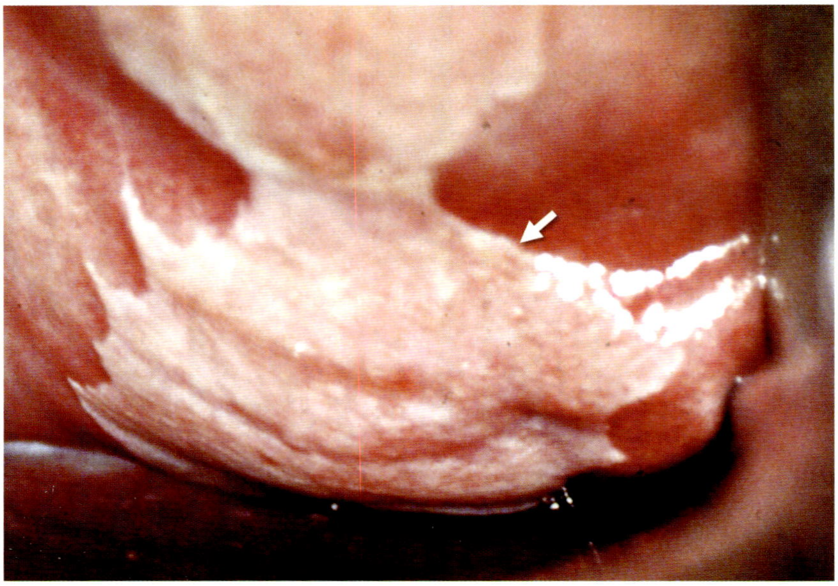

Figure 203 - Congenital metaplasia produces a thick acetowhite area in the posterior vaginal fornix, with very sharp borders (arrow) but with no significant histologic changes.

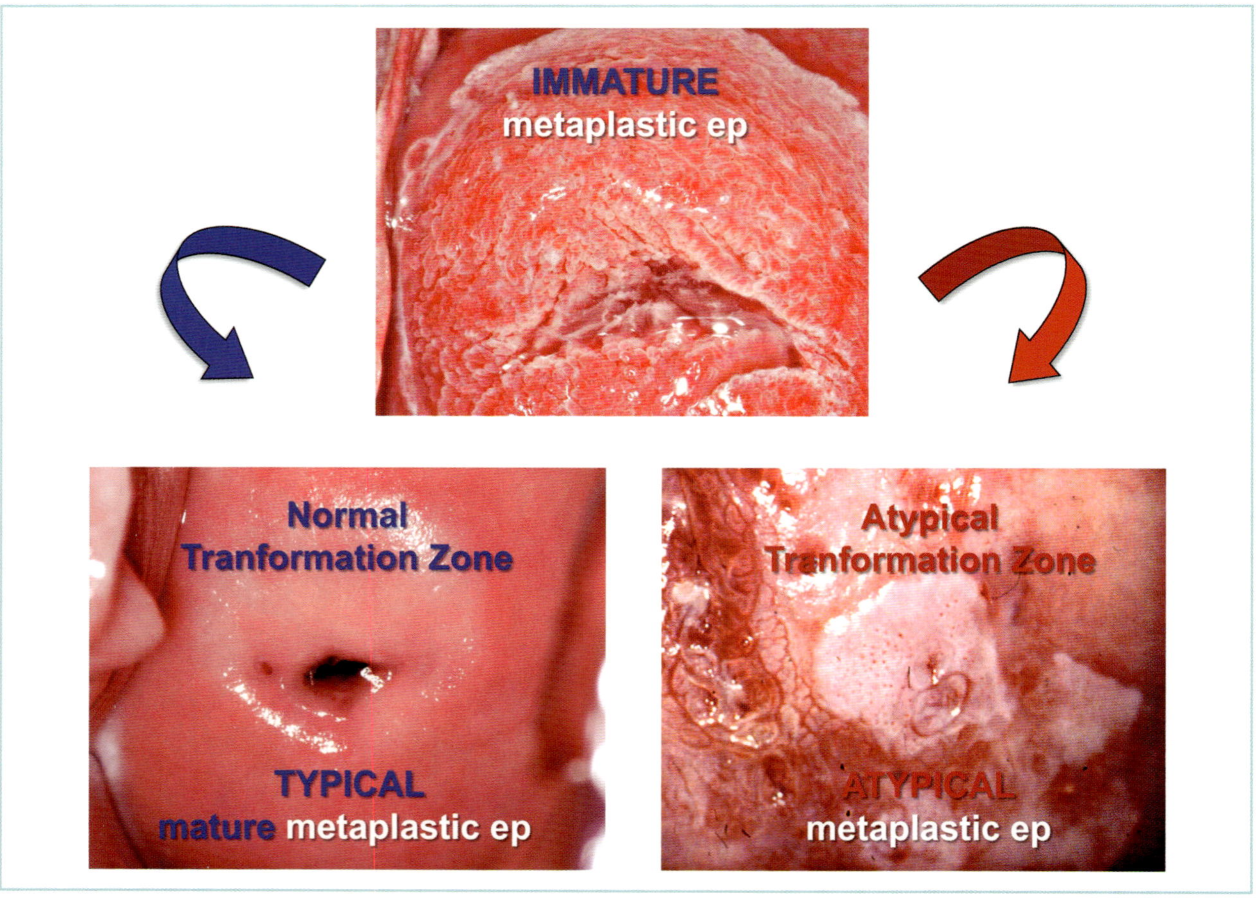

Figure 204 - Immature metaplastic epithelium may take two directions: a typical mature metaplastic epithelium, within a normal transformation zone, and an atypical metaplastic epithelium which occurs in the atypical transformation zone.

into three groups: mild, moderate and severe. The Bethesda System (TBS) has created the term squamous intraepithelial lesion (SIL) which comprehends low-grade (L-SIL) and high-grade (H-SIL) lesions. HPV lesions and CIN 1 are included in L-SIL whereas CIN 2, CIN 3 and in situ carcinoma (ISC) belong to high-grade SIL.

In low-grade SIL, most of the atypical protein-rich cells are located in the lower third of the epithelium where acetic acid can penetrate (Figure 206). Ace-

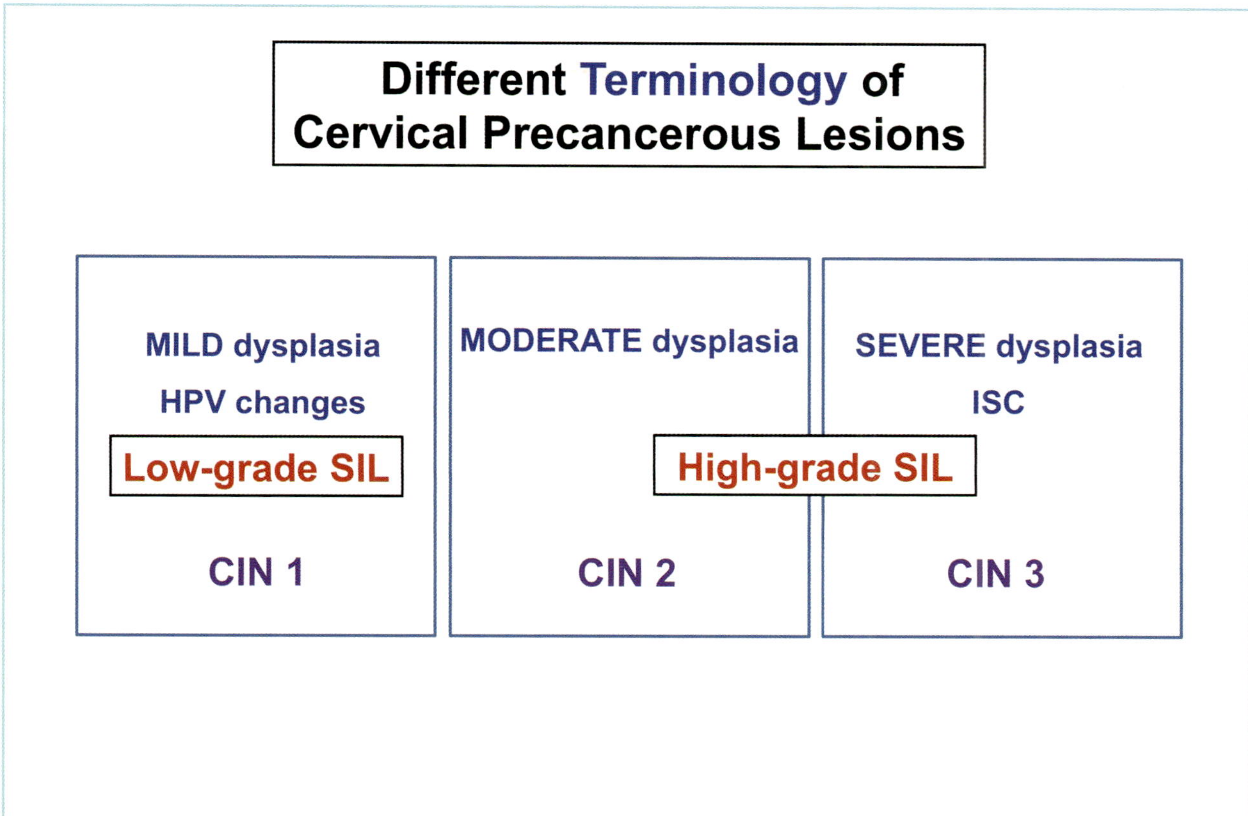

Figure 205 - Different terminology of cervical precancerous lesions.

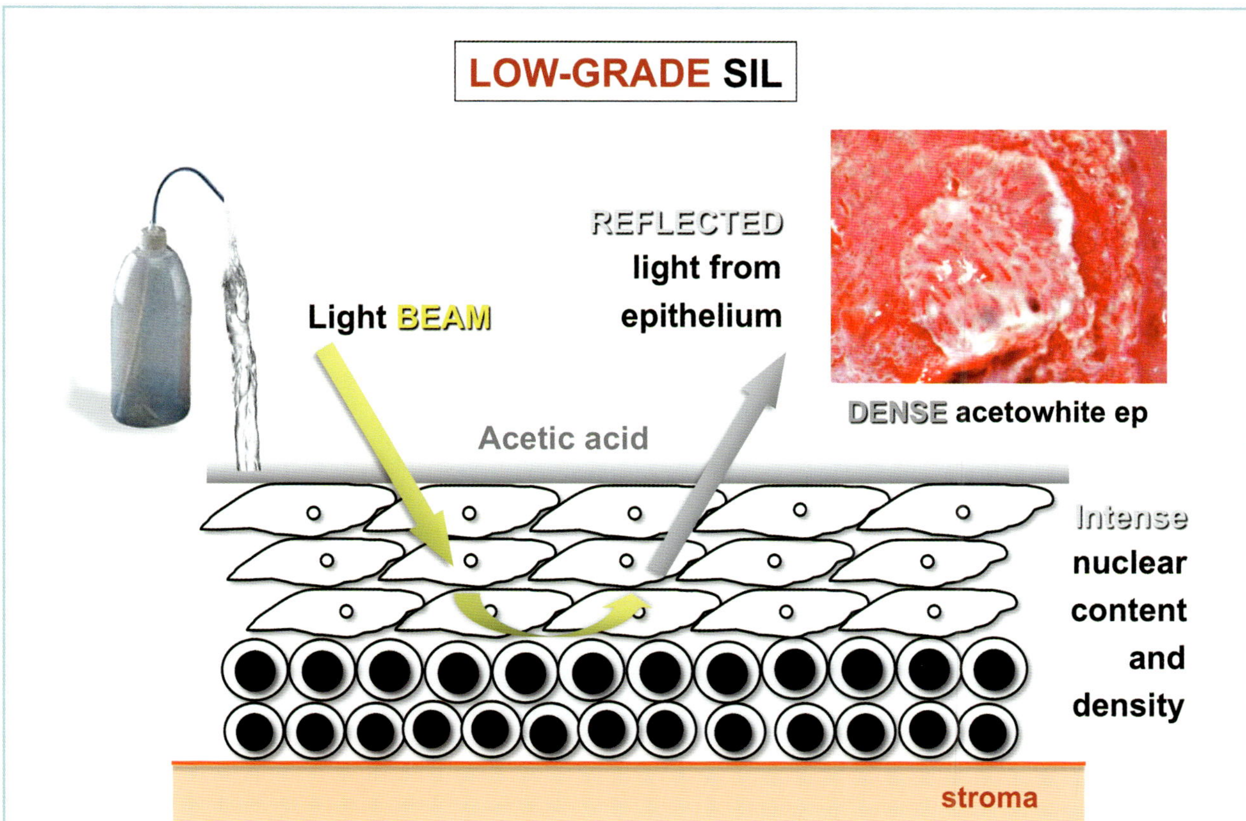

Figure 206 - Diagrammatic representation of the light pathway, through a dysplastic epithelium, after application of acetic acid. The cervix in the colpophotograph shows a dense acetowhite epithelium (low-grade SIL).

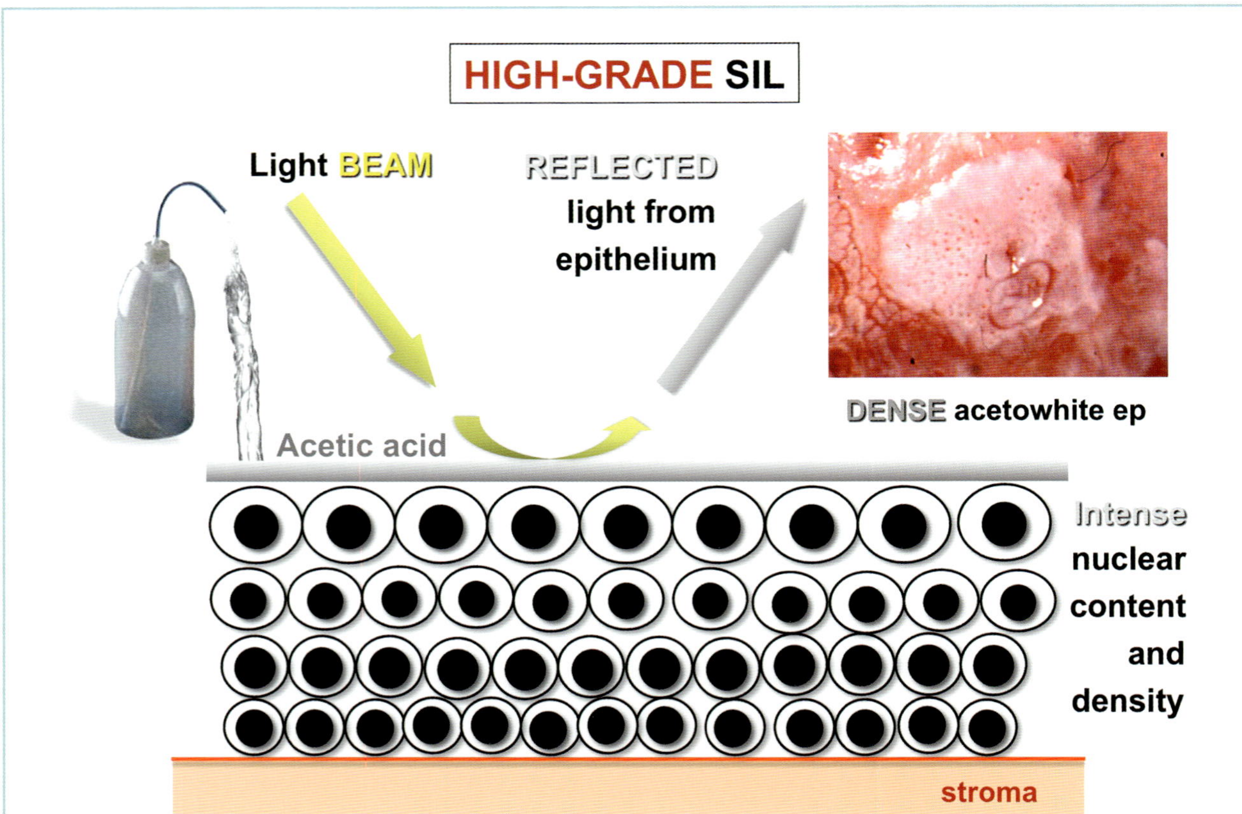

Figure 207 - Diagrammatic representation of the light pathway, through a dysplastic epithelium, after application of acetic acid. The cervix in the colpophotograph shows a dense acetowhite epithelium (high-grade SIL).

towhitening is delayed and less intense compared to high-grade SIL or early invasive carcinoma. The acetowhite epithelium associated with low-grade SIL is more dense, thick and opaque compared to areas with immature metaplastic epithelium and turns white more quickly. Acetowhite lesions associated with SIL point away from the external os and spread centrifugally.

In high-grade lesions and preclinical invasive cancer, a large number of dysplastic cells, abnormally loaded in nucleoproteins, reach the superficial layers of the epithelium (Figure 207). After acetic acid treatment, the direct light is quickly reflected by the dense epithelium, giving an opaque, grey-white (Figure 208) or snow-white appearance (Figure 209). The acetowhite change quickly appears and persists for more than one minute. These lesions usually have regular and well-defined margins which may sometimes be raised and rolled-out.

High-grade dysplastic epithelium shows a more or less complete absence of maturation of the cell layers and disappearance or very marked decrease of glycogen content. Consequently, the application of Lugol's iodine solution will give a mustard or saffron yellow color (Figure 210). High-grade lesions that do not stain with iodine are known as positive Schiller's test or iodine negative areas.

Acetowhite lesions may be associated with characteristic vascular patterns such as punctation and/or mosaic. Changes in vascular patterns are closely related to histologic changes.

In an atypical transformation zone, dysplastic epithelium starts to grow in buds or blocks. Due to the dysplastic process, the nutritional requirements of the tissue increase, and individual stromal papillae do not flatten but instead are broadened, elongated and more irregular in size and shape. They sometimes lift the epithelium, giving a micropapillary or warty appearance. A thin layer of epithelium remains on top of the capillaries that may be trapped within the elongated stromal papillae. These histologic abnormalities occurring in the atypical transformation zone are essential for the understanding of punctate and mosaic patterns. Punctation and mosaic patterns may be classified as either fine or coarse.

Capillaries within stromal papillae may undergo dilatation and proliferation near the surface, where they are seen in a stippled pattern as red dots on a

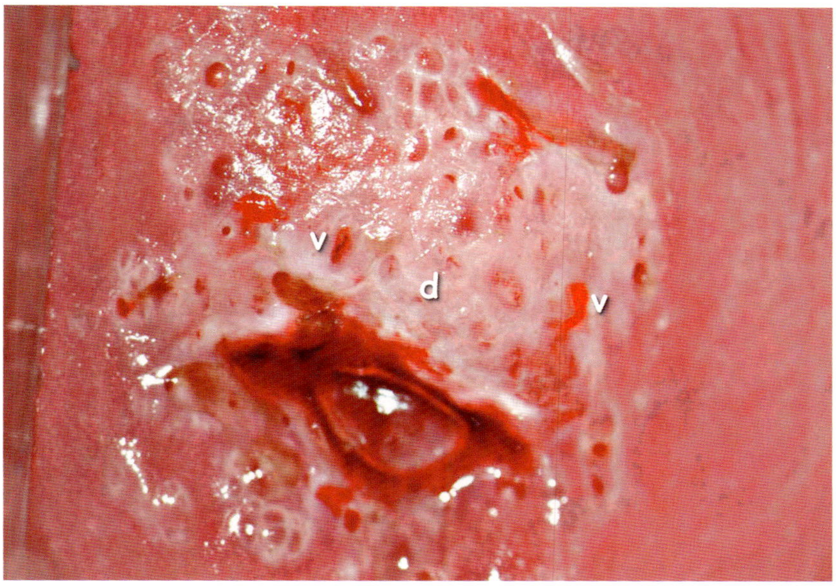

Figure 208 - Dense acetowhite epithelium (d), with atypical vessels that appear and disappear abruptly (v). Histology revealed this lesion to be CIN III/CIS.

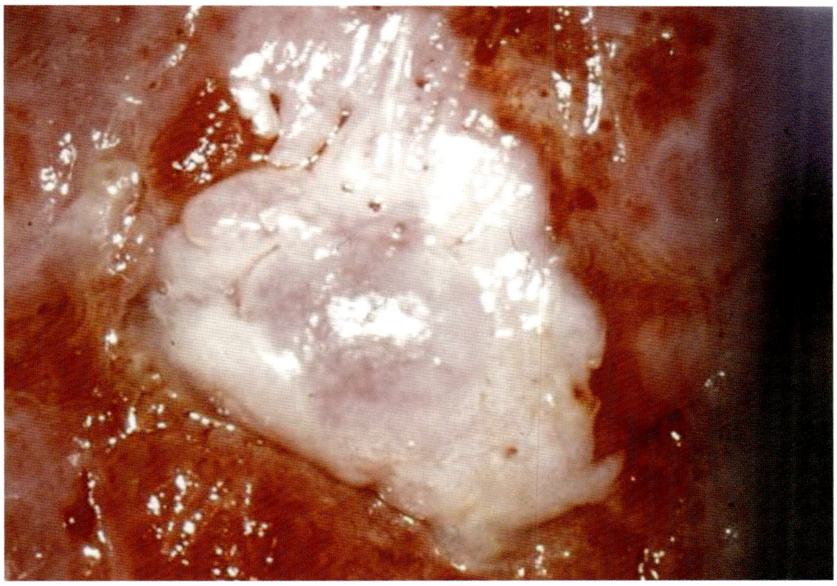

Figure 209 - Dense acetowhite lesion with snow-white appearance (CIN III).

white or opaque background after application of acetic acid. This atypical architecture gives rise to so-called **punctation** (Figure 211).

Punctation may be fine or coarse (2011 IFCPC Nomenclature) (Table 1), based on the intercapillary distance and the size of dilated vessels which reflect the severity of the lesion. In *fine* punctation, the delicate dots are close together (Figure 212), whereas in *coarse* punctation, petechiae are larger and widely separated (Figure 213). Low-grade SIL produces intermediate forms of punctation, with varying degree of intercapillary distance, so that sometimes it is difficult to classify the punctate as fine or coarse.

Dilated hairpin capillaries (Figure 214) or clustered in patches (Figure 215) are generally observed diffusely across the ectocervix in inflammatory conditions. Inflammatory capillary effusions may also involve vagina (Figure 216), inner aspect of the labia minora (Figure 217) or the whole vestibulum (Figure 218). These capillaries lie close together, without any sharp border between normal and abnormal epithelium. The red spots, scattered (Figure 219) or clustered in patches (Figure 220), vary in shape and distribution, and are due to patchy infiltration of the stroma, associated with dilated capillaries.

Patched capillaries and vascular effusions may also be observed in the presence of severe dystrophy in menopause (Figure 221) or in pharmacologically induced conditions (Figure 222). Direct microscopy may assist in reaching a correct diagnosis, displaying

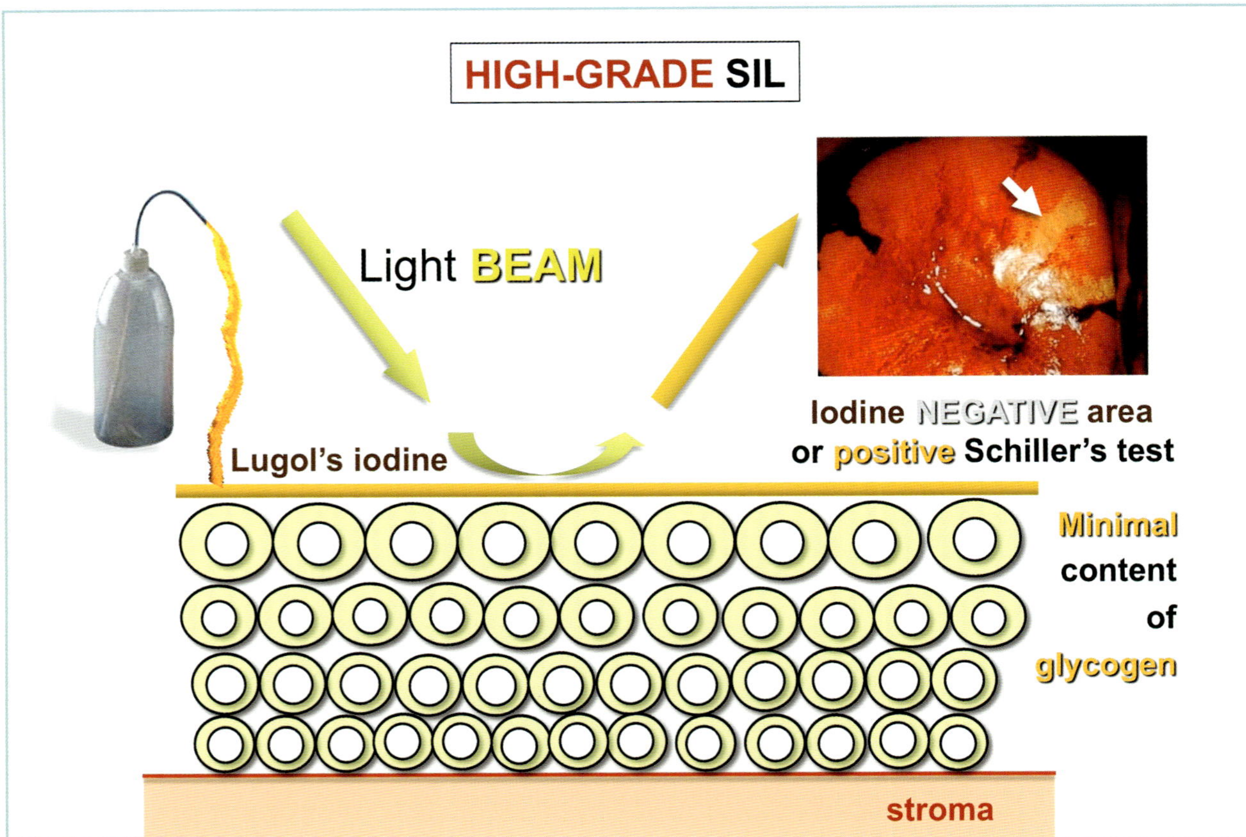

Figure 210 - Diagrammatic representation of the light pathway, through a dysplastic epithelium, after Lugol's iodine application. The colpophotograph displays an iodine negative area (arrow) (high-grade SIL).

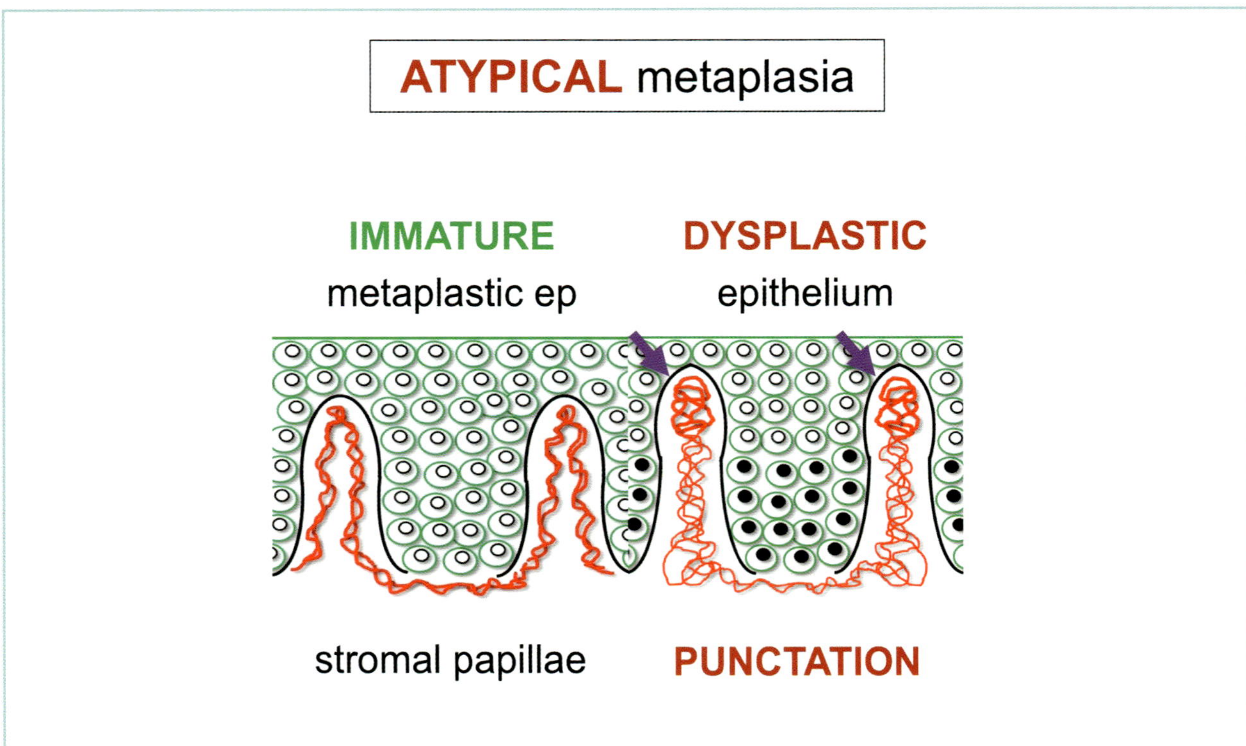

Figure 211 - Diagrammatic representation of the behavior of stromal papillae in immature metaplastic epithelium and in dysplastic epithelium. The arrows indicate capillaries within stromal papillae which underwent dilatation and proliferation near the surface, giving rise to punctation.

Table 1 - 2011 IFCPC Nomenclature - Accepted in Rio World Congress, July 5, 2011
(Nomenclature Committee chairman: Jacob Bornstein MD)

2011 IFCPC colposcopy terminology of the cervix			
General assessment		• Adequate/inadequate for the reason ... (i.e.: cervix obscured by inflammation, bleeding, scar) • Squamo-columnar Junction visibility: completely visible, partially visible, not visible • Transformation zone types 1,2,3	
Normal colposcopic findings		Original squamous epithelium: • Mature • Atrophic Columnar epithelium • Ectopy Metaplastic squamous epithelium • Nabothian cysts • Crypt (gland) openings Deciduosis in pregnancy	
Abnodrmal colposcopic findings	**General principles**	**Location of the lesion:** Inside or outside the T-zone, Location of the lesion by clock position **Size of the lesions:** Number of cervical quadrants the lesion covers, Size of the lesion in percentage of cervix,	
	Grade 1 Minor	Thin aceto-white epithelium Irregular, geographic border	Fine mosaic Fine punctation
	Grade 2 (Major)	Dense aceto-white epithelium Rapid appearance of acetowhitening, Cuffed crypt (gland) openings	Coarse mosaic, Coarse punctation, Sharp border, Inner border sign Ridge sign
	Non specific	Leukoplakia (keratosis, hyperkeratosis), Erosion Lugol's staining (Schiller's test): stained/non-stained	
Suspicius for invasion		Atypical vessel **Additional signs:** Fragile vessels, Irregular surface, Exophytic lesion, Necrosis, Ulceration (necrotic), tumor/gross neoplasm	
Miscellaneous finding		Congenital transformation zone, Condyloma, Polyp (Ectocervical/endocervial) Inflammation,	Stenosis, Congenital anomaly, Post treatment consequence, Endometriosis

an atrophic cell pattern characterized by basal and parabasal cells, without any evidence of inflammation (Figure 223).
Fine or coarse punctation may be also observed in association with respectively low-grade and high-grade anal intraepithelial neoplasia (AIN) (Figure 224).
In histologic abnormalities, punctation is usually confined in a well-delimited area, sharply separated from normal epithelium. In high-grade lesions, coarse punctation may rise up from the plane of the surrounding abnormal epithelium, appearing in the form of papillae (Figure 225). This colposcopic change is known as *papillary punctation*.
In the **mosaic** pattern, vessels arborize within the stromal papillary ridges, form a basket-like structure around buds of abnormal epithelium and run pa-

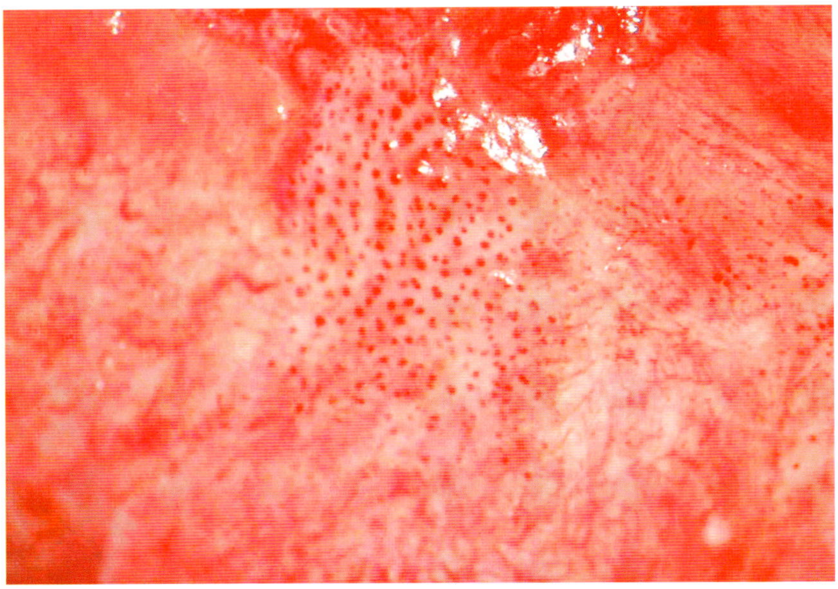

Figure 212 - Fine punctation pattern showing fine dots with regular intercapillary distance.

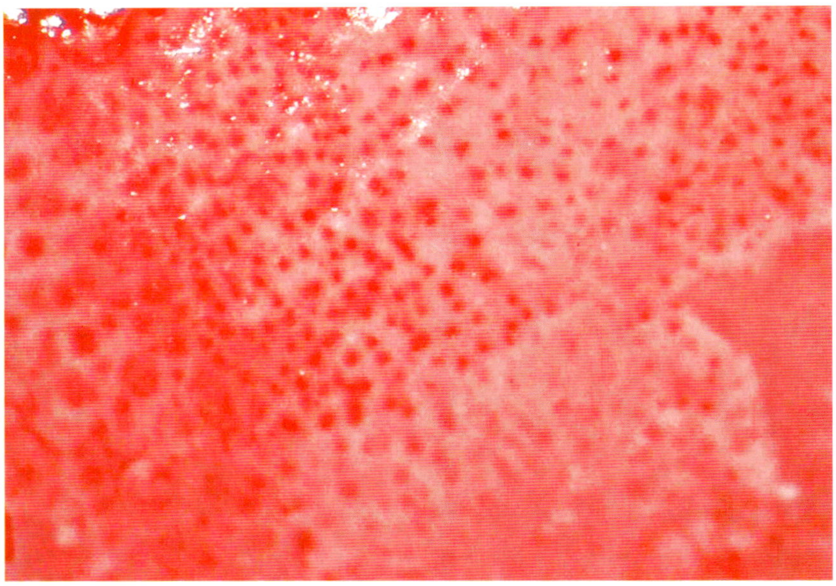

Figure 213 - Coarse punctation with large, widely separated petechiae.

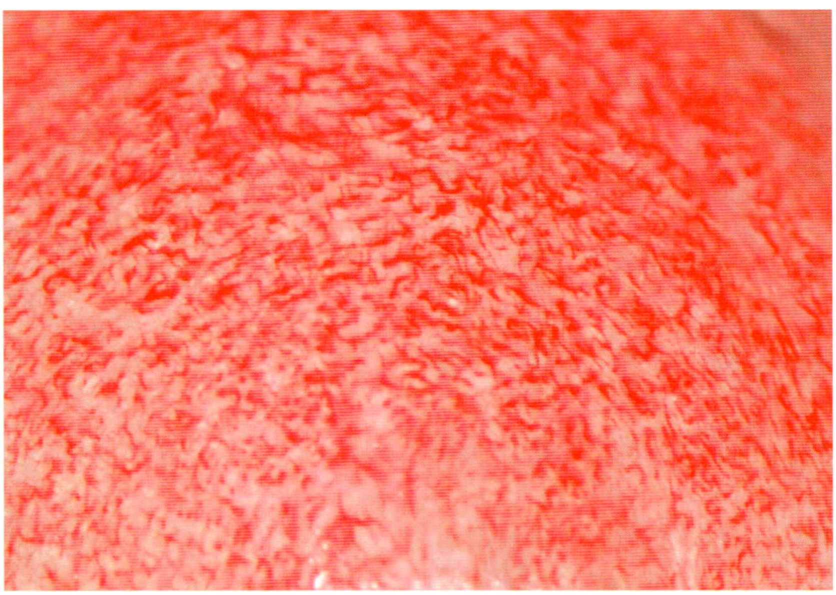

Figure 214 - Patched capillaries, scattered on the cervix.

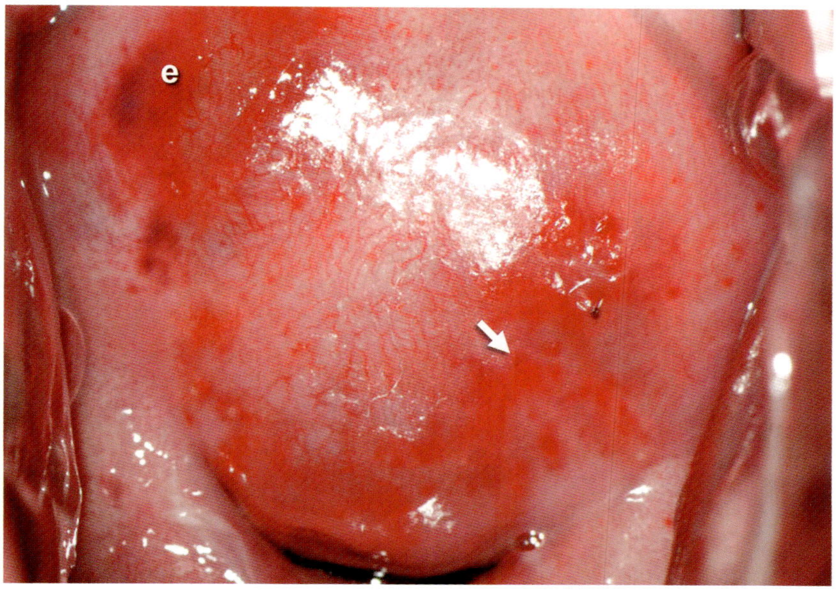

Figure 215 - Candida infection induced patched capillaries (arrow), scattered on the cervix. Vascular effusion (e).

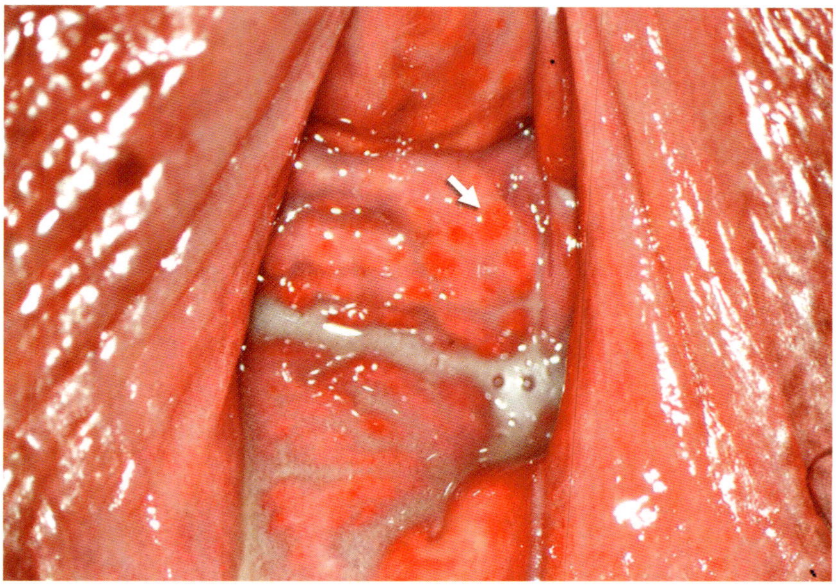

Figure 216 - Patches of dilated capillaries (arrow) involve the vaginal walls, due to an infection by Trichomonas vaginalis.

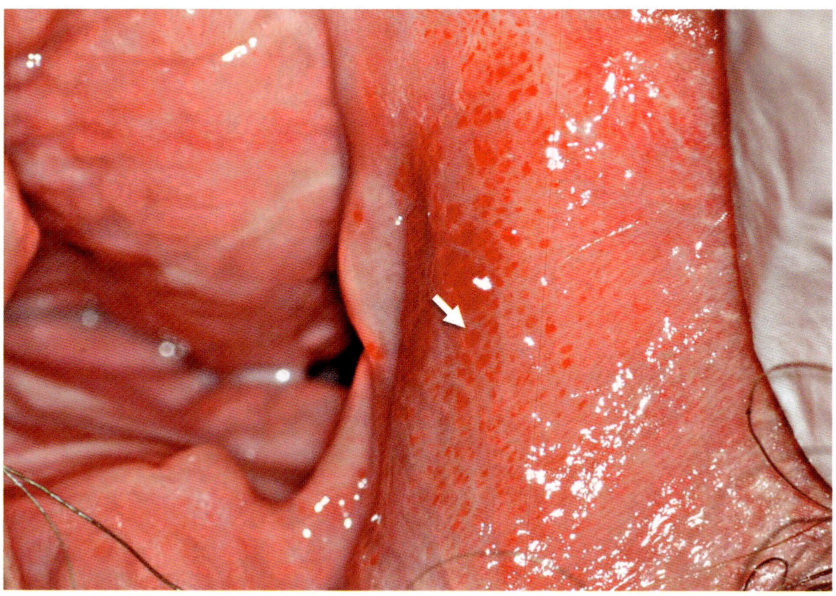

Figure 217 - Inflammatory patched capillaries (arrow) involve the inner aspect of the left labium minor.

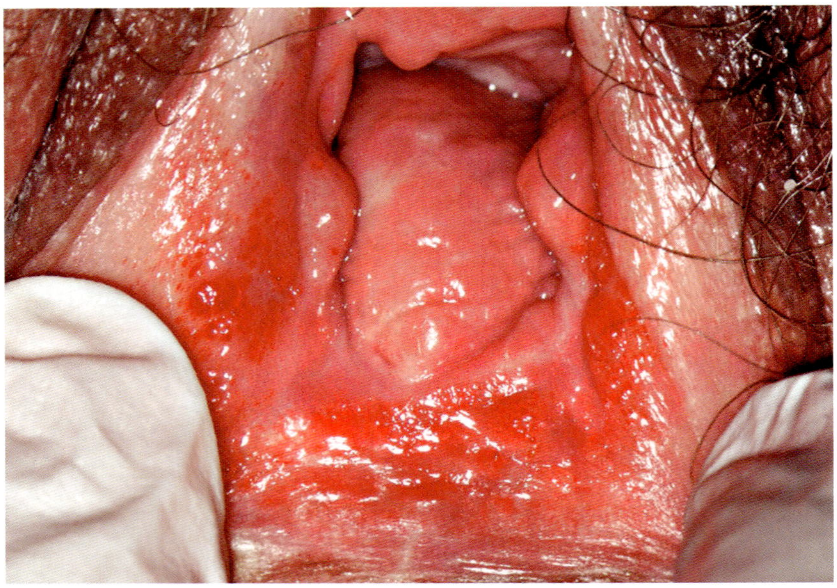

Figure 218 - Candida vulvitis has produced widespread patches of dilated capillaries on the mucosal surface of labia minora and on fourchette.

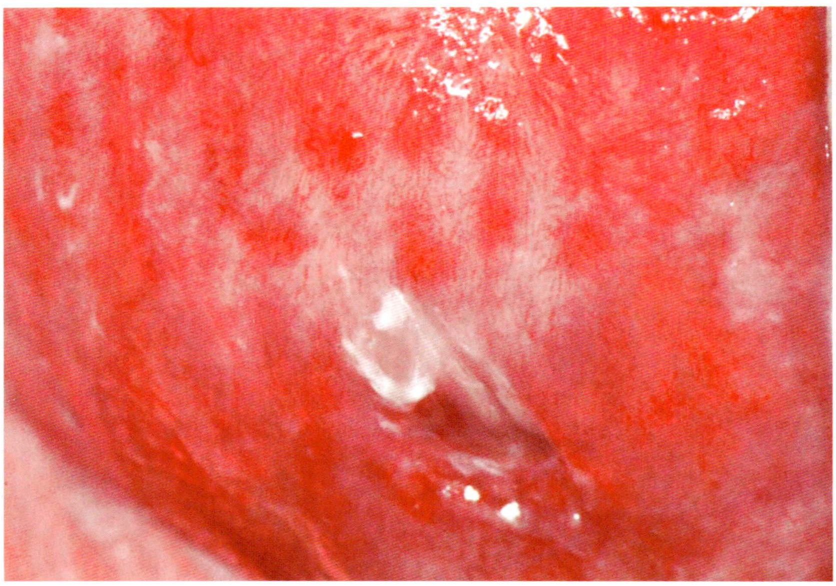

Figure 219 - Spots of dilated capillaries, caused by candidiasis, are scattered on the cervix.

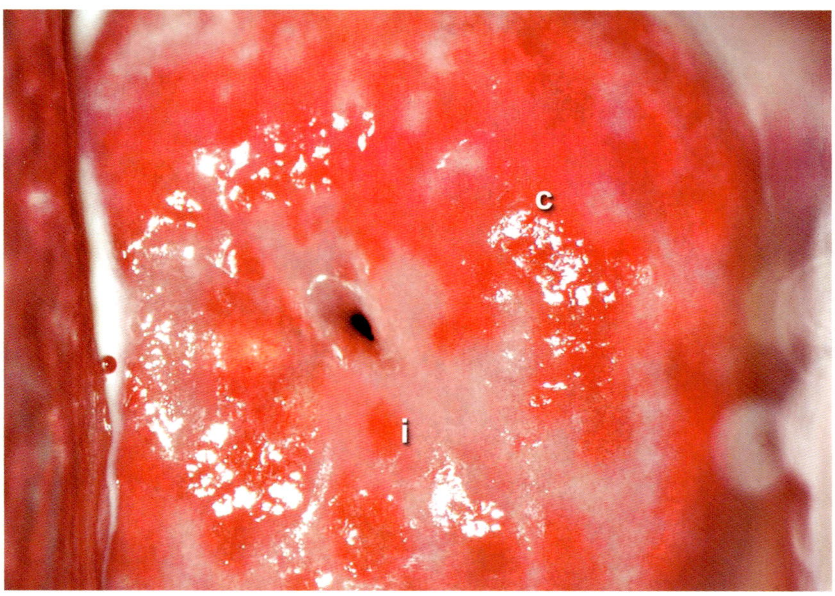

Figure 220 - Spots of dilated capillaries appear isolated (i) or confluent (c). Direct microscopy revealed Candida infection.

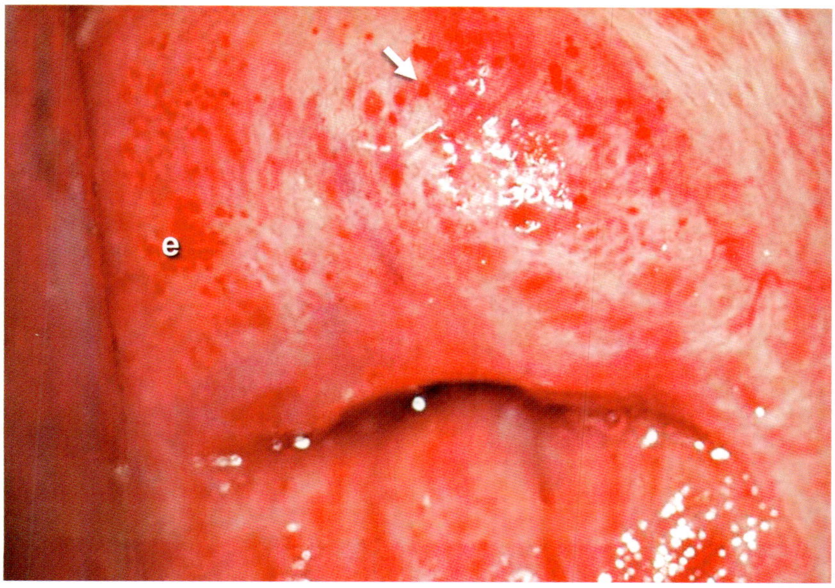

Figure 221 - Dystrophic cervix in menopause showing patched capillaries (arrow) and vascular effusions (e).

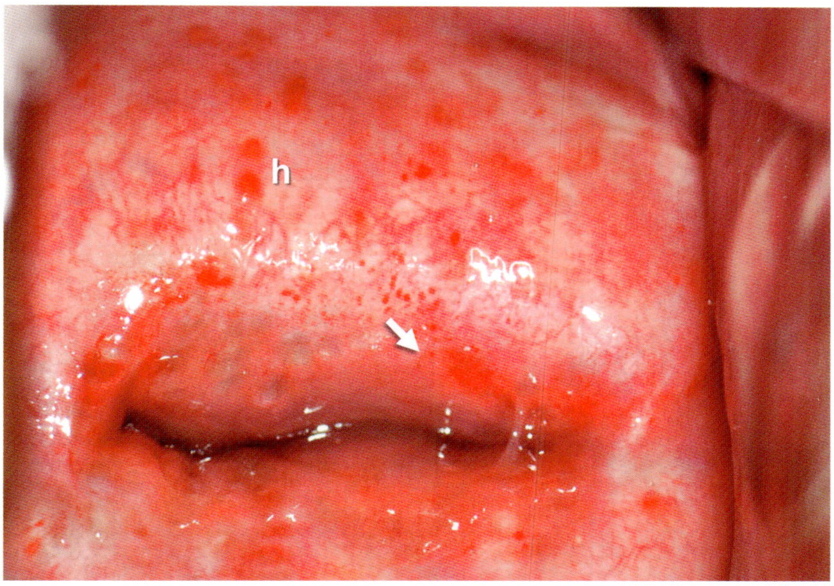

Figure 222 - Cervical atrophy induced by Tamoxifen. Scattered subepithelial hemorrhages (h) of varying size can be seen. The squamocolumnar junction is barely recognizable (arrow).

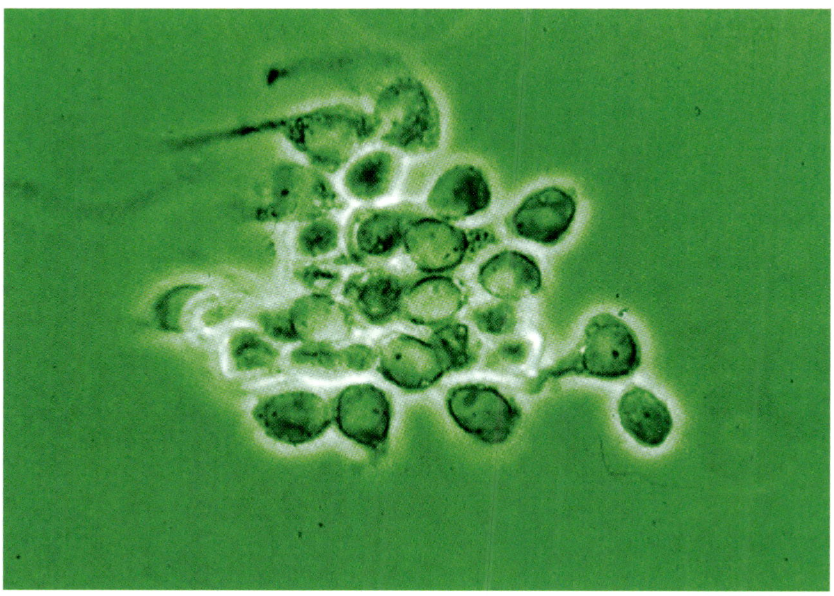

Figure 223 - The microphotograph shows an atrophic cell pattern, characterized by a cluster of basal cells.

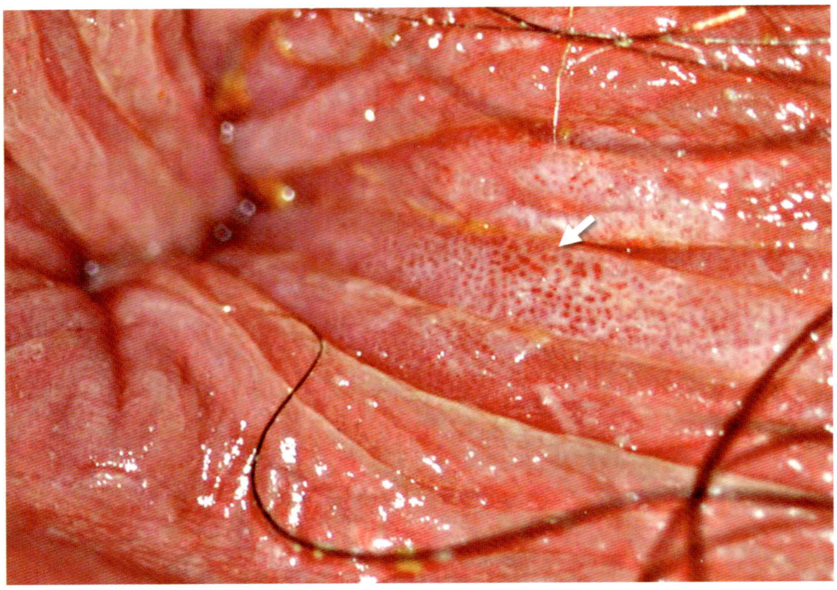

Figure 224 - Perianal acetowhite area with coarse mosaic (arrow). Punch biopsy disclosed a high-grade anal intraepithelial neoplasia.

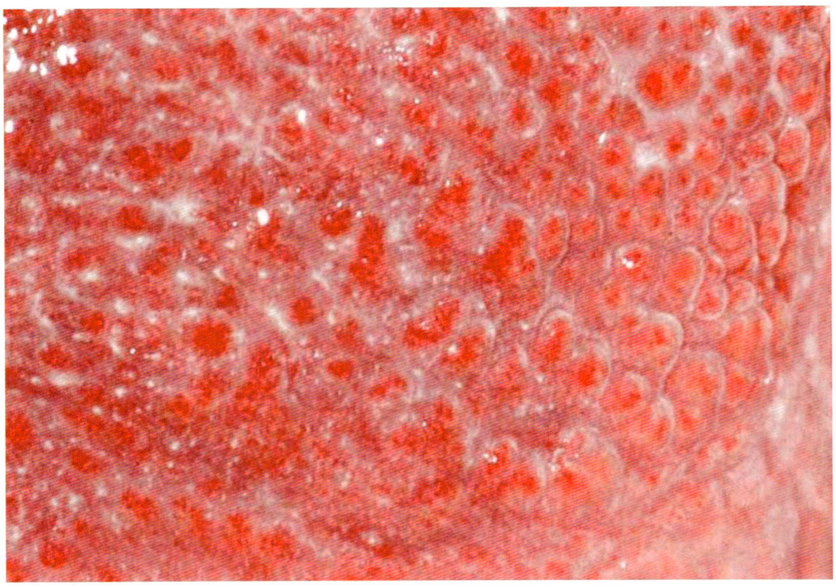

Figure 225 - Papillary punctation in high-grade lesion. Coarse punctation rises up from the plane of the surrounding abnormal epithelium, appearing in the form of papillae.

rallel with the surface, demarcating mosaic-like avascular fields (Figure 226). After acetic acid treatment, the epithelial buds appear as small white cobbles, surrounded by the aforementioned blood vessels, defining mosaic-like avascular fields. The cobbles may be regular in size and shape, or irregular, depending on the degree of the underlying abnormality. These two colposcopic findings, which include intermediate degrees of altered vessels, distinguish fine mosaic from coarse mosaic (2011 IFCPC Nomenclature).

In *fine* mosaic pattern, the blood vessels in the stroma are visible as a network of fine capillaries of uniform caliber in close proximity to one another, enclosing regular epithelial cobbles (Figure 227). Fine mosaic may still turn into a nonacetowhite mature metaplastic epithelium. In the progressing change, a fine vascular texture may be observed over a faint acetowhite epithelium or a fully mature metaplastic epithelium. This finding is referred to as *mosaic base* (Figure 228).

Coarse mosaic is characterized by a greater irregularity of the epithelial cobbles which appear bigger and more variable in size (Figure 229). Intercapillary distance depends upon the severity of the lesion. The furrows between the epithelial cobbles are more widely spaced and intensely red. The blood vessels may not be traced completely and are lost in places ("broken" or "open" mosaics). The epithelial tiles are often seen raised (Figure 230). After the effect of the acetic acid wearing off, coarse mosaic patterns are more clearly visible (Figure 231).

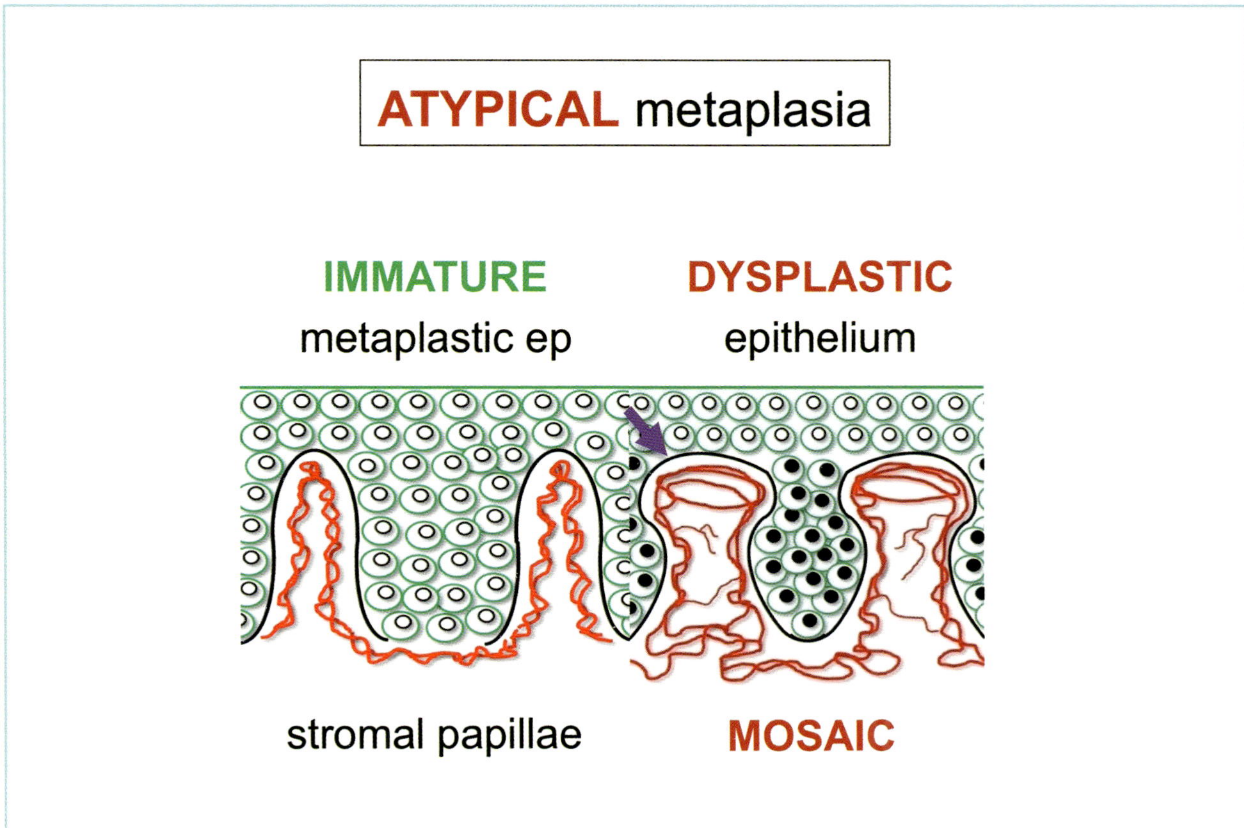

Figure 226 - Diagrammatic representation showing the different behaviour of vessels within papillae, between immature metaplastic epithelium and dysplastic epithelium (arrow).

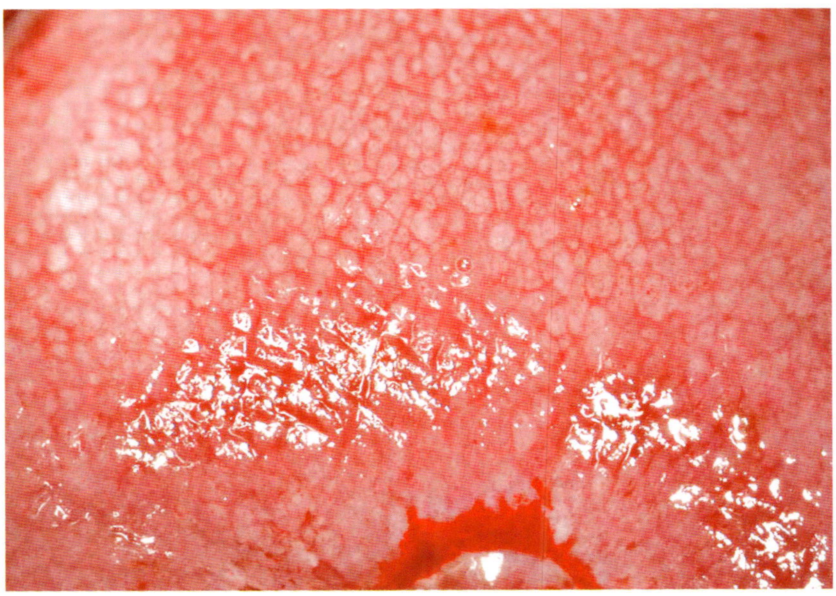

Figure 227 - Regular epithelial cobbles, delimited by fine capillaries of uniform caliber, define fine mosaic.

Coarse punctation and coarse mosaic often occur in high-grade SIL and early preclinical invasive cancer. When the two vascular patterns are overlapped in the same area, the dilated capillary loop can be seen in the center of each mosaic tile, defining the so-called *umbilication* (Figure 232).

Reverse mosaic is a rare colposcopic finding because it is short-lived and indicates the beginning of atypical metaplasia (Figure 233). It is characterized by small red islands corresponding to the tips of former columnar papillae, circumscribed by white metaplastic squamous epithelium. When atypical epithe-

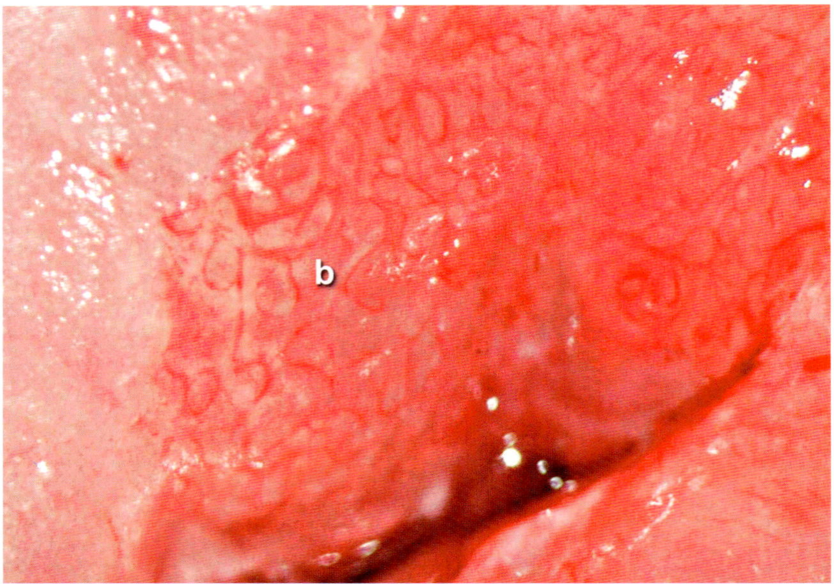

Figure 228 - Mosaic base (b) is characterized by a fine vascular texture over a faint acetowhite epithelium or a fully mature metaplastic epithelium.

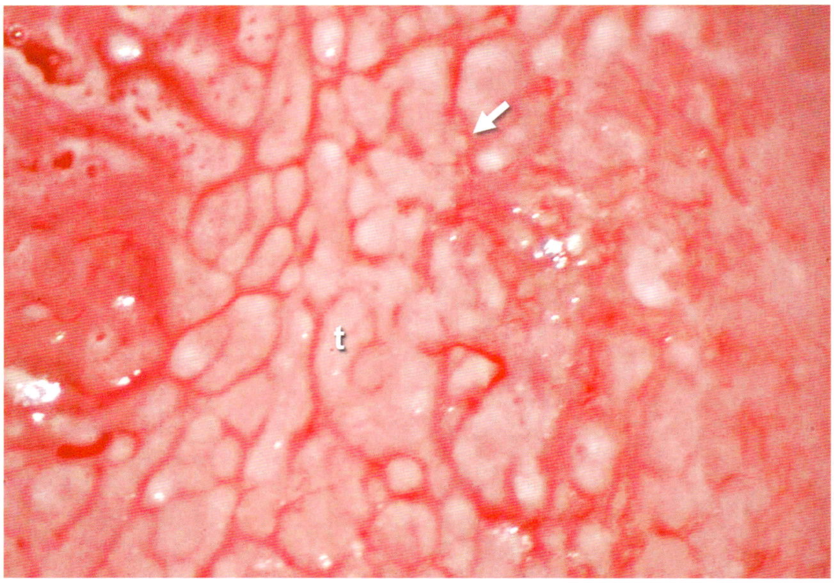

Figure 229 - Coarse mosaic with irregular tiles (t) and capillaries of different caliber. The arrow indicates the place where the coarse mosaic appears broken.

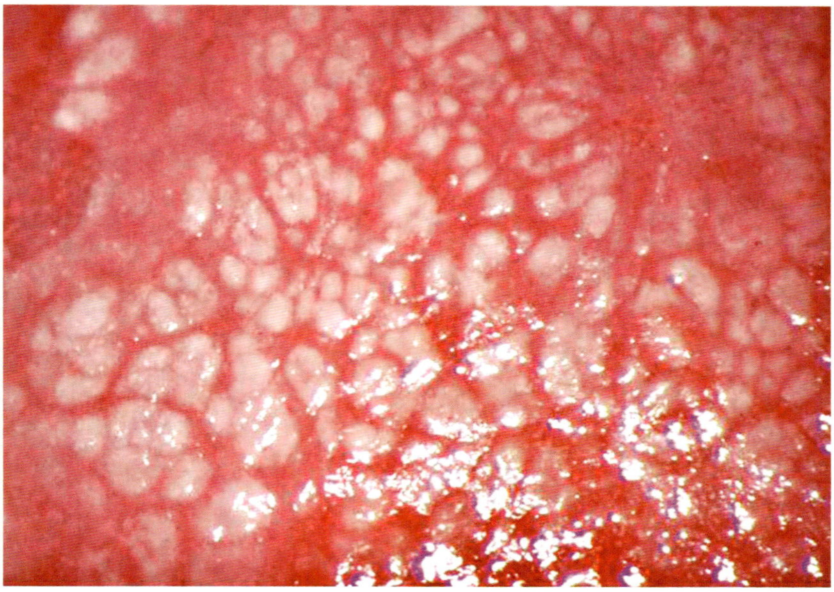

Figure 230 - The tiles of this coarse mosaic appear variable in size and are raised. Histology showed CIN 3.

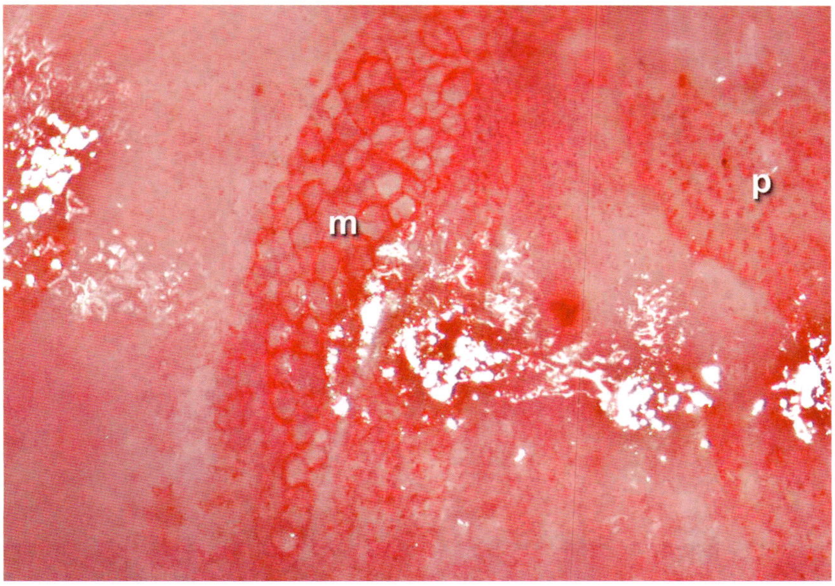

Figure 231 - The intensely red furrows between the cobbles of the coarse mosaic (m) appear more evident after the effect of the acetic acid wearing off. Histology disclosed an HPV/CIN III epithelium. Punctation (p).

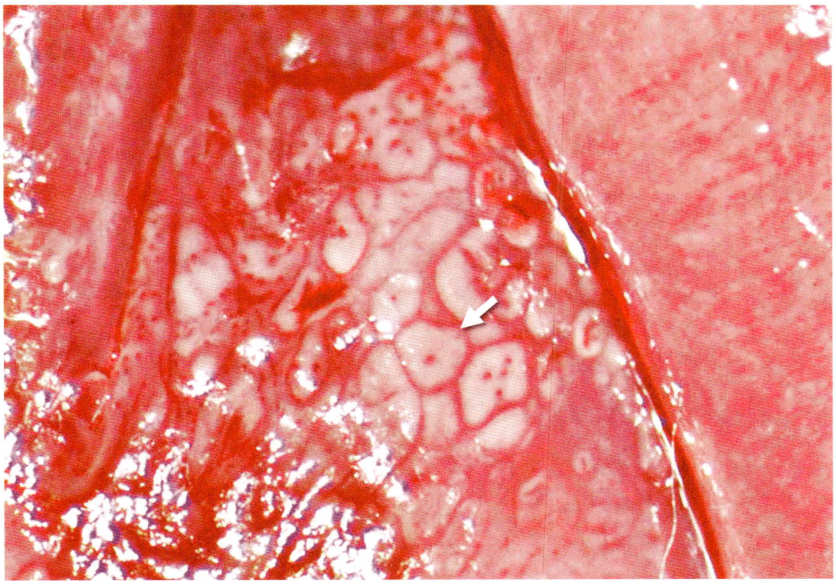

Figure 232 - Coarse mosaic and punctation vascular pattern are overlapped (arrow). This colposcopic appearance is named umbilication. This lesion was shown to be composed of HPV/CIN III epithelium.

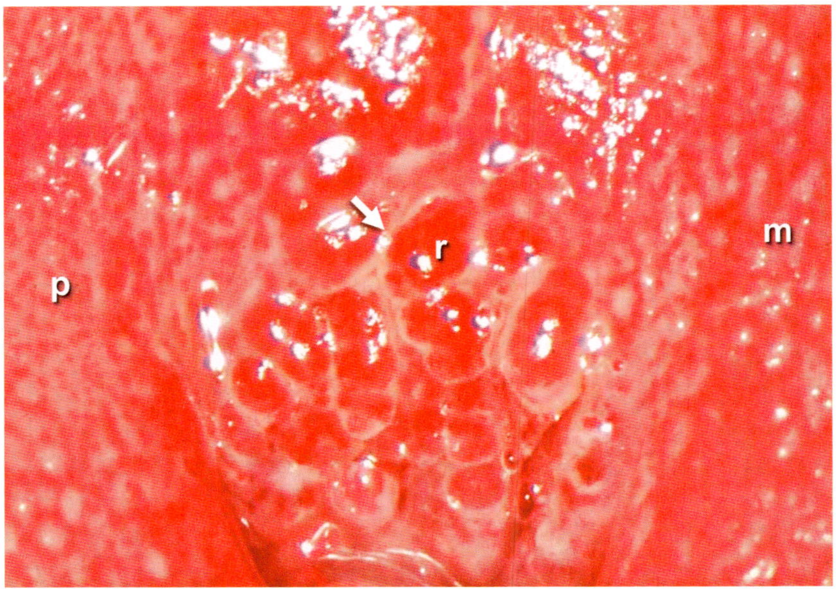

Figure 233 - Reverse mosaic characterized by raised small red areas (r), circumscribed by acetowhite metaplastic epithelium (arrow). This colposcopic appearance is associated with punctation (p) and mosaic vascular pattern (m).

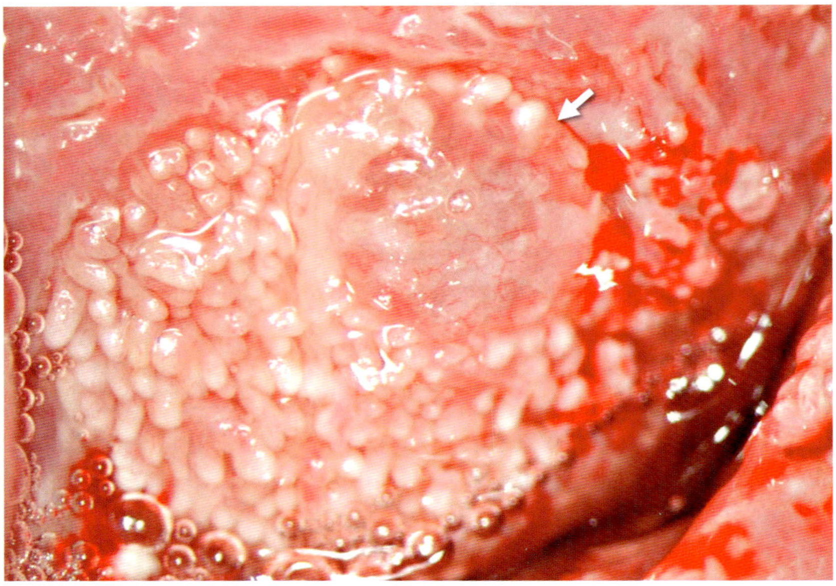

Figure 234 - Despite the absence of any atypical vessels, the smooth raised area (arrow) over acetowhite papillae proved to be adenocarcinoma in situ.

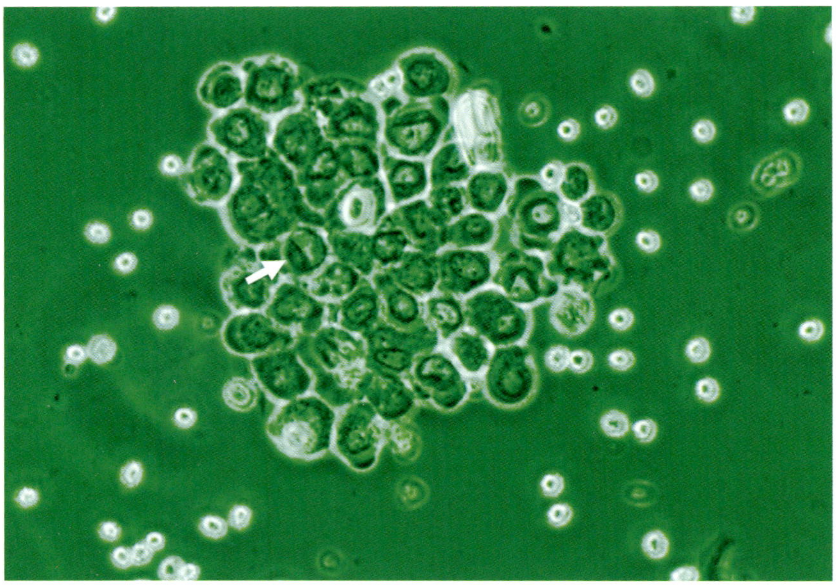

Figure 235 - Wet mount appearance showing a cluster of neoplastic cells in adenocarcinoma in situ. The nuclei appear different in size (anisokaryosis) and characteristically eccentric (arrow).

lium progresses, reverse mosaic soon turns into either punctation or mosaic.

Fine punctation is often combined with equally fine mosaic and coarse punctation may coexist with coarse mosaic in the same lesion.

This finding is not surprising because both punctation and mosaic patterns develop in a similar atypical direction within the transformation zone. Even if vascular alterations represent the first morphologic feature in the development of cervical neoplasia, it is useful to point out that punctation and mosaic may also be found in normal epithelium and outside the transformation zone but the same vascular patterns within the TZ are more likely to represent epithelial atypia

On the other hand, many squamous intraepithelial lesions and glandular atypia do not have colposcopically atypical vessels (Figures 234, 235).

Colposcopy is of great value for the diagnosis of early or preclinical invasive lesions -mostly preceded by cervical intraepithelial neoplasia- when neoplastic cells have invaded the stroma underlying the epithelium, without symptoms and/or gross physical signs. Unfortunately, there is sometimes a surprising paucity of colposcopic changes. Most invasive foci originate from CIN within cervical glands and less frequently from the surface epithelium. Colposcopic detection of small areas of *early stromal invasion* (ESI) depends on their extension. The predominance of the proliferating component, epithelial or connective tissue, in the atypical area gives rise to different colposcopic findings. Newly formed vessels, due to the increased metabolic demand of the rapidly proliferating cells, are responsible for localized hyperemia and a decrease in intercapillary distance. At this stage, a colposcopy may reveal localized, rough, hyperemic areas which bleed on touch. Focal collections of atypical vessels are highly suspicious for ESI.

When a **red area** intensely whitens after the application of acetic acid, a more serious histologic lesion is expected (Figure 236), whereas a merely inflamed area becomes white only to some extent, with indistinct margins. Suspicious red areas must be distinct from inflammatory papules which appear as well circumscribed and raised red lesions (Figure 237). Histologically, the infiltrate is mainly composed of lymphoplasma cells, eosinophils and spindle cell proliferation. Some red areas are due to detachment of epithelium, so that the well-defined red area represents the exposed stroma and the vascular network (Figure 238).

As abnormal cell proliferation progresses, irregular blocks of the expanding neoplastic epithelium on the vascular spaces, compress and distort the vessels, some of which disappear. The resulting ischemic necrosis is responsible for the loss of mucosal integrity. On colposcopy, these architectural disorders result in thick acetowhite areas with slightly uneven or nodular surfaces, capillary oozing or contact bleeding. Sometimes, it may be impossible to designate chalky white areas to punctation or mosaic. If the lesion is predominantly exophytic, microinvasive carcinoma may produce a small bulge on the surface

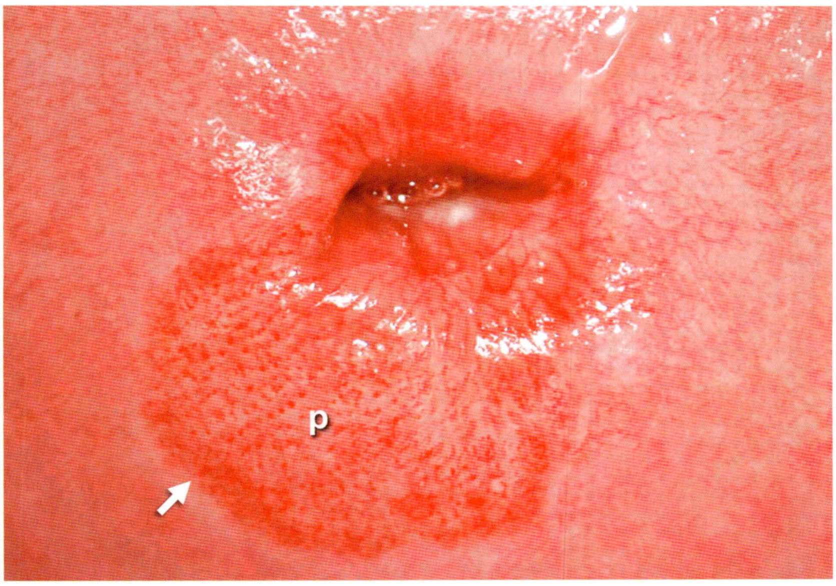

Figure 236 - The arrowed intensely red area displays a punctation pattern (p) with irregularly spaced dots. On histology, carcinoma in situ was reported.

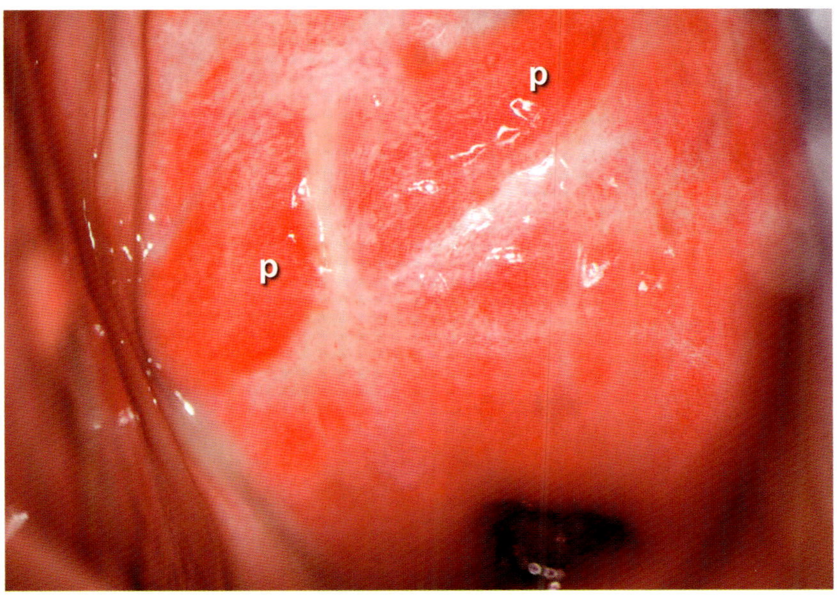

Figure 237 - Inflammatory papules (p) appear as well circumscribed and raised red lesions.

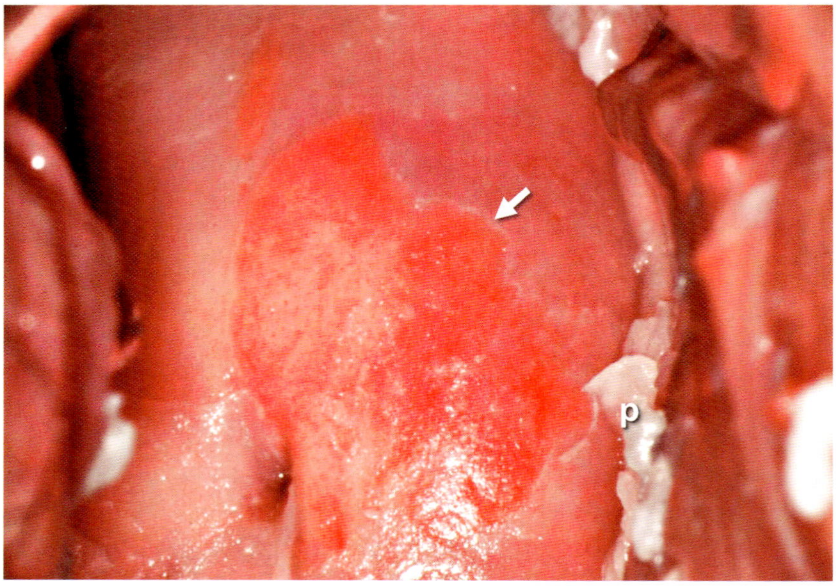

Figure 238 - The arrow indicates an exposed stroma with evident vascular network. Peeled off epithelial sheet (p).

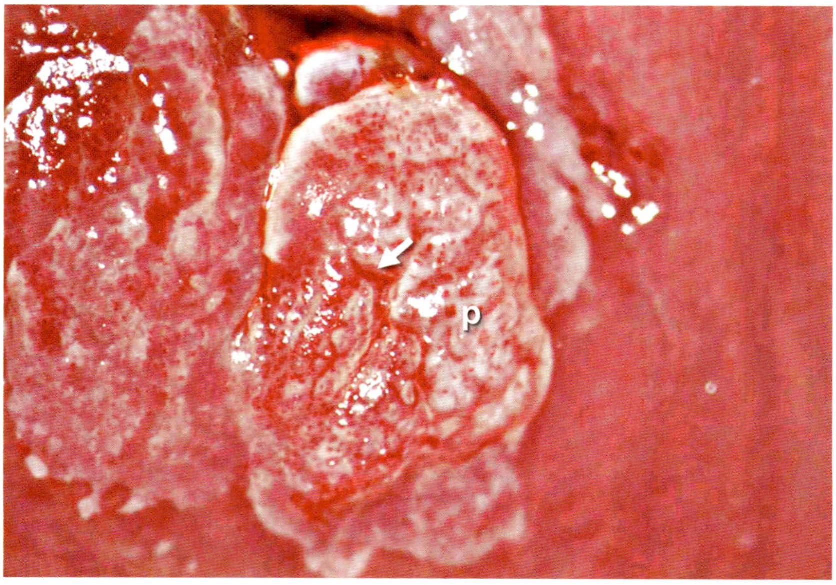

Figure 239 - Bulging acetowhite lesion with atypical vessels (arrow) and coarse punctation (p). Histology showed a microinvasive carcinoma.

(Figure 239). Larger tumors can produce a confined polypoid lesion showing atypical vessels (Figures 240, 241).

These epithelial derangements are associated with widened intercapillary distance, large avascular area, ulceration and vascular abnormalities. Atypical blood vessels show haphazard distribution, are strikingly irregular in caliber, shape, size, course and mutual arrangement, and intercapillary distance is substantially greater and more variable than that seen in normal epithelium and low-grade dysplasia. There is no steady decrease in the diameter of the tree-like dividing branches which suddenly become smaller and then abruptly open up again into larger vessels. Atypical vessels may show sharp, irregular bends, gross fluctuations in width, angular changes in direction, constriction and dilatation, and may appear and disappear abruptly. Bizarre vessels in the forms of wide hairpins, spaghetti, threads, roots, tendrils, corkscrews, commas and tadpoles may be seen.

The appearance of atypical blood vessels usually indicates the first sign of invasion, but it should be pointed out that in endophytic lesions where the cervix is retracted, vascular abnormalities may not be seen even in the presence of thick and chalky white areas after the application of acetic acid.

Most cases of *invasive* carcinoma can be detected on naked-eye inspection and the use of the colposcope is not necessary. Advanced invasive carcinoma may show nodular (Figure 242) or polypoid surface, with or without exophytic growth pattern. In *exo-*

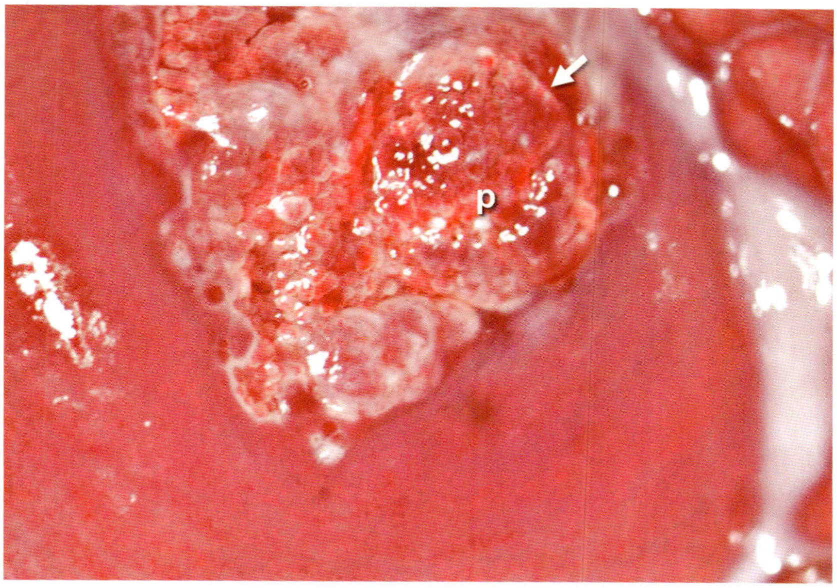

Figure 240 - The arrowed lesion can be mistaken for a polyp, but the coarse punctation (p) may assist in reaching a correct diagnosis. Histology disclosed a microinvasive carcinoma.

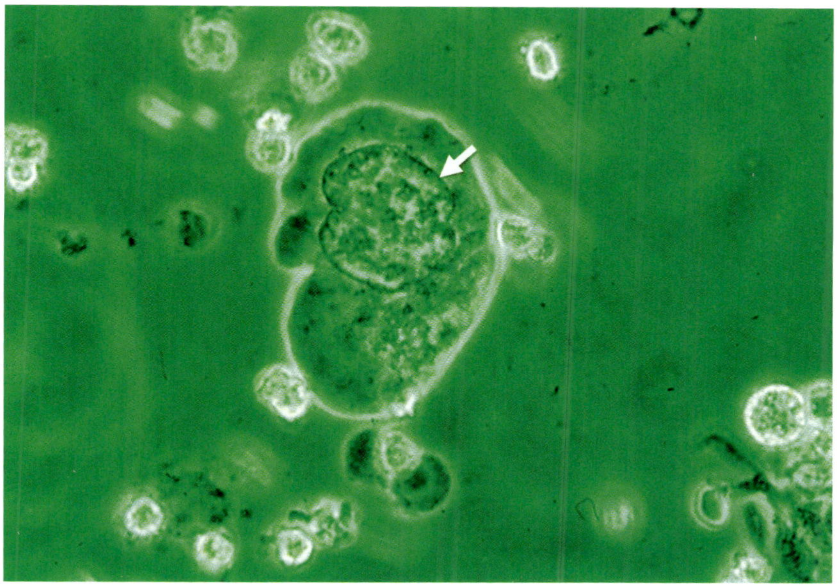

Figure 241 - The wet mount finding shows a giant nucleus with irregular outline (arrow) in microinvasive carcinoma.

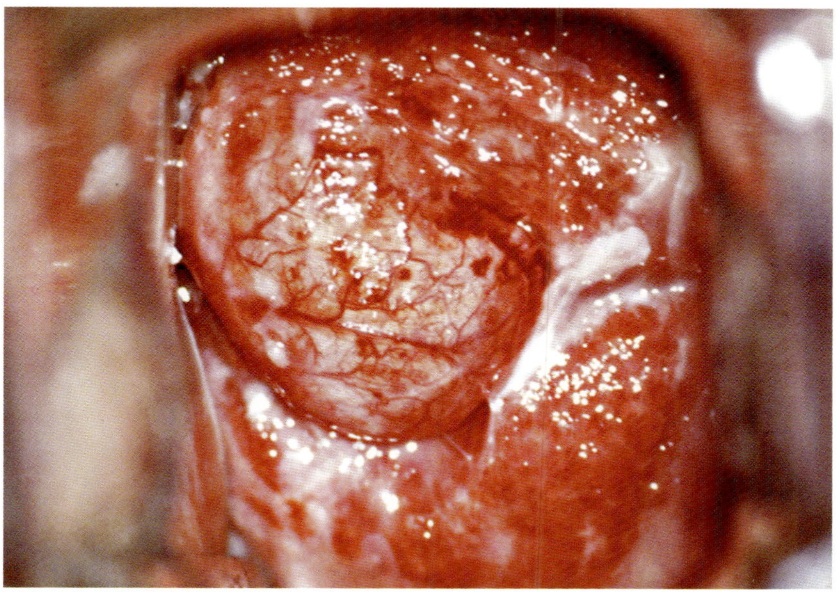

Figure 242 - The lesion exhibits a nodular surface with bizarre blood vessels and capillary effusions. The diagnosis was invasive squamous cell carcinoma.

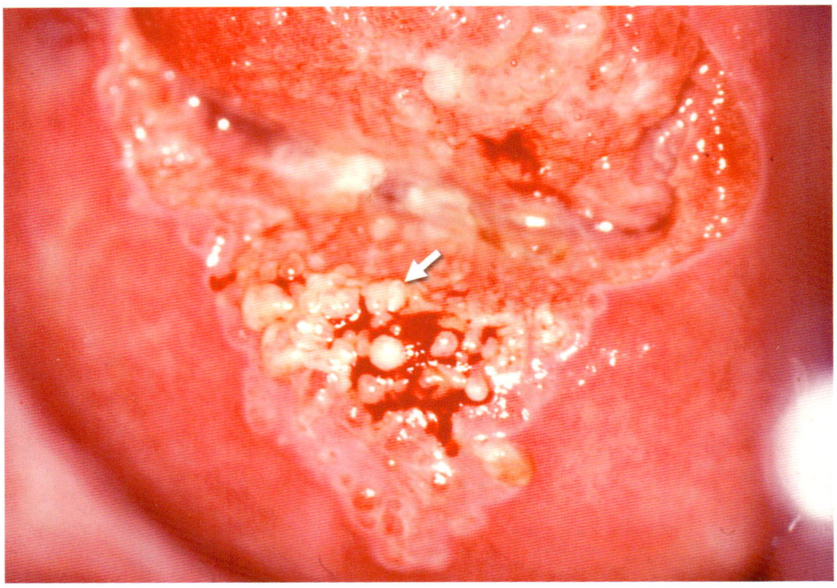

Figure 243 - Once acetic acid has been applied, stromal papillae appear intensely white (arrow) and partially fused. The tissue is friable and fragile, with capillary oozing. Histology showed invasive squamous cell carcinoma. Malignancy may mimic a hypertrophic exposed epithelium.

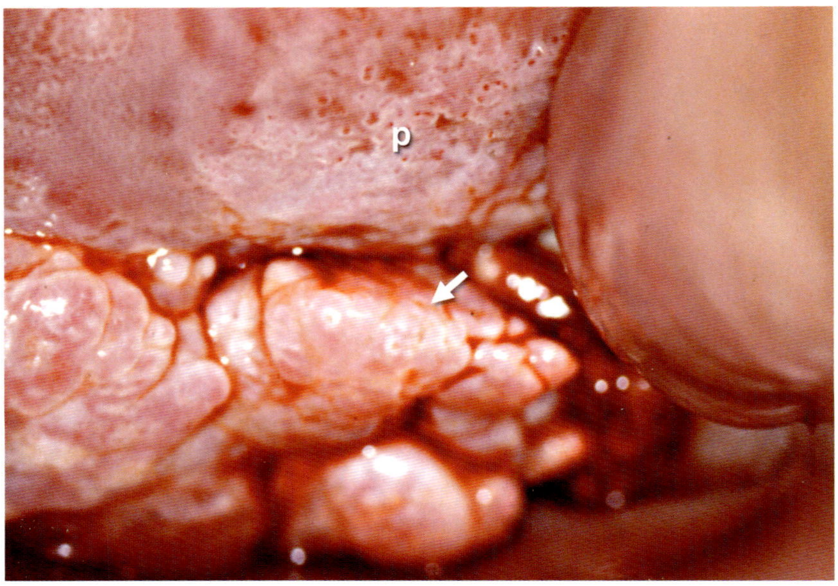

Figure 244 - Polypoid invasive squamous cell carcinoma (arrow) can mimic a large benign cervical polyp. The anterior lip of the cervix shows a dense acetowhite epithelium with coarse punctation. The red dots appear irregular in size and distance among punctations (p).

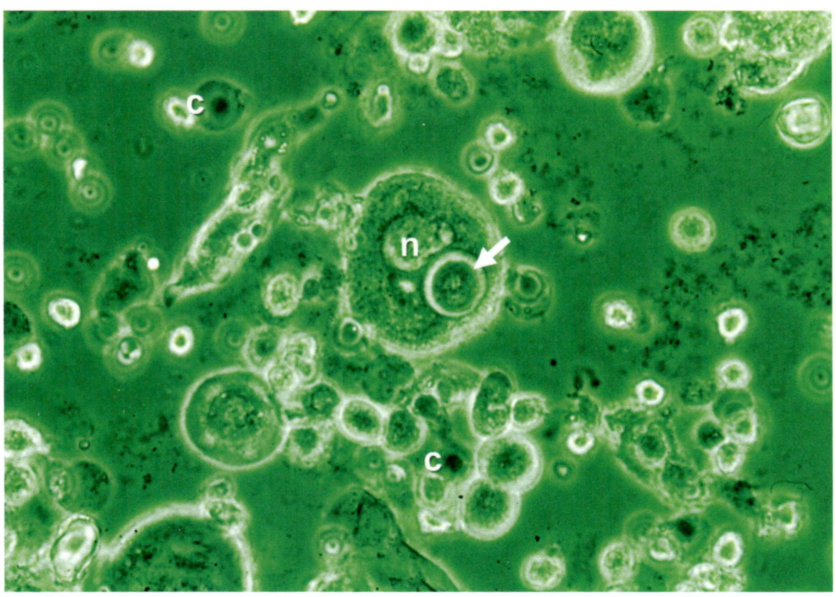

Figure 245 - The wet mount microphotograph exhibits a cell cannibalism. A malignant cell with irregularly edged nucleus (n) has phagocytosed a smaller cell (arrow). Associated cells are different in size and contain nuclei with clumped chromatin (c).

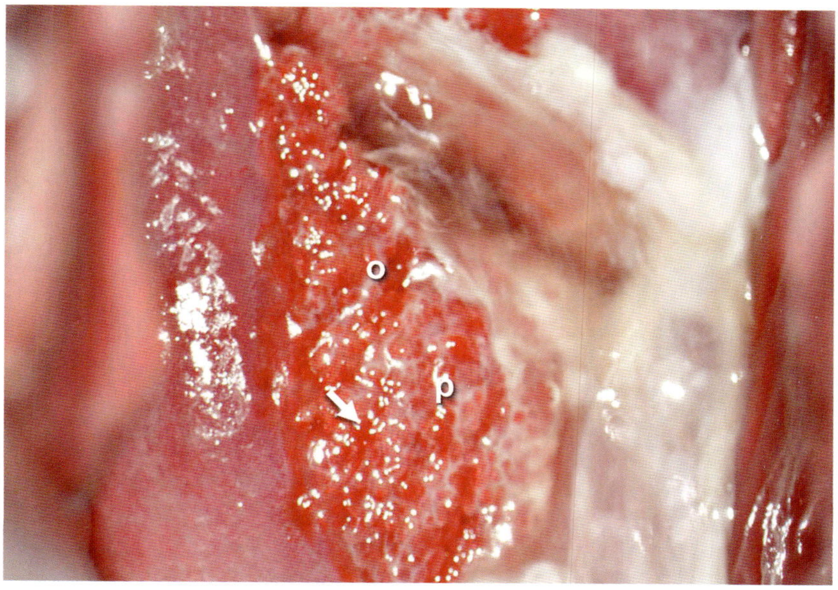

Figure 246 - The exophytic adenocarcinoma inside the transformation zone can mimic simple ectopy, but the atypical vessel with abrupt disappearance (arrow), coarse punctation (p) and capillary oozing (o) may raise the doubt of malignancy.

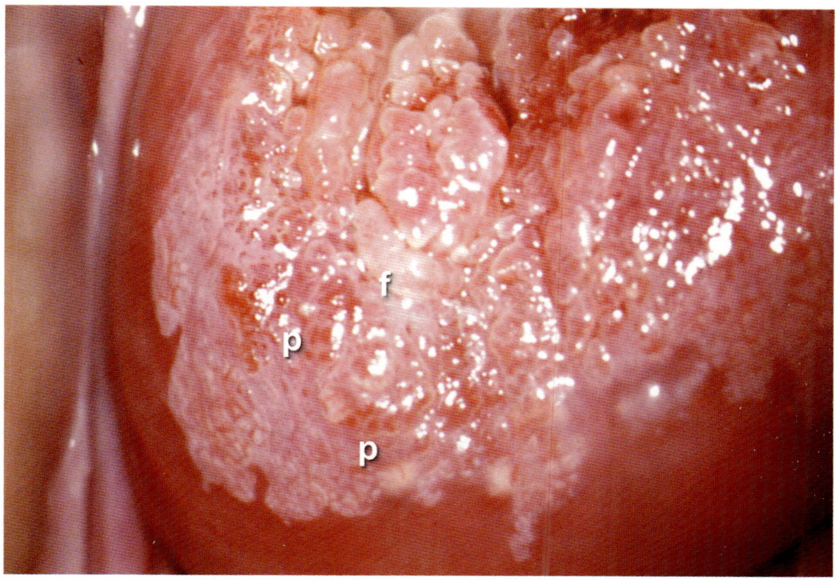

Figure 247 - After application of acetic acid, enlarged and fused papillae (f) turn strongly whitish. The lesion exhibits coarse punctation (p). Histology disclosed adenocarcinoma.

phytic invasive carcinomas, the surface contour is uneven and usually irregularly fissured like a cauliflower. Exophytic growth displaying a cauliflower-like surface is the most common pattern (75% of cases). The tissue is often friable, and the vessels appear atypical and fragile. Stromal papillae appear intensely white in response to acetic acid and may fuse together giving rise to irregular blocks. When the papillae are finer and more regular, malignancy may mimic a hypertrophic exposed epithelium (Figure 243). Polypoid invasive squamous cell carcinoma could be mistaken for a large, benign cervical polyp (Figures 244, 245). In this case, vascular pattern and the use of a thin probe (Chrobak's probe) may assist in reaching a correct diagnosis. In contact with a benign polyp, the probe encounters elastic resistance, whereas it advances into malignant lesions as into butter.

Flat *endophytic* invasive carcinomas with ulcerated surfaces or associated with hyperkeratosis, may pose diagnostic problems in colposcopy. An unusual transformation zone with well-defined and easily injured superficial ulcerations, must raise the doubt of invasive carcinoma.

Adenocarcinoma in situ (AIS) and microinvasive adenocarcinoma do not show any characteristic colposcopic appearance. Diagnostic difficulties for these glandular lesions are greater than for squamous cell carcinoma. For this reason, most glandular lesions are usually an incidental finding in ablative procedures for CIN, although they are increasingly detected by cytology. Moreover, in some cases, it is

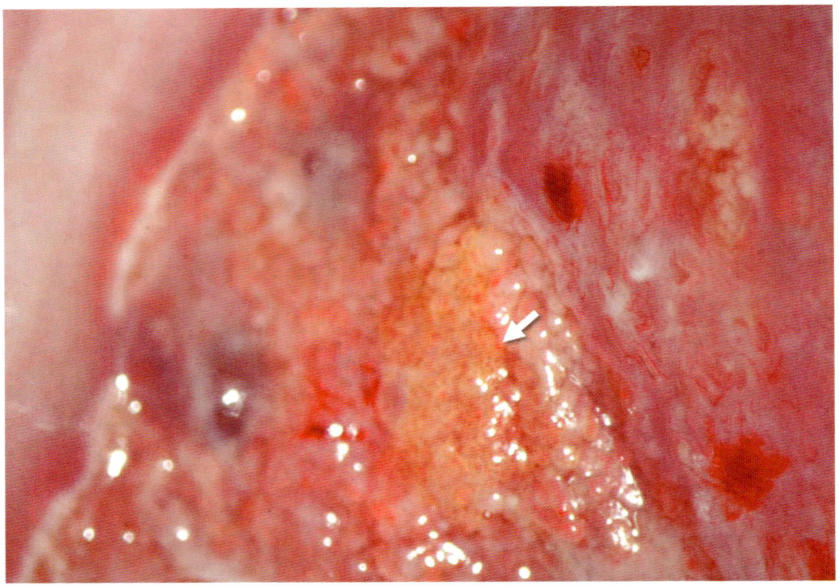

Figure 248 - Circumscribed yellow area (arrow), in stark contrast to the surrounding pinkish white columnar villi. Excision biopsy and resultant histology revealed adenocarcinoma.

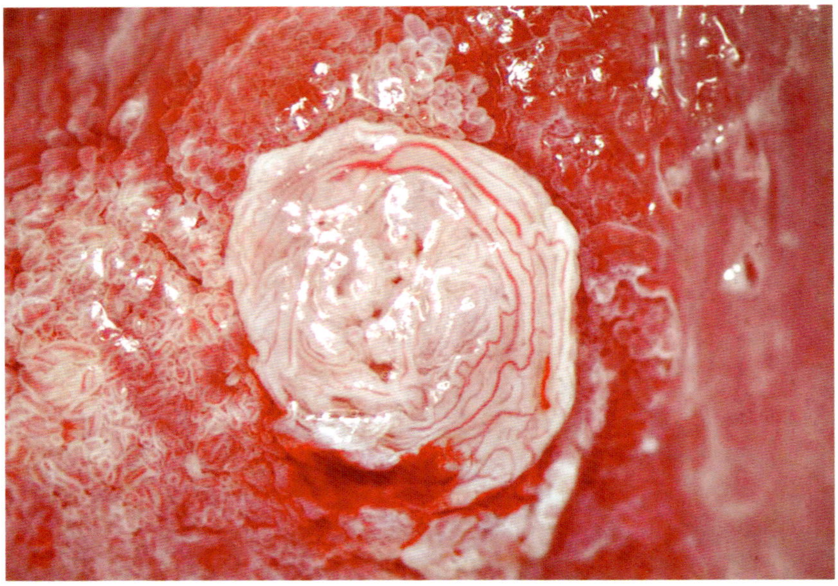

Figure 249 - Twenty-eight-year-old woman. Adenocarcinoma appears as an elevated acetowhite lesion in the form of a papillary lesion, associated with atypical vessels showing bizarre course, in stark contrast to the surrounding columnar epithelium. Pap smear gave a false negative result.

difficult to distinguish between AIS and microinvasive cancer even by histology. Often adenocarcinoma in situ coexists with CIN.

Most glandular lesions originate in the transformation zone, so small areas of early exophytic adenocarcinoma may mimic simple ectopy (Figure 246). Glandular lesions must be suspected in the presence of individual or fused enlarged papillae of columnar epithelium (Figure 247), in discrete patches, that turn strongly whitish after the application of acetic acid, or with the detection of a circumscribed yellow area, in stark contrast to the surrounding pinkish white columnar villi (Figure 248).

Colposcopic suspicion is also justified in the presence of closely placed, multiple cuffed gland openings in a dense acetowhite area with an uneven surface, or with the detection of large gland openings in the columnar epithelium or in the presence of a variegated patchy red and white lesion, harboring small papillary excrescences. Adenocarcinoma can be indicated by elevated acetowhite lesions in the form of polypoid or papillary lesions associated with atypical vessels showing varying calibers, changes of direction, bizarre courses (Figure 249), corkscrew and comma-like forms. It should be pointed out that in early stages of adenocarcinoma, vessels may not show any atypical pattern and intercapillary distance usually remains normal. Sometimes no vascular pattern can be observed (see Figure 118).

REFERENCES

- Burghardt E, Pickel H, Girardi F. Primary Care Colposcopy: Textbook and Atlas. Thieme, 2005.
- Chow C, Singer A. Colposcopic appearances of mature squamous, metaplastic and glandular epithelium, p. 37. EAGC Course Book on Colposcopy. Primed-X Press, 2003.
- Cibas ES, Ducatman BS. Cytology. Diagnostic Principles and Clinical Correlates. Elsevier Saunders, 2014.
- Das SK, Nigam S, Batra A, Chandra M. An Atlas of Colposcopy, Cytology and Histopathology of lower Female Genital Tract. Jaypee Brothers Medical Publishers Ltd, 1995.
- Dexeus S, Cusido MT, Carach M. The colposcopic appearances of invasive lesions of the cervix (squamous cell carcinoma and adenocarcinoma), p. 99. EAGC Course Book on Colposcopy. Primed-X Press, 2003.
- Donders G, Bellen G, Rezeberga D. Aerobic vaginitis in pregnancy.BJOG, Sep; 118(10):1163, 2011.
- Etherington IJ. The colposcopic appearances of CIN, p. 89. EAGC Course Book on Colposcopy. Primed-X Press, 2003.
- Eurocytology Courses. Cervical Cytology (Up to date, 2016).
- Girardi F, Reich O, Tamussino K. Burghardt's Colposcopy and Cervical Pathology. Textbook and Atlas. Thieme, 2015.
- Glab G. HPV w ginekologii. Innowacje 2020. Mobile SCANMED Systems.
- Gupta N, Chandra M. Colposcopy Made Easy. Jaypee Brothers Medical Publishers LTD, 2009.
- Herbeck G, Ondrus J, Dvorak V, Mortakis A. Atlas Kolposkopie. Maxdorf, 2011.
- Hillier SL. Diagnostic microbiology of bacterial vaginosis. Am J Obstet Gynecol. Aug;169(2 Pt 2):455-9, 1993.
- International Agency for Research on Cancer. Atlas of Colposcopy: Principlas and Practice, 2021.
- Koneman EW, Allen SD, Dowel VR-J, Janda WM, Sommers HM, Winn WC-J. Color atlas and textbook of diagnostic microbiology; JB Lippincott Company, 1988.
- Miniello G. Citogramma Vaginale - Vaginal Cytogram. CIC Edizioni Internazionali, 1994.
- Miniello G. Colposcopia e Microscopia a fresco – Colposcopy and Phase Contrast Microscopy. CIC Edizioni Internazionali, 1998.
- Miniello G. Le Micosi Vaginali in microscopia a fresco. Vaginal Fungal Infections by phase contrast microscopy. CIC Edizioni Internazionali, 2001-2012.
- Miniello G, Saraiya U. Color Atlas of Cytology and Colposcopy. CBS Publishers, New Delhi, 1999.
- Miniello G. Direct Microscopy in Gynecologic Practice. Edra, Milano 2017.
- Miniello G. Easy Colposcopy. Full Immersion. Edra, Milano 2019.
- Pickel H. The histology and cytology of atypical colposcopic lesions, p. 53. EAGC Course Book on Colposcopy. Primed-X Press, 2003.

- Prendiville W, de Camargo MJ. Treatment of cervical intraepithelial neoplasia, p. 105. EAGC Course Book on Colposcopy. Primed-X Press, 2003.
- Reich O, Girardi F, Tamussino K, Pickel H. Burghardt's Primary Care Colposcopy. Thieme, 2017.
- Saraiya UB, Miniello G. HPV Infections and its Role in Cervical Cancer. From: Principles & Practice of Obstetrics and Gynecology for Postgraduates. Ch. 111, p. 1006, Jaypee Brothers Medical Publishers LTD, 2008.
- Saraiya UB, Miniello G. Atlas of Cytology and Colposcopy. Jaypee Brothers Medical Publishers, 2009.
- Sellors JW, Sankaranarayanan R. Colposcopy and Treatment of Cervical Intraepithelial Neoplasia: A Beginners' Manual. IARC Press, 2003.
- Singer A, Monaghan JM: Lower Genital Tract Precancer. Colposcopy, Pathology and Treatment. Blackwell Science, Inc, 2nd edition, april 2008.
- Stoll P, Dallenbach-Hellweg G. Cytology in Gynecological Practice. An Atlas of Phase Contrast Microscopy - Gynäkologische Vitalzytologie in der Praxis. Atlas der Phasenkontrastmikroskopie. Springer-Verlag, 1993.
- Suresh A, Rajesh A, Bhat RM, Rai Y. Cytolytyc vaginosis. Indian J Sex Transm Dis. Jan;30(1):48, 2009.
- Syrjanen KJ. The colposcopy, cytology and histology of genital HPV infections, p.71. EAGC Course Book on Colposcopy. Primed-X Press, 2003.
- Szalay L : Cytolology of the Uterine Cervix. Wilhelm Maudrich-Medical Publishers, 1990.
- TEMPERA G, FURNERI PM. Management of aerobic vaginitis. Gynecol Obstet Invest, Oct70(4):244, 2010.
- Winter-Roach B, Monaghan JM, de B. LOPS A. Colposcopy of the vagina, p.119. EAGC Course Book on Colposcopy. Primed-X Press, 2003.
- Wojciech R. The diagnostic value of cytology and colposcopy in women with cervical intraepithelial neoplasia. Ginecol Pol. Aug;82(8):607, 2011.

FULL IMMERSION

The second session of this Atlas, termed as Full Immersion, contains colpophotographs which do not follow any particular order or etiological scheme, but are presented as they may routinely be observed by both novice and advanced colposcopists, in daily gynecological practice.

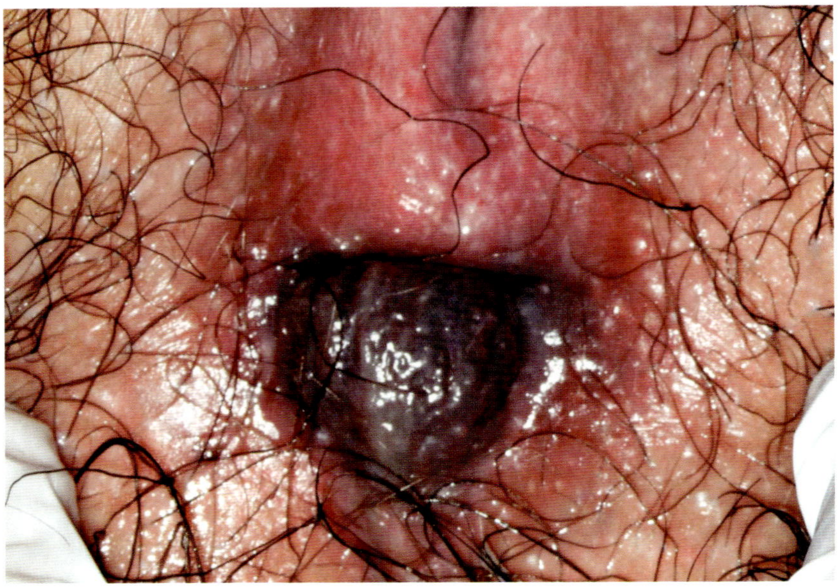

Figure 250 - Abnormal soft and painful growth at the fourchette in a 13-year-old girl. Positive transillumination and a Doppler ultrasonography suggest a cavernous hemangioma.

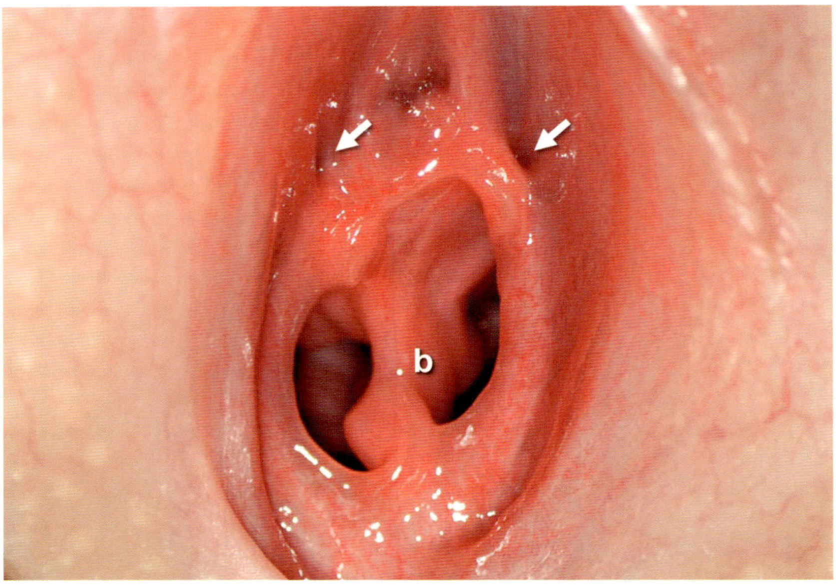

Figure 251 - Septate hymen. A band of extra tissue in the middle (b) creates two small vaginal openings. Posterolateral to the urethral meatus there are two dimples (arrows) which denote the main position of Skene's ducts.

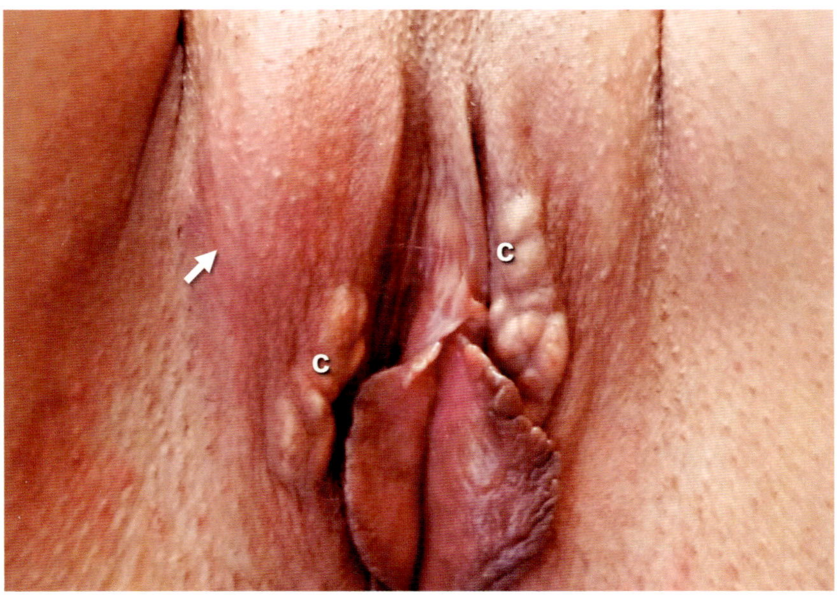

Figure 252 - Multiple voluminous sebaceous cysts (c) and abscess of the right labium majus (arrow).

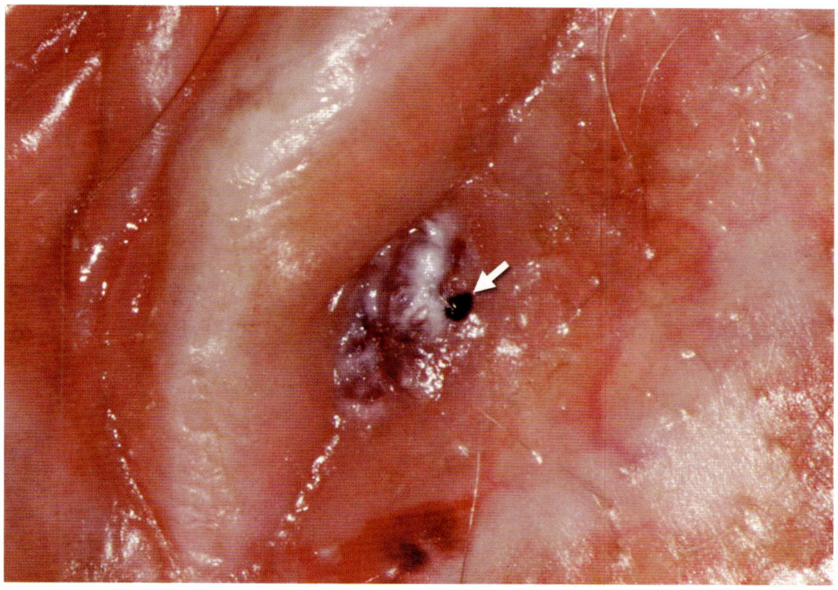

Figure 253 - The purple papule in the left interlabial sulcus (angiokeratoma) shows a rough scaly surface. It is composed of dilated blood vessels. A clot has formed in the lesion (thrombosis), changing the colour to black overnight (arrow).

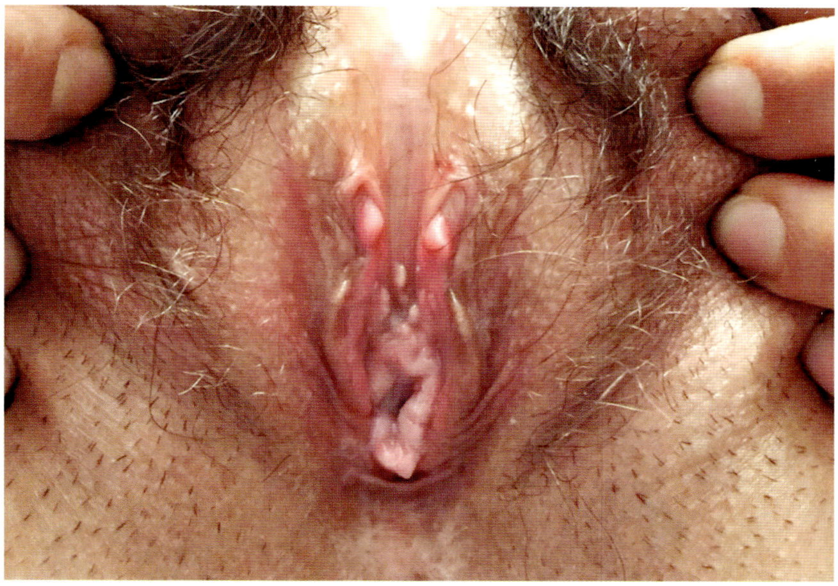

Figure 254 - Double clitoris.

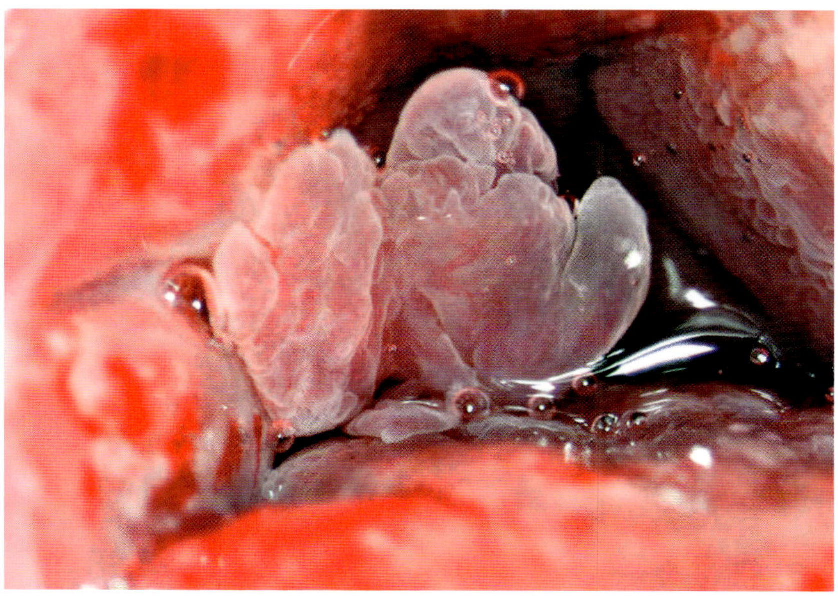

Figure 255 - Endocervical polyps.

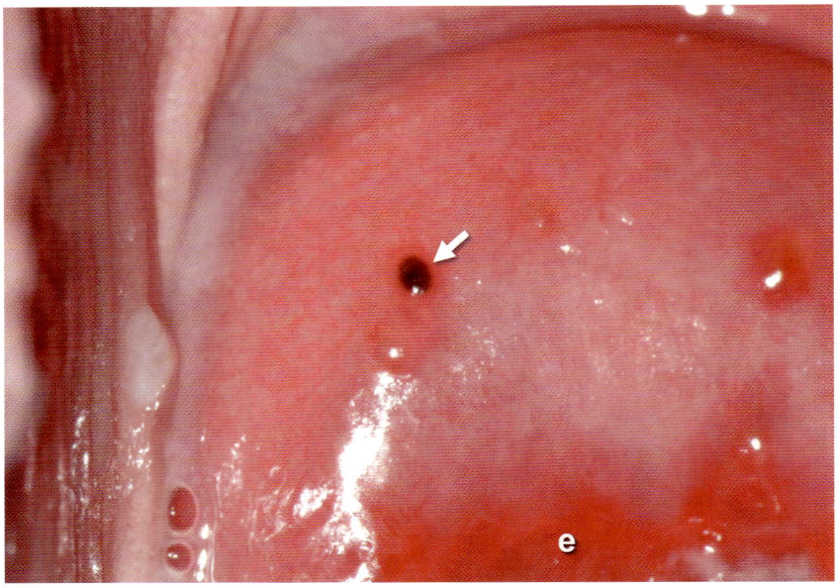

Figure 256 - The arrow indicates an endometrial focus. Exposed columnar epithelium (e).

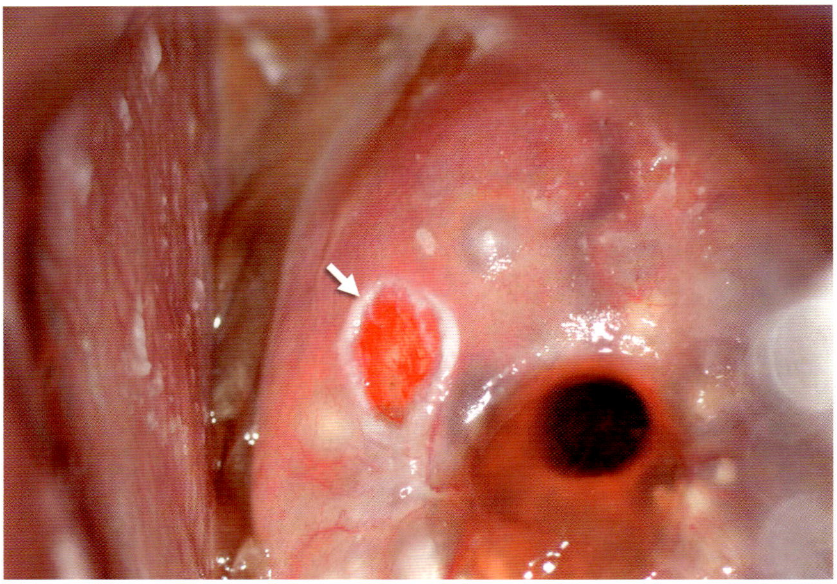

Figure 257 - Syphilitic cervical sore, known as a chancre (arrow).

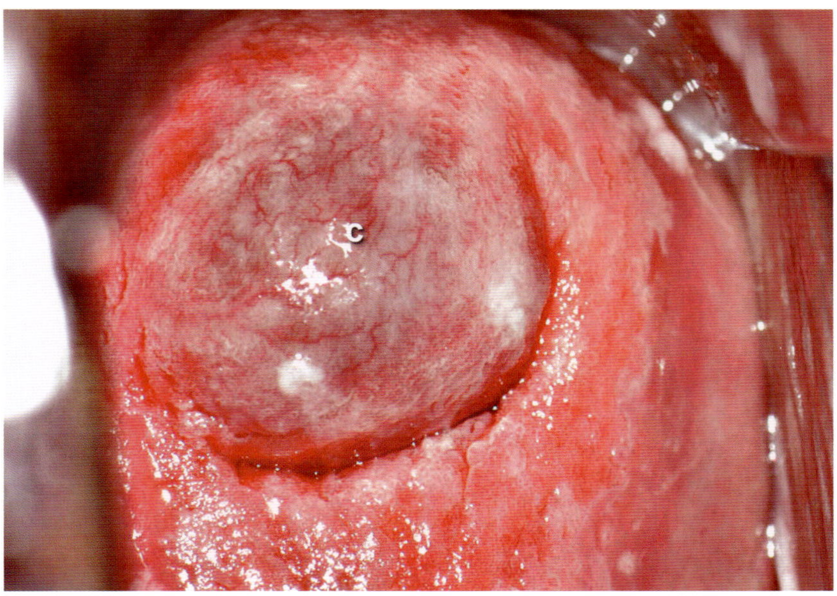

Figure 258 - A voluminous serous cyst (c), coated with acetowhite immature metaplastic epithelium, involves the distal extremity of the hypertrophic stem of arbor vitae and completely occludes the external os.

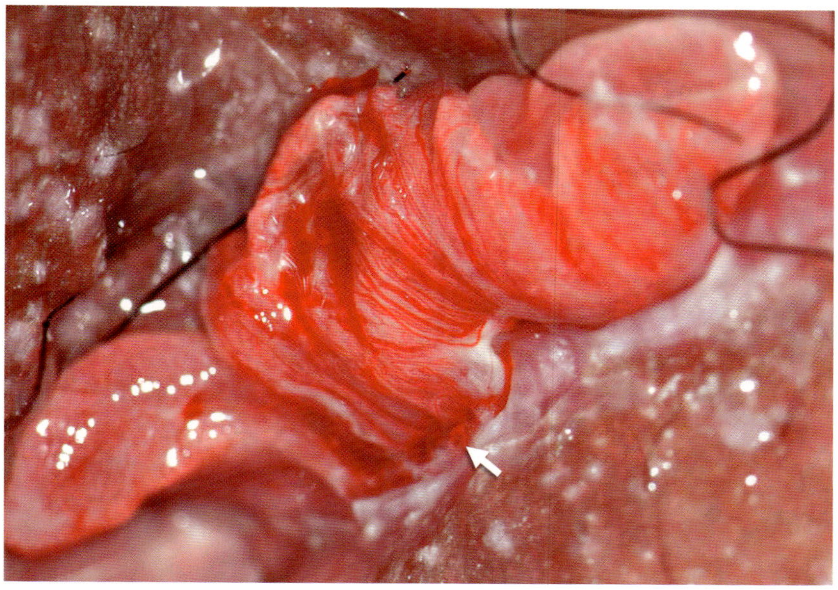

Figure 259 - A polypoid granulation tissue comes out from the breach (arrow) of a healed episiorrhaphy.

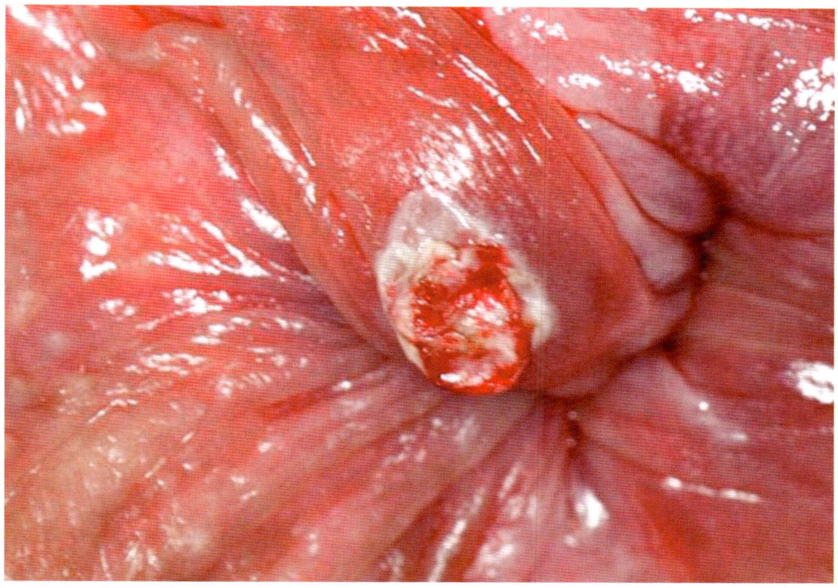

Figure 260 - Perianal hard ulcer with an eroded center (chancre).

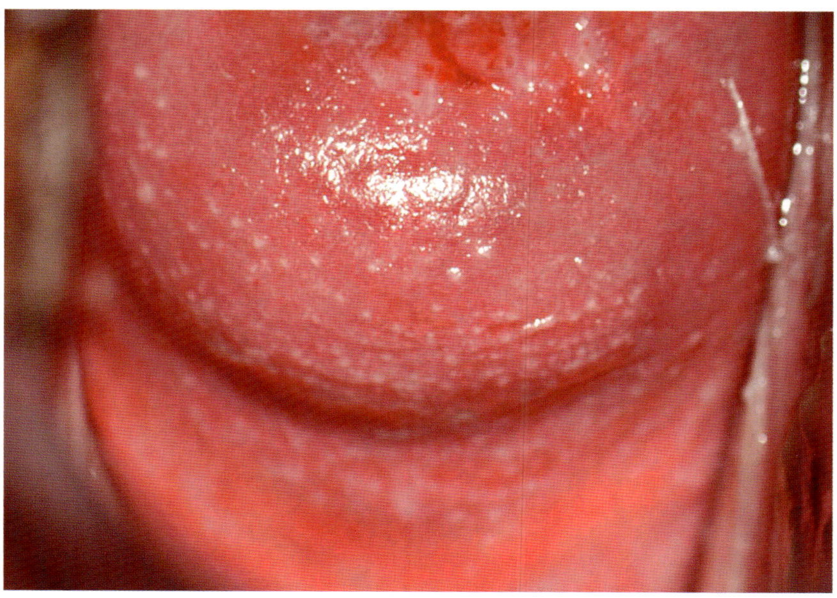

Figure 261 - Fungal white punctation induced by Candida infection involves both cervix and vaginal walls.

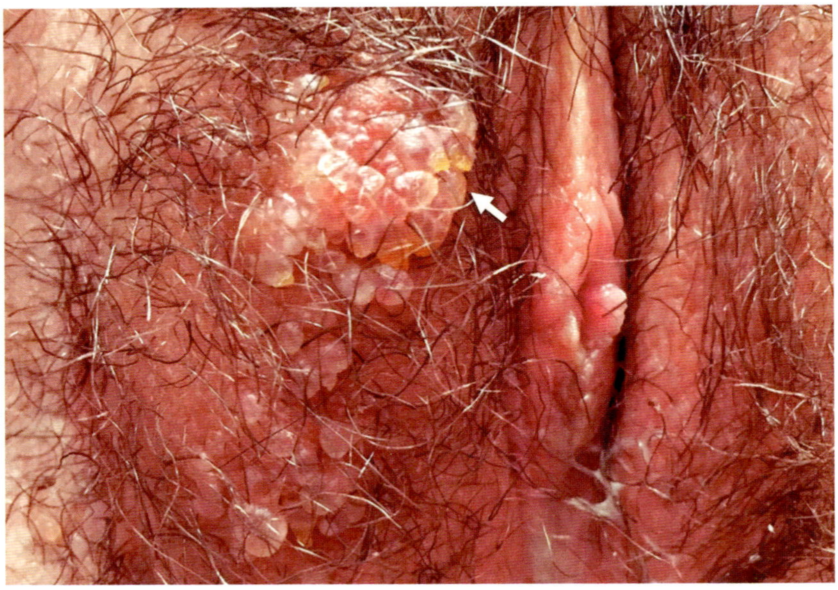

Figure 262 - The multiple confluent vesicles (arrow) are due to a lymphatic vascular malformation.

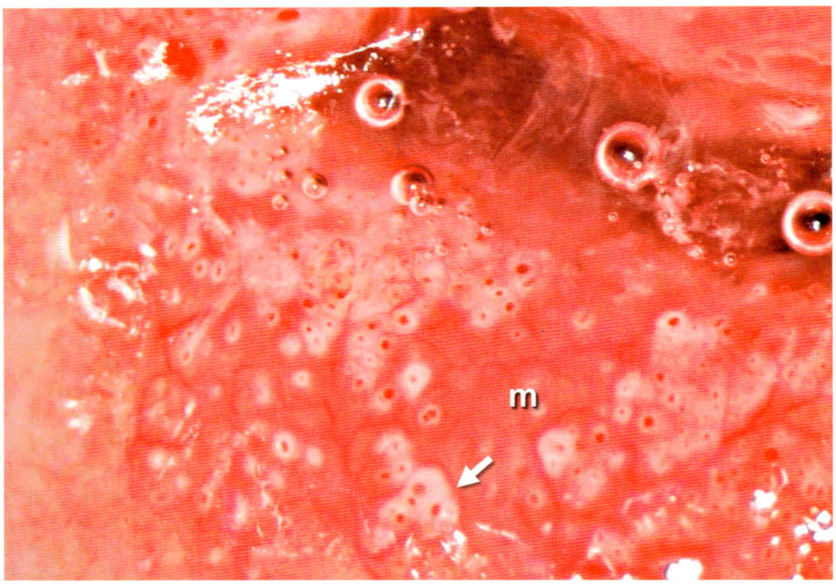

Figure 263 - Numerous gland openings of different grades are scattered over a mature metaplastic epithelium. Despite the presence of grade IV gland openings (arrow), no atypia is present. Mosaic base (m).

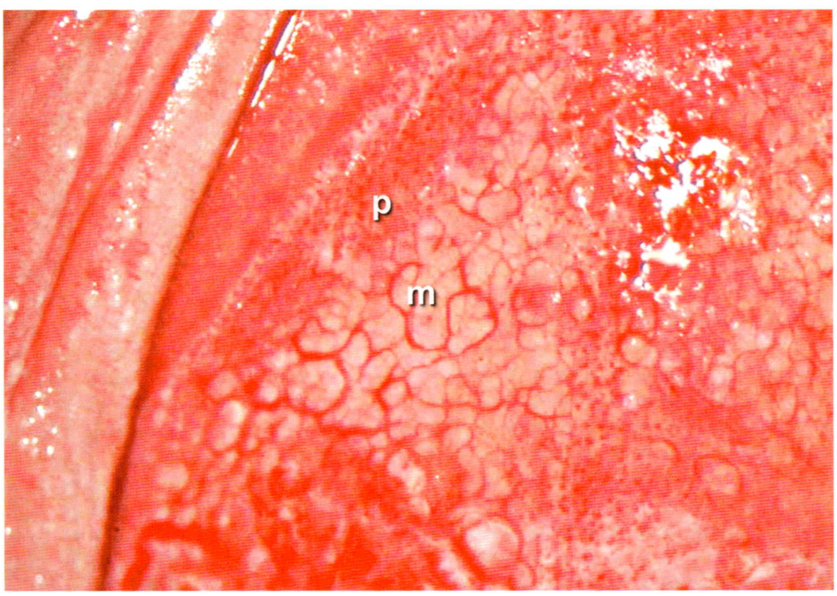

Figure 264 - Coarse mosaic (m) and fine punctation (p).

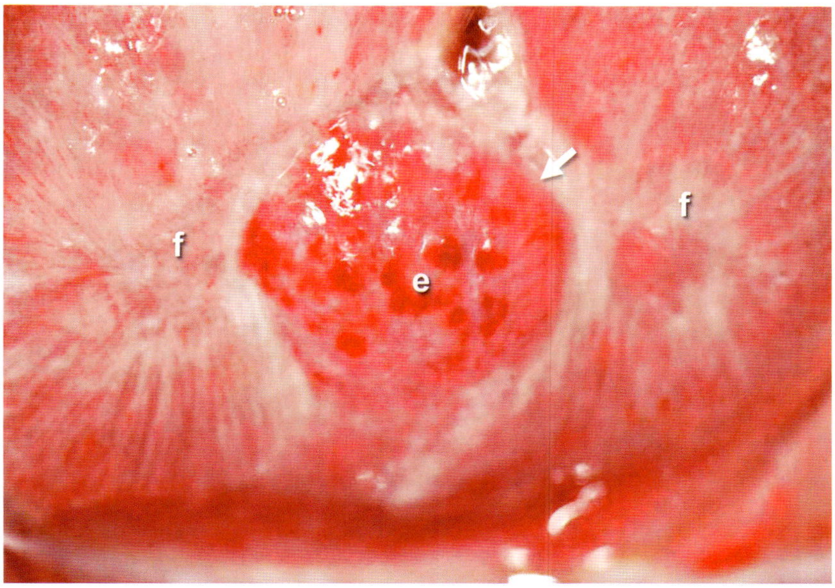

Figure 265 - The arrow indicates an inflammatory papule with hemorrhagic effusions (e). Subepithelial fibrosis (f), following diathermy, is seen as white areas before the application of acetic acid.

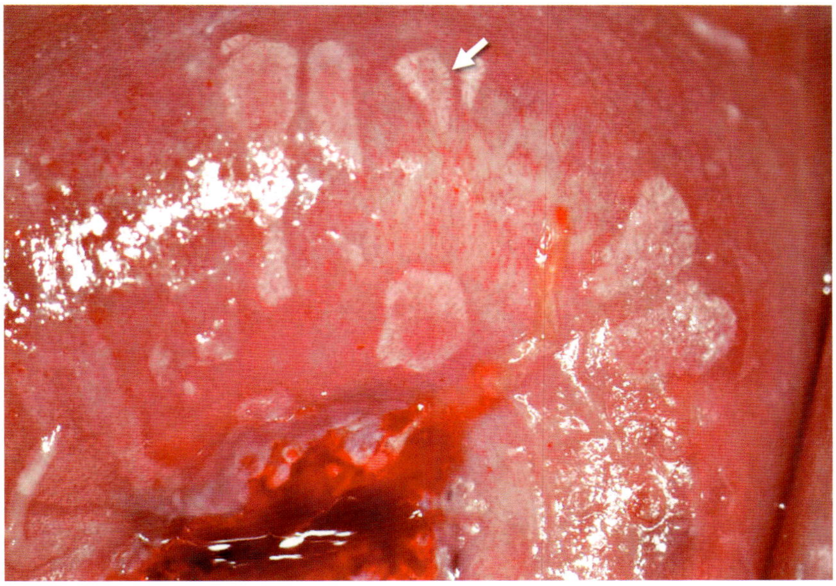

Figure 266 - Widespread raised acetowhite lesions (arrow) (HPV flat condylomas).

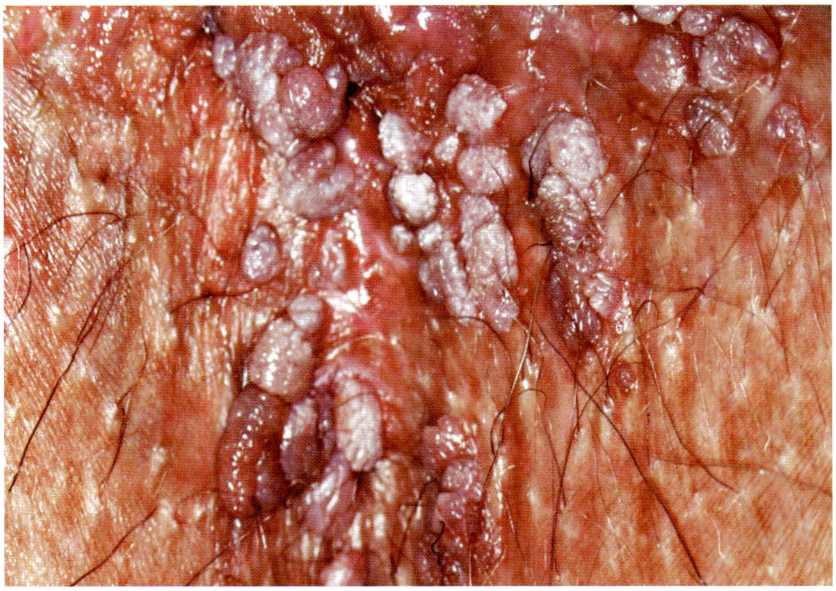

Figure 267 - Perineal warts.

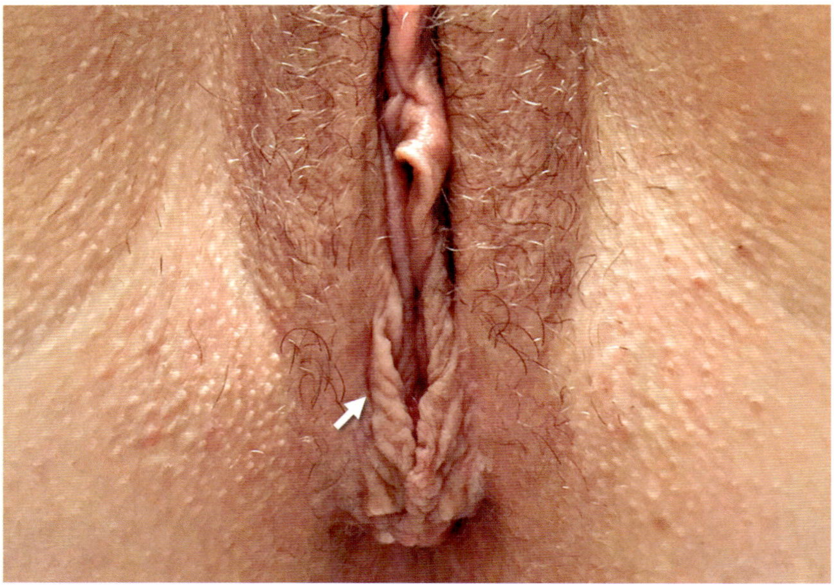

Figure 268 - Hypertrophy of the lower portion of labia minora (arrow) ("inferior prepuce").

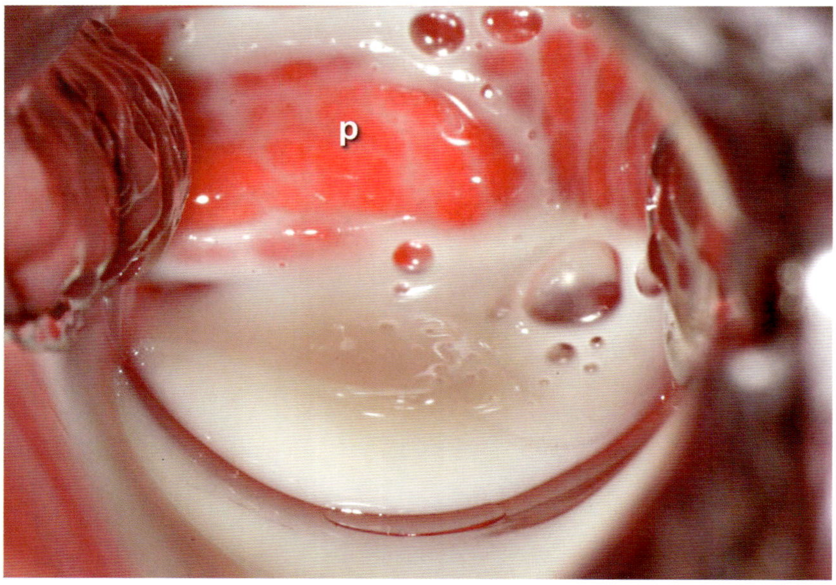

Figure 269 - Trichomonas infection is responsible for the abundant white-yellowish discharge which fills the posterior valve of the speculum, and causes erythematous patches on the cervix (p).

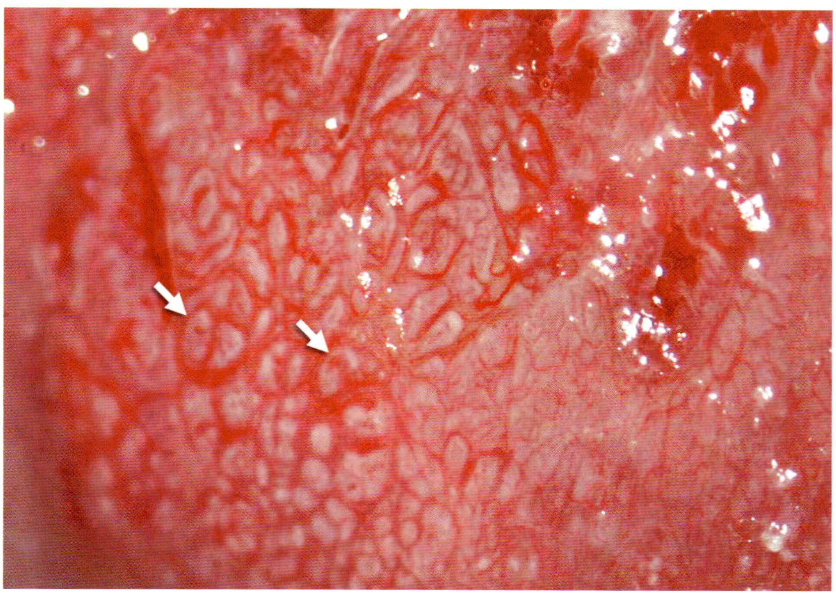

Figure 270 - This coarse mosaic exhibits a great irregularity of the epithelial tiles. The furrows between the epithelial cobbles are widely spaced and intensely red. The arrows indicate umbilication.

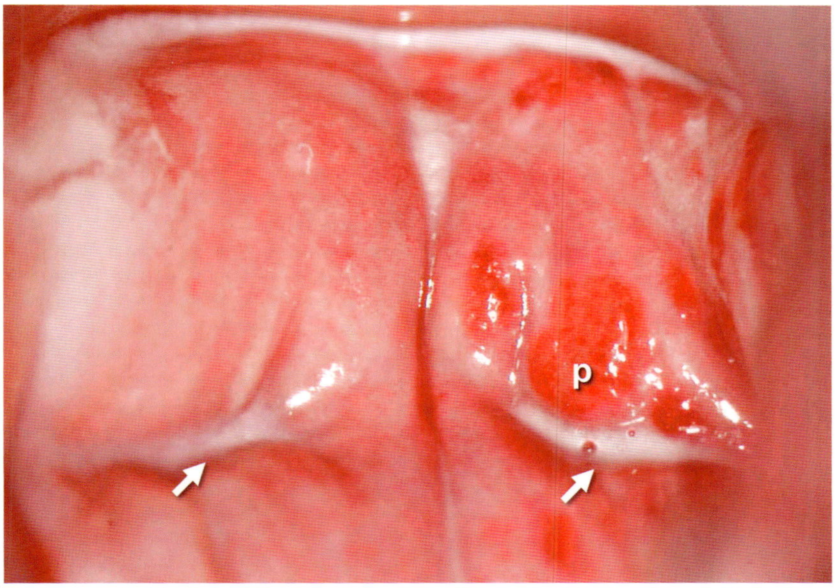

Figure 271 - Vaginal vault following hysterectomy, shows lateral recesses (dog ears) (arrows) and erithematous papules (p), due to fungal infection.

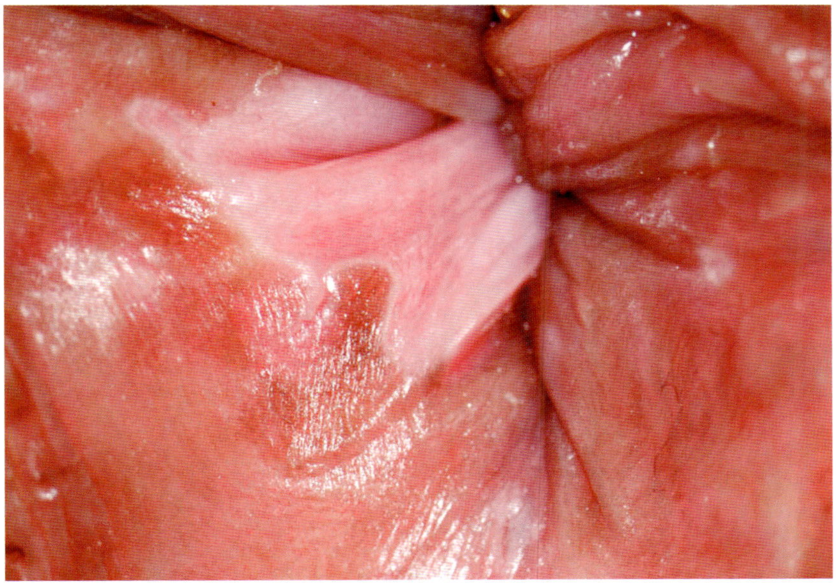

Figure 272 - Perianal vitiligo.

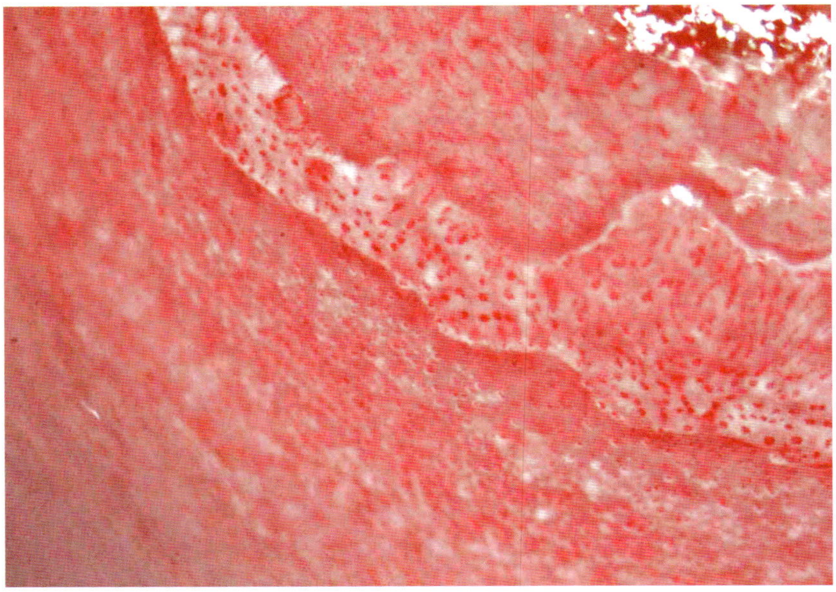

Figure 273 - The coarse punctation displays widely separated red dots irregular in size, over a faint acetowhite epithelium. Histology showed a low-grade HPV-CIN lesion.

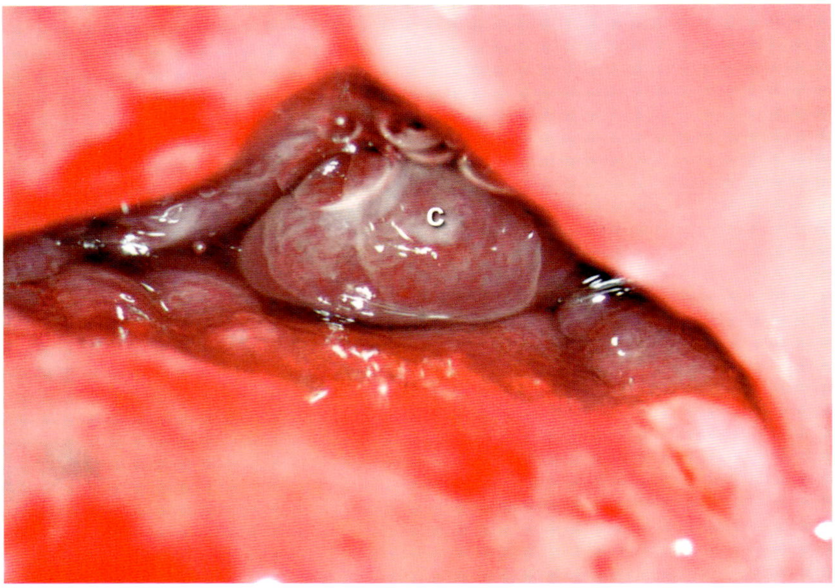

Figure 274 - Endocervical cysts (c) could be mistaken for polyps.

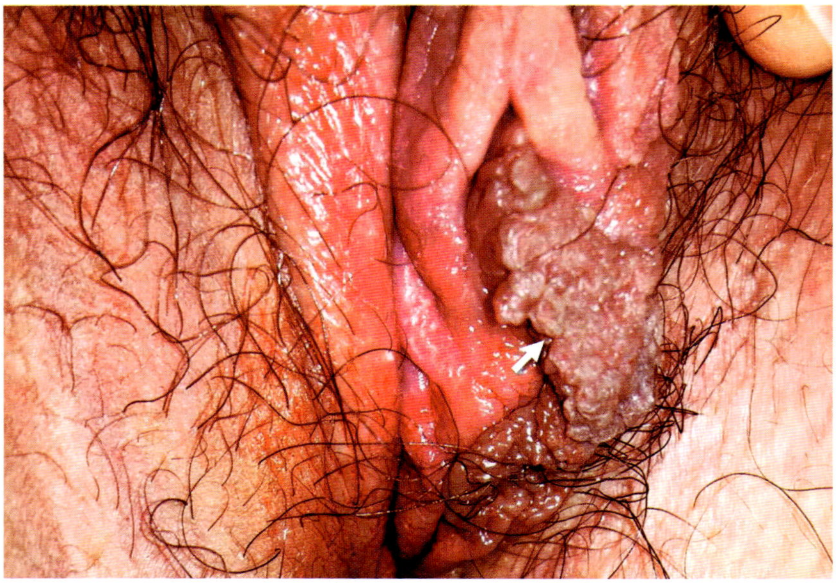

Figure 275 - Hypertrophy of the left inner labium (arrow).

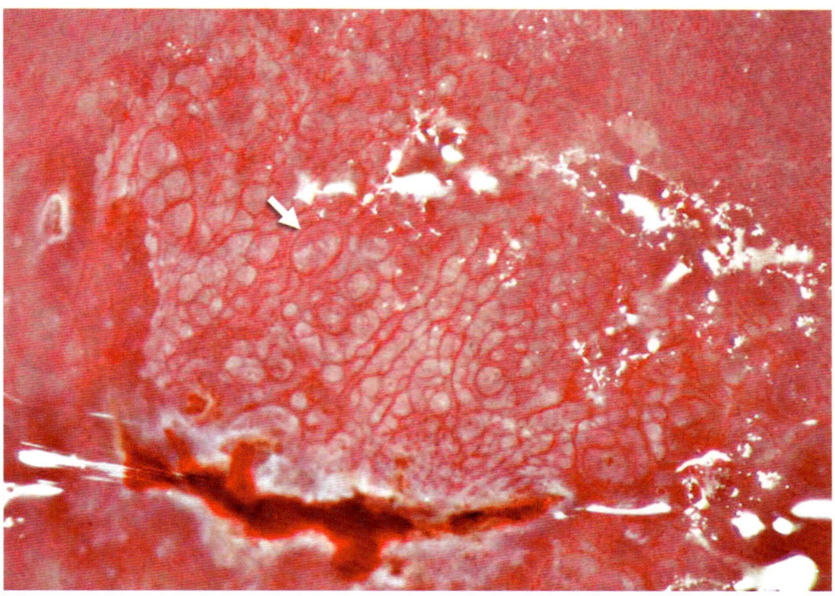

Figure 276 - This irregular mosaic pattern shows a network of convoluted blood vessels defining oval tiles (arrow). Histology revealed no atypical epithelium.

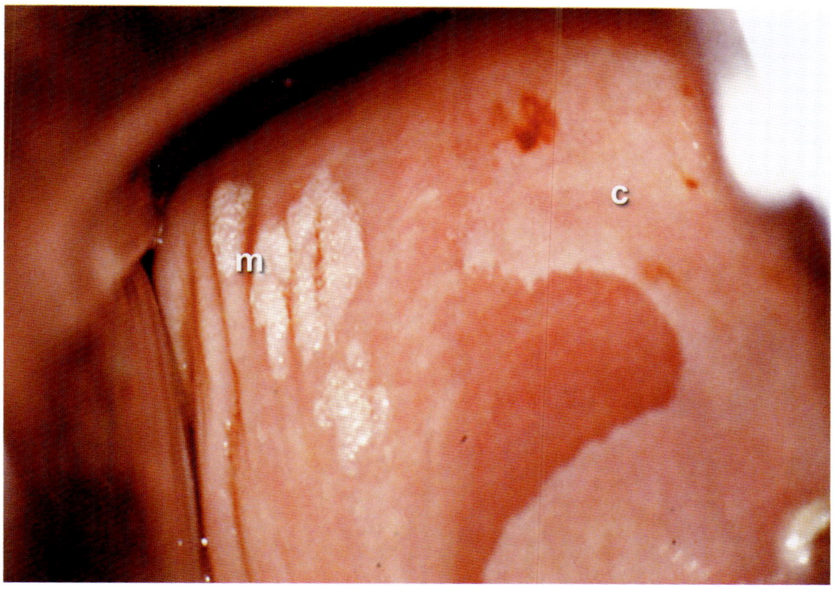

Figure 277 - Vaginal HPV micropapillary lesions (m) are associated with a faint acetowhite epithelium in a congenital transformation zone (c).

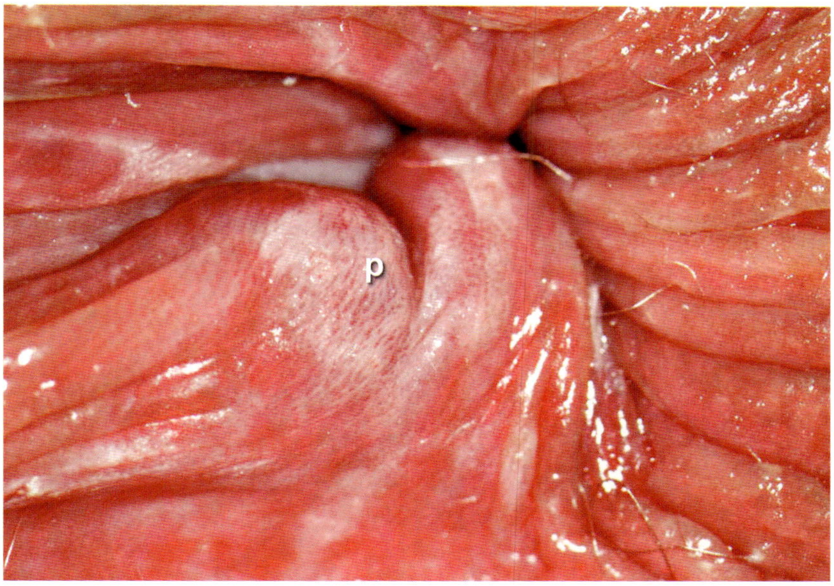

Figure 278 - Perianal acetowhite areas harbour fine punctation (p) in HPV infection.

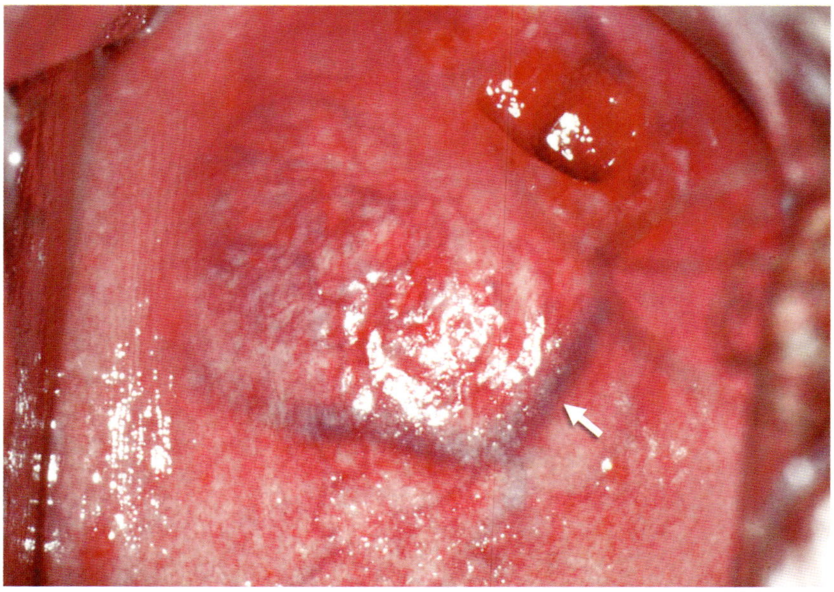

Figure 279 - Cervical varices (arrow).

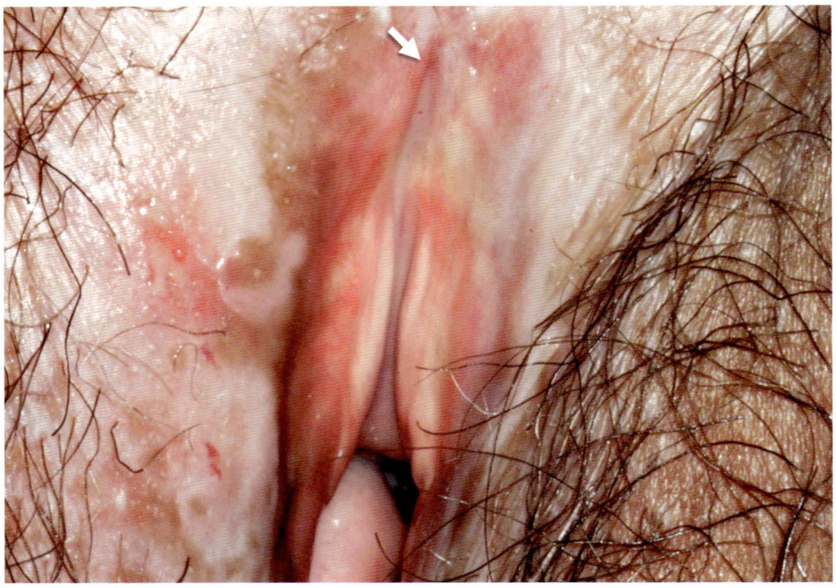

Figure 280 - Severe genital atrophy with disappearance of clitoris (arrow).

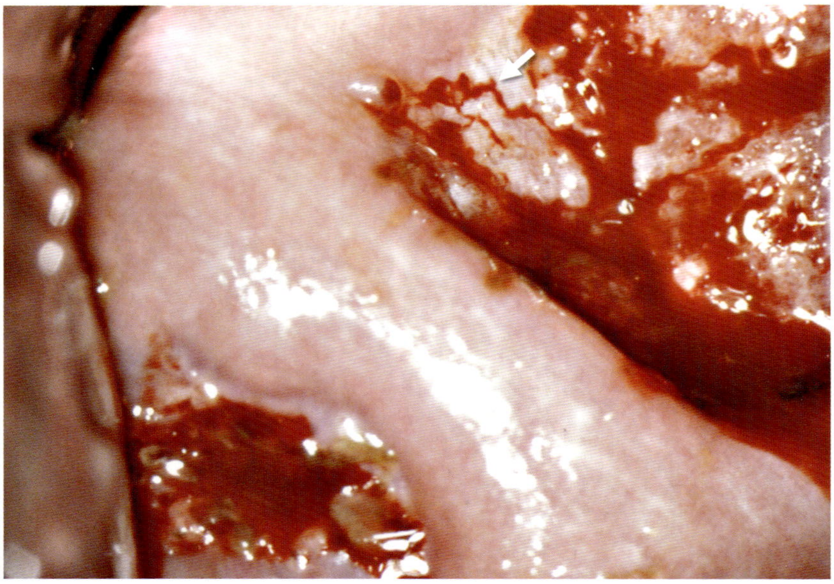

Figure 281 - Uterus didelphys unicollis. The arrow indicates an atypical vessel which runs over an ulcerated and friable surface. These ulcerated areas may be mistaken for ectopic columnar epithelium. Histology revealed an endophytic invasive carcinoma. An unusual transformation zone with well-defined and easily injured superficial ulcerations, must raise the doubt of invasive carcinoma.

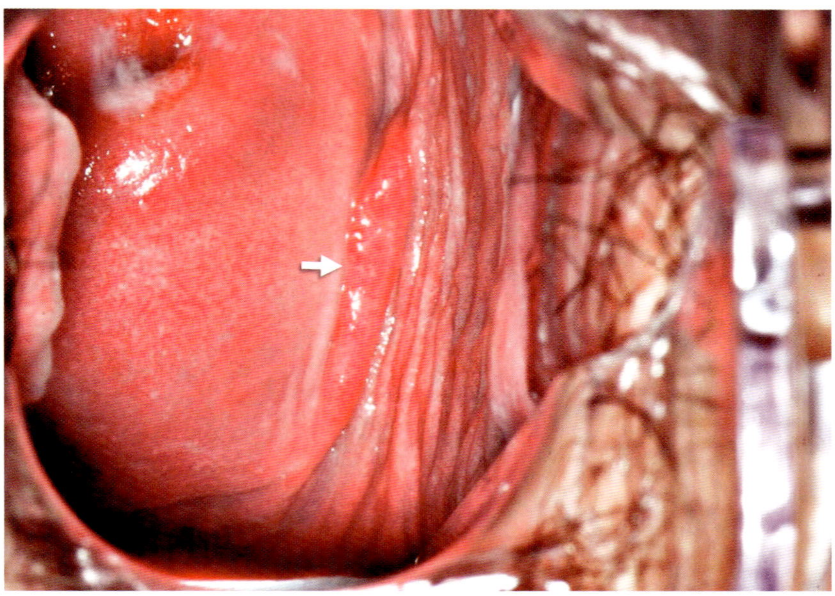

Figure 282 - A congenital tissue brindle (arrow) fixes the cervix to the lateral vaginal wall.

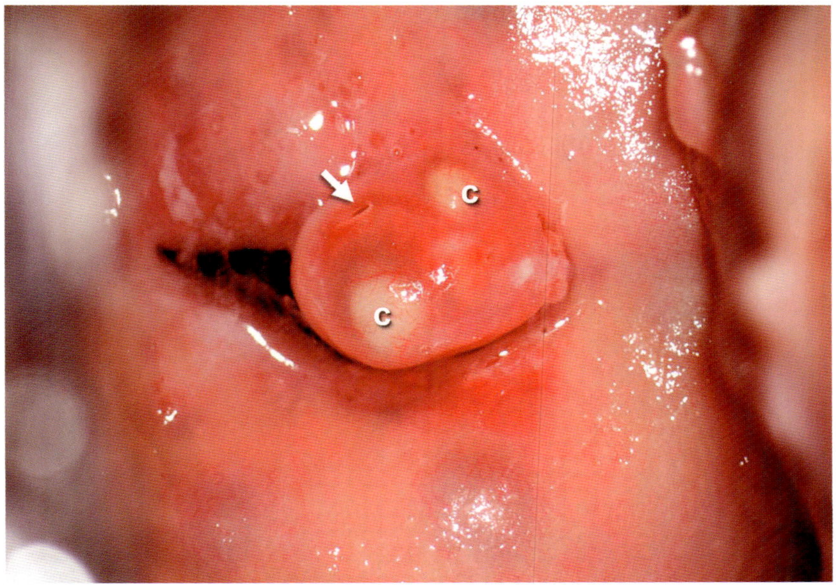

Figure 283 - Localized hypertrophy of the anterior lip of the cervix, showing nabothian cysts (c) and a gland opening (arrow).

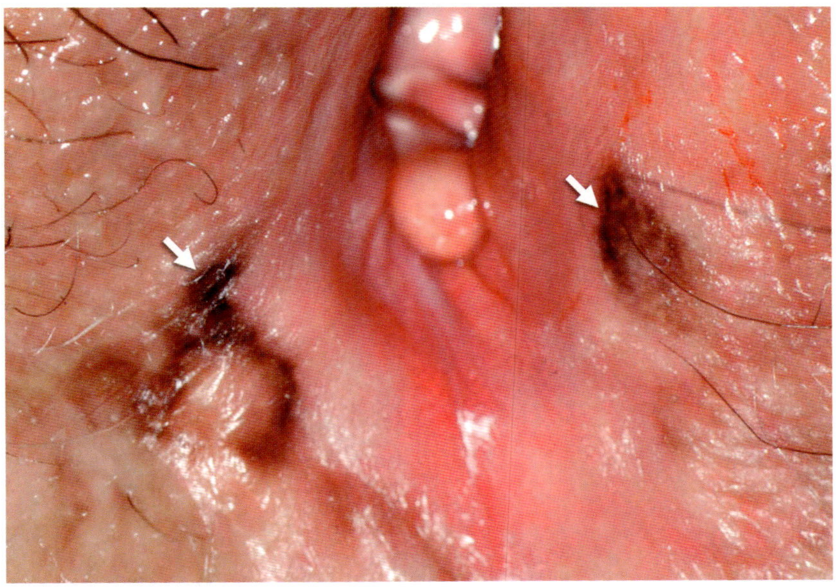

Figure 284 - Agenesis of the labia minora. The pigmented areas (arrows) correspond to the inferior insertion of the missing labia.

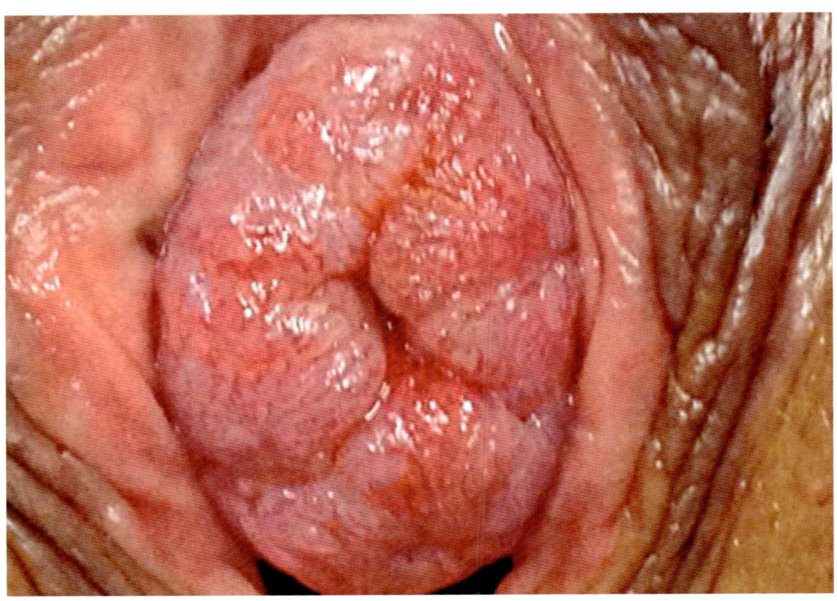

Figure 285 - Urethral florid condyloma in a HIV positive patient.

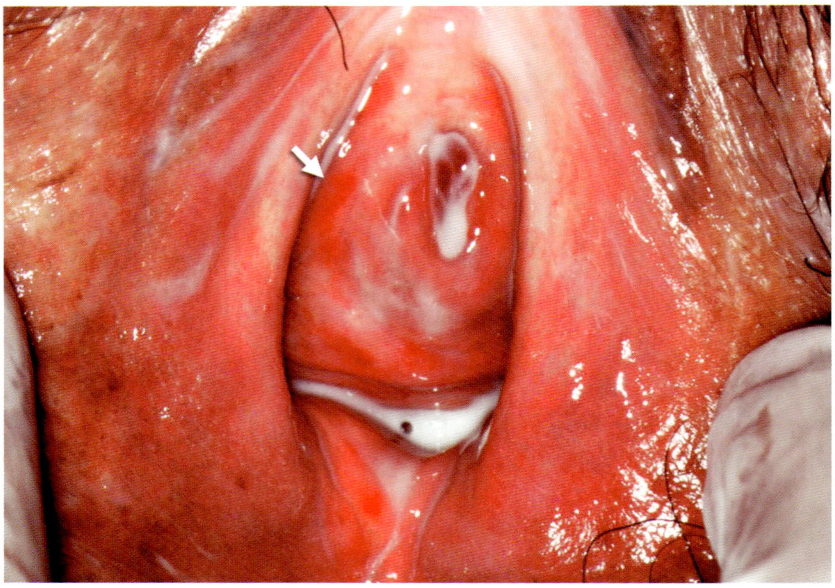

Figure 286 - Paraurethral area shows patches of dilated capillaries (arrow), due to Candida infection which produces a frothy creamy discharge.

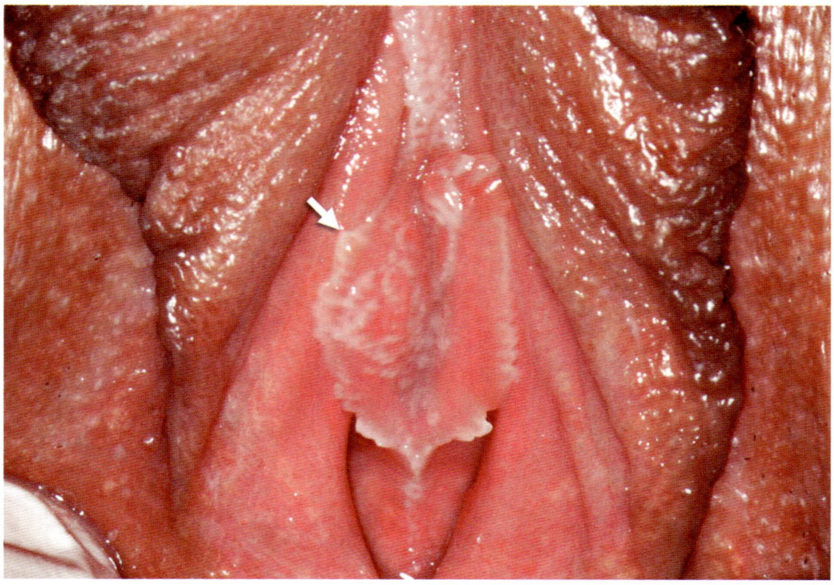

Figure 287 - Periurethral hypertrophic mucosal folds (arrow).

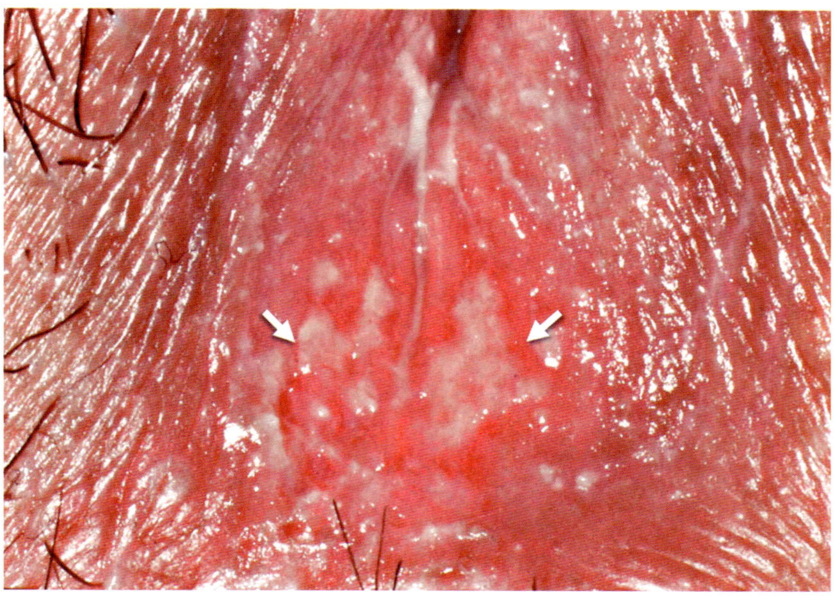

Figure 288 - Genital herpes. The arrows indicate two "kissing" ulcers.

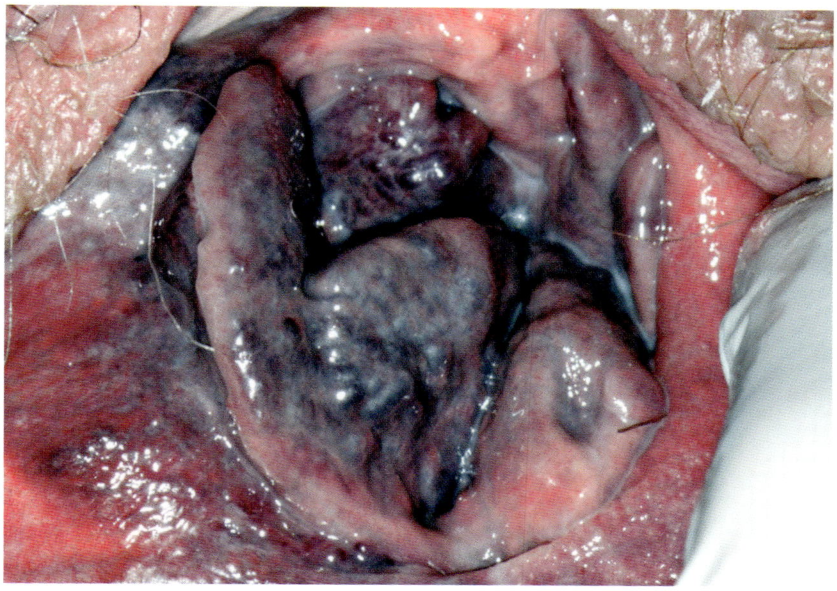

Figure 289 - Vestibular varices at 20th week of gestation.

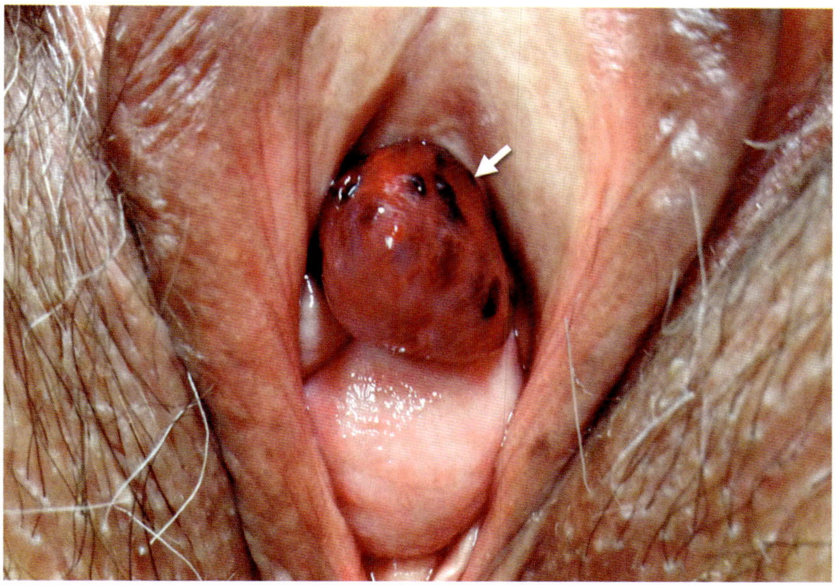

Figure 290 - Urethral polyp (arrow) with dilated and thrombosed capillaries.

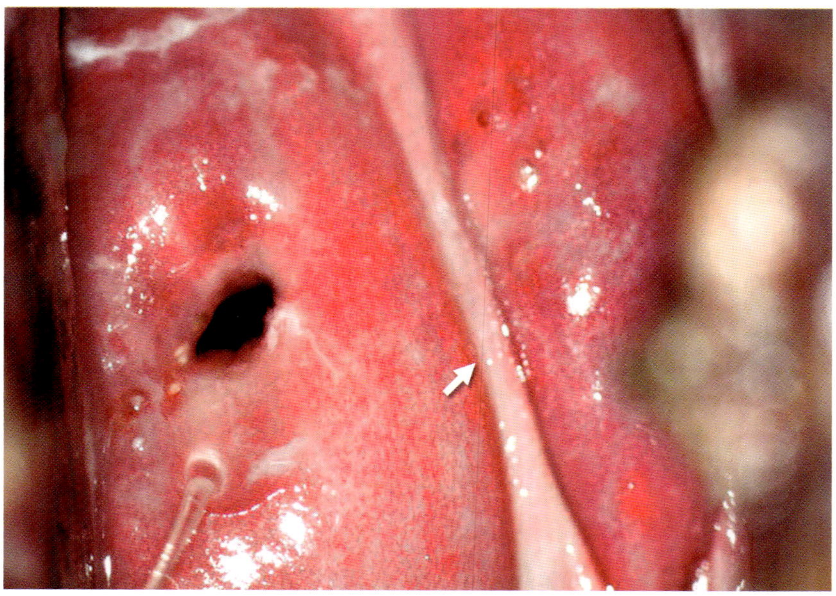

Figure 291 - Uterus bicollis bicornis. A fibrous band (arrow) divides the two cervices.

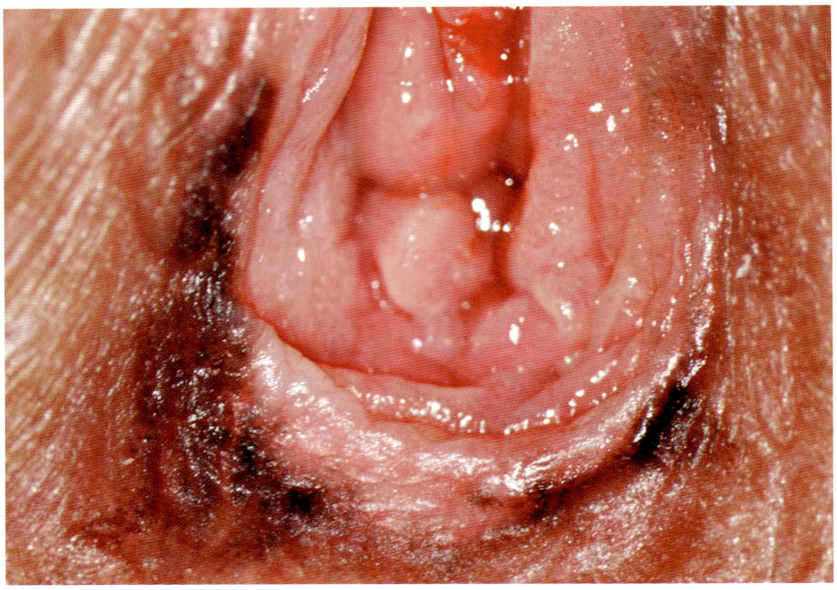

Figure 292 - Agenesis of the labia minora. Pigmented areas at the fourchette.

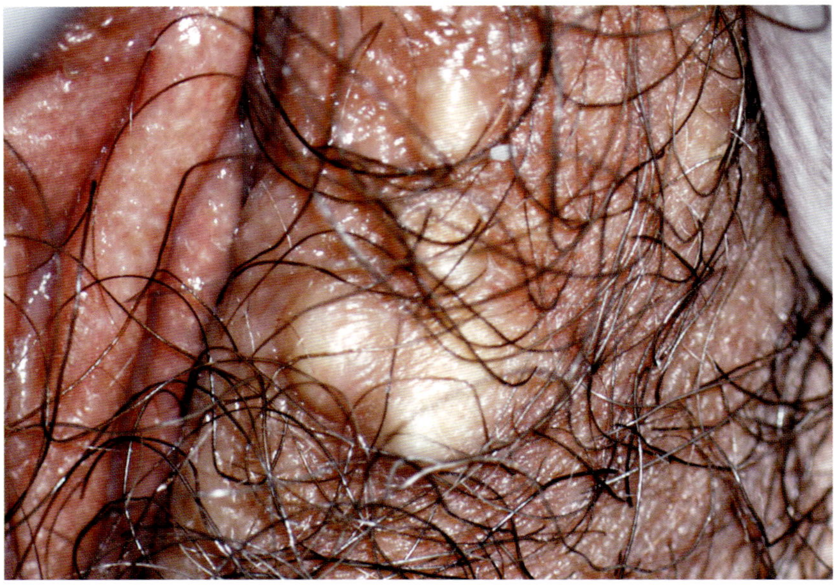

Figure 293 - Vulvar sebaceous cysts.

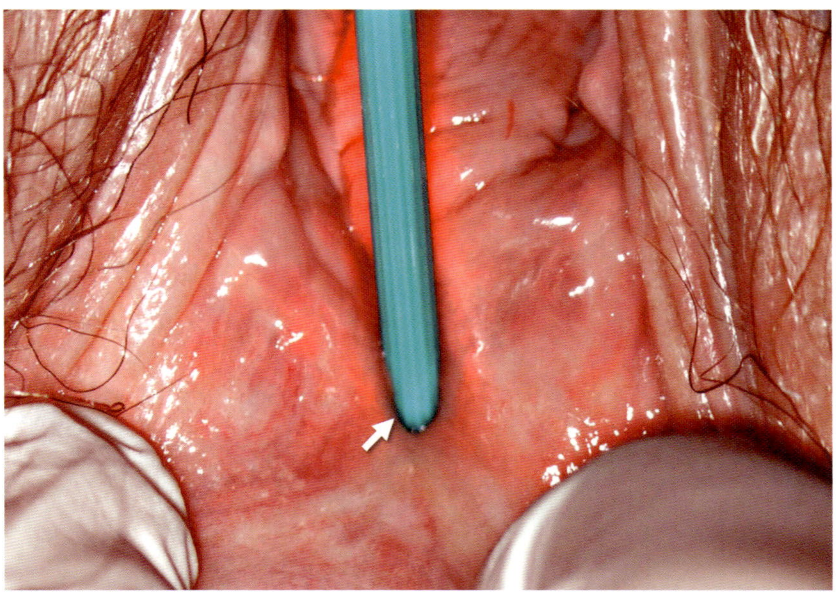

Figure 294 - The extremity of a cytobrush (arrow) passes through the opening of a rectovaginal fistula resulting from Crohn's disease.

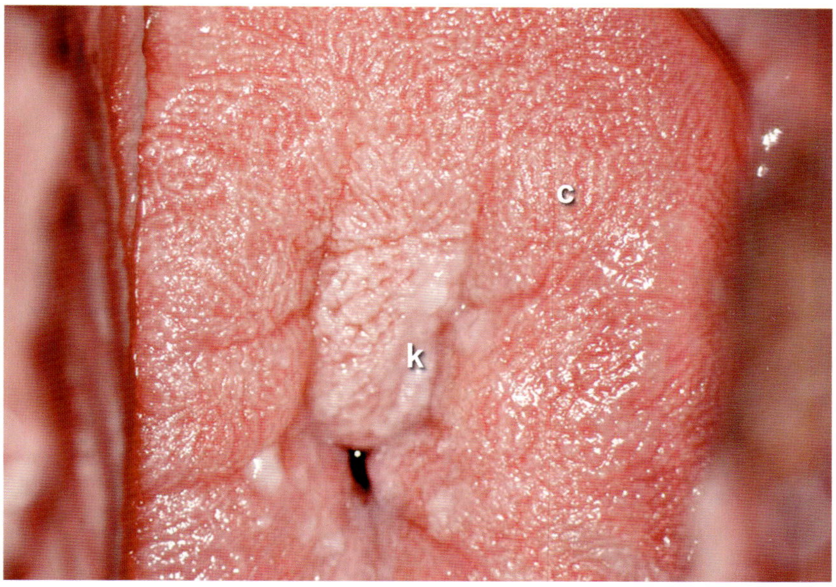

Figure 295 - Extensive scarring after cold-knife conization and Sturmdorf suture for hemostasis, obscure the SCJ, thus making the follow-up more difficult. Keratosis (k) and mucosal crinkling (c).

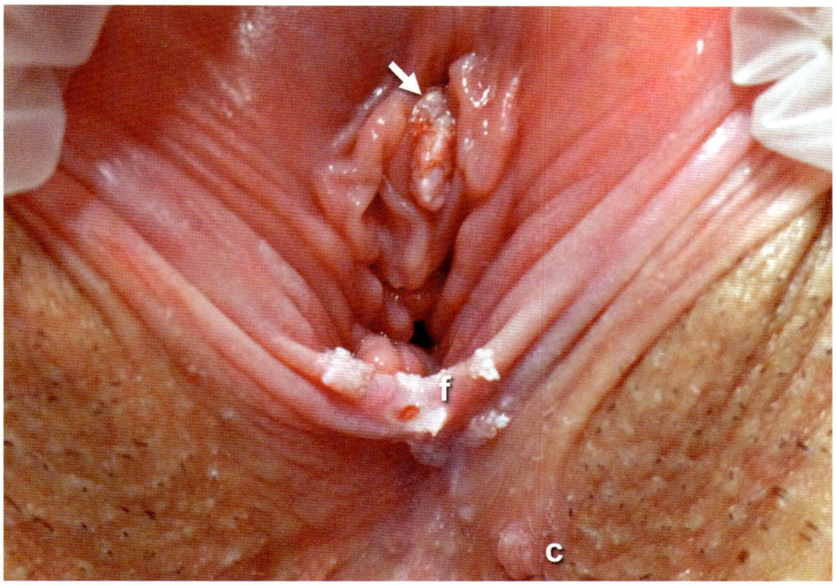

Figure 296 - This colpophotograph exhibits florid condylomas (f) at the fourchette, a flat condyloma (c) at the perineum and HPV micropapillary lesions (arrow) close to the external urethral orifice.

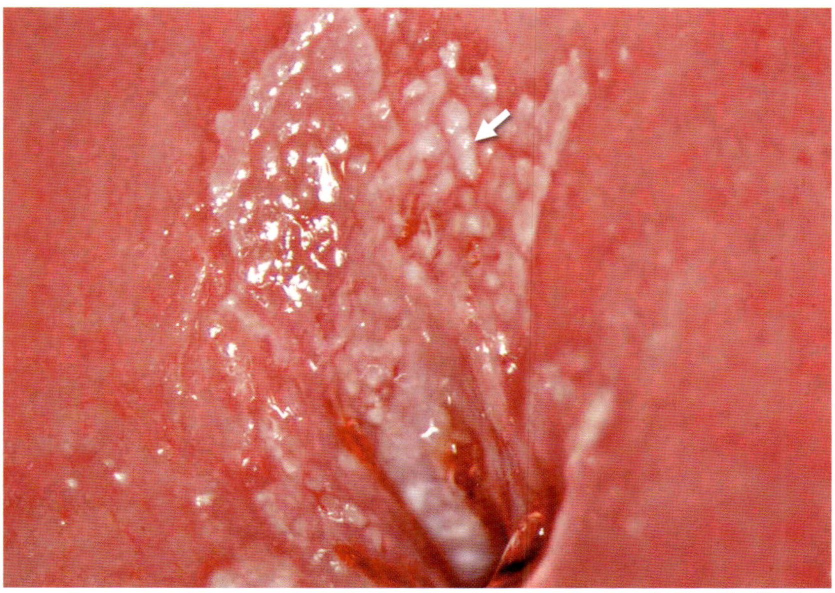

Figure 297 - A coarse mosaic with raised cobbles (arrow) involves the anterior lip of the cervix and enters the cervical canal. Histology confirmed a high-grade HPV lesion.

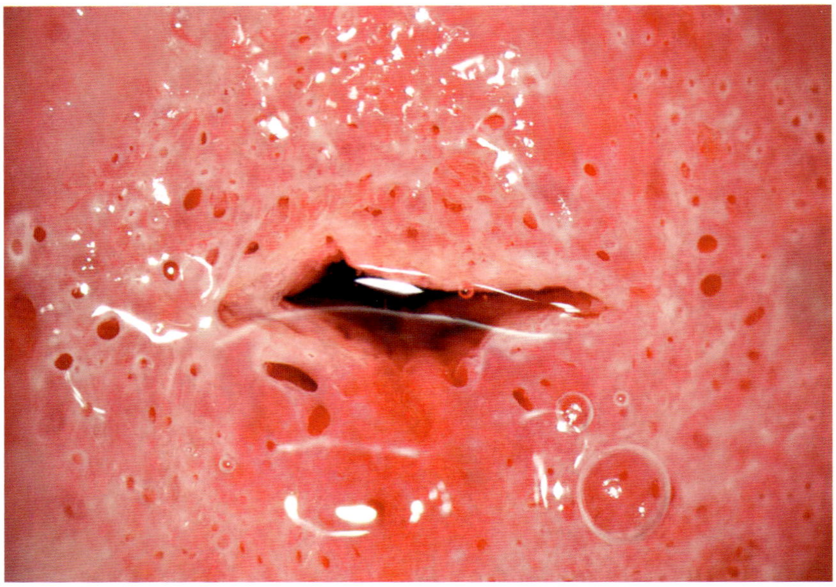

Figure 298 - Maturing metaplastic epithelium showing scattered grade I gland openings.

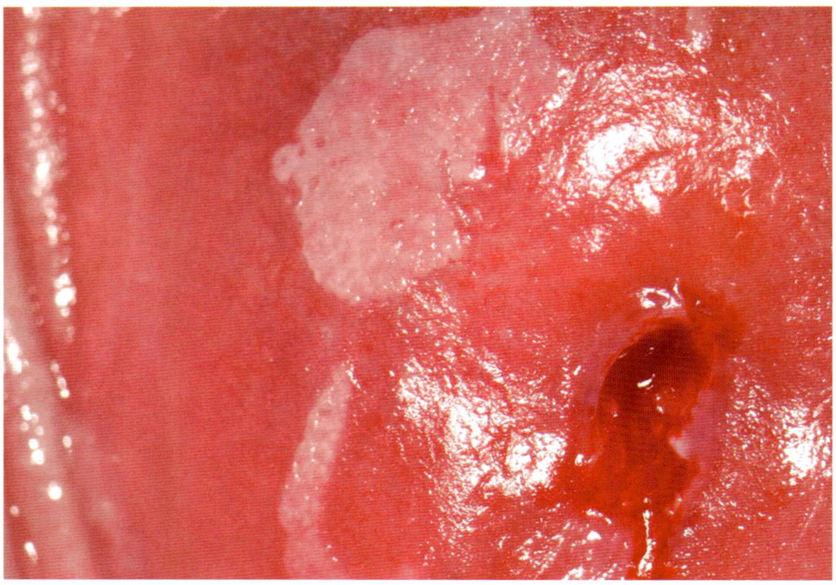

Figure 299 - Well-defined dense acetowhite and slightly raised areas in HPV infection.

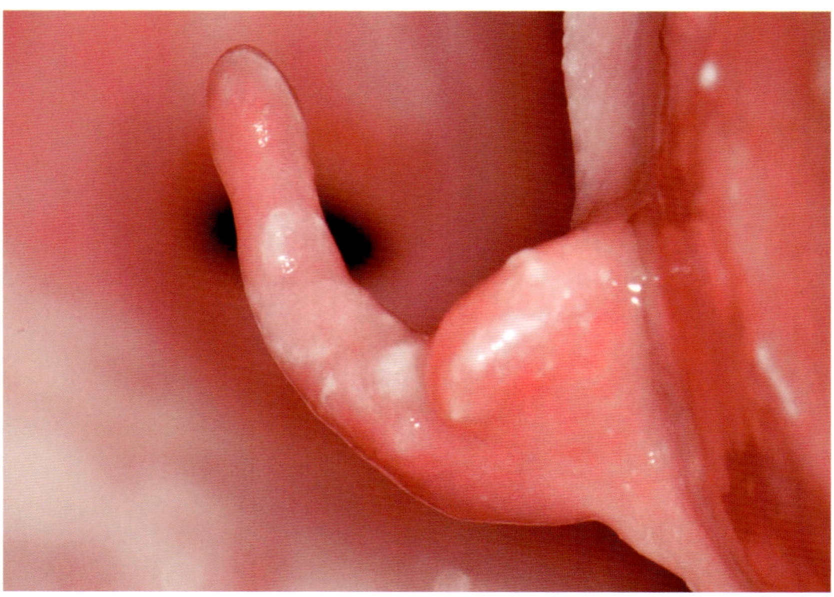

Figure 300 - A finger-shaped fibroid rises from the vaginal wall.

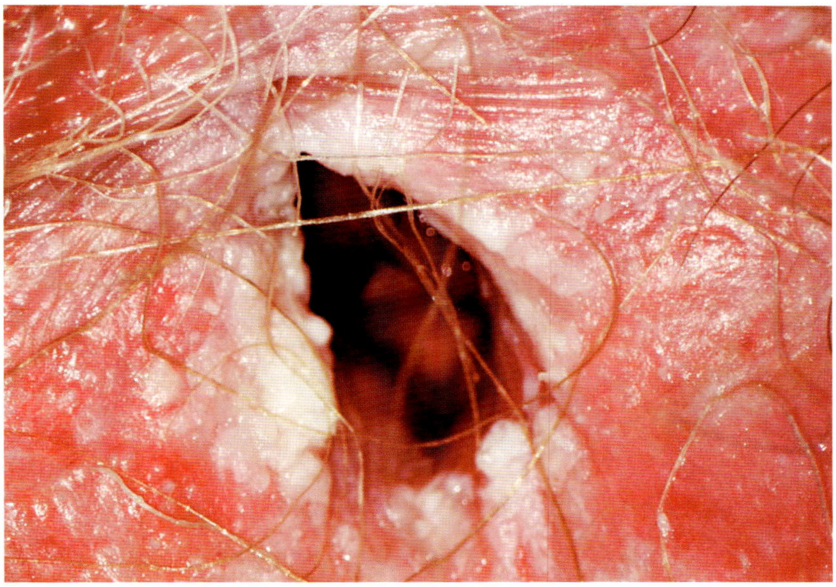

Figure 301 - Severe vulvar atrophy with intraoital constriction.

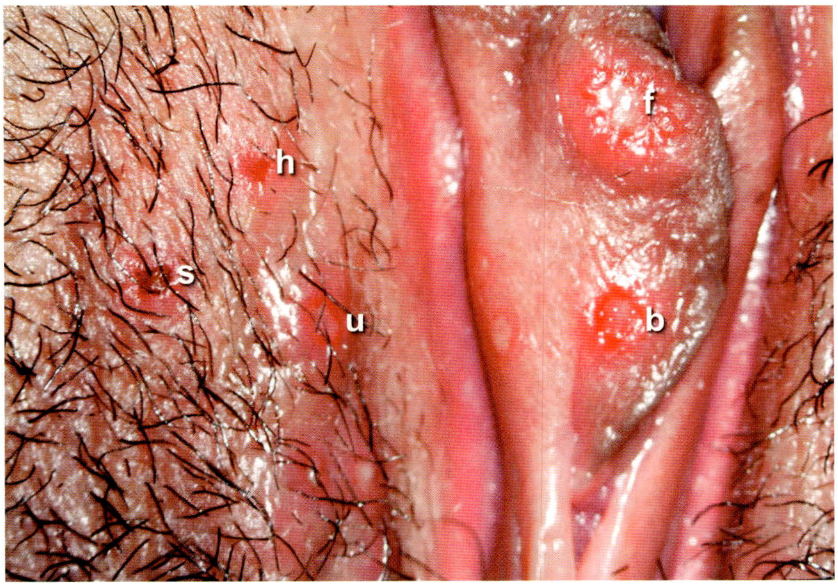

Figure 302 - Vulvar herpetic lesions in different stages of maturation: blister (b), ulcer (u), ulcer covered with fibrin (f), scab (s), healing lesion (h).

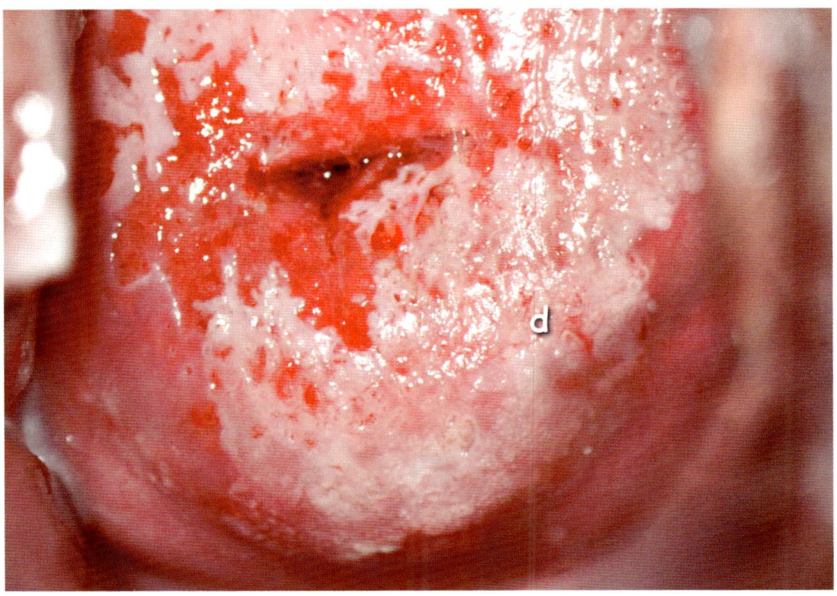

Figure 303 - Dense acetowhite epithelium (d) due to immature metaplastic epithelium.
Despite the colposcopic appearance, no atypia is present.

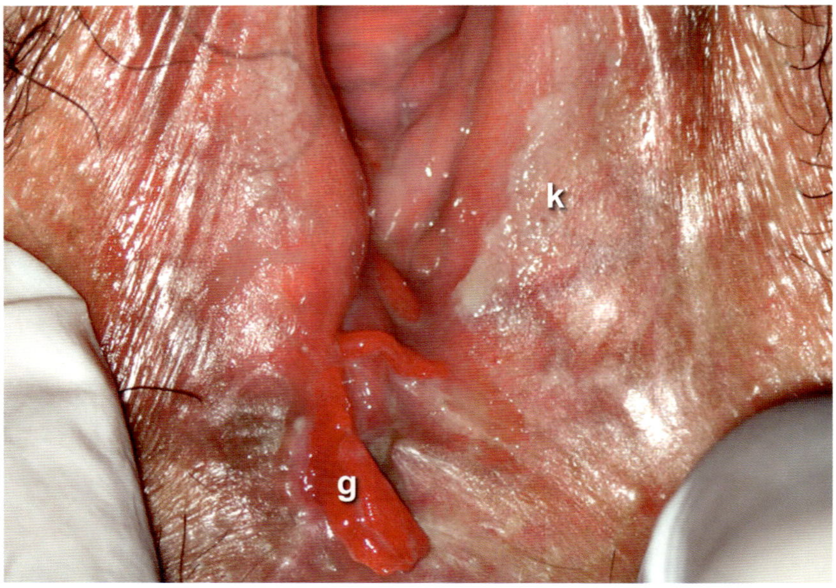

Figure 304 - Polypoid granulation tissue (g) along the suture following episiorrhaphy. The external surface of labia minora and the fourchette are involved by thin keratosis (k).

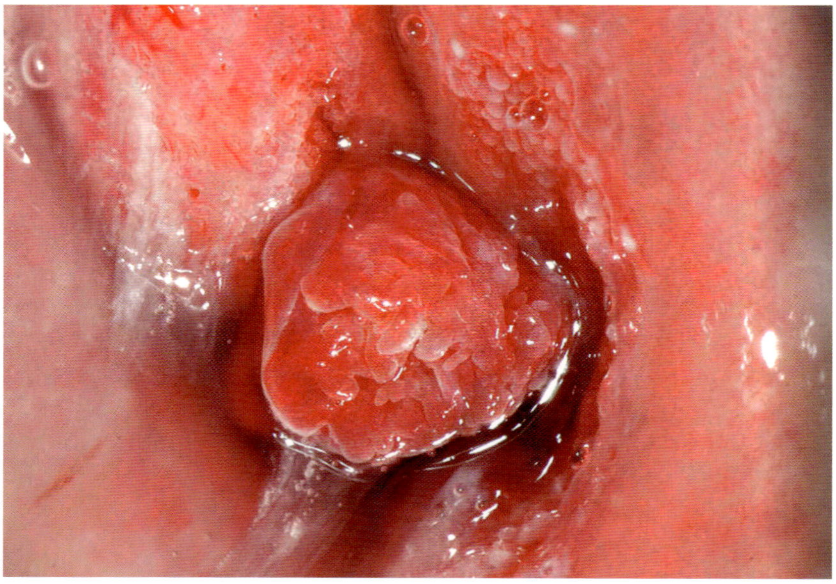

Figure 305 - A pedunculated submucosal fibroid protrudes from the cervical canal.

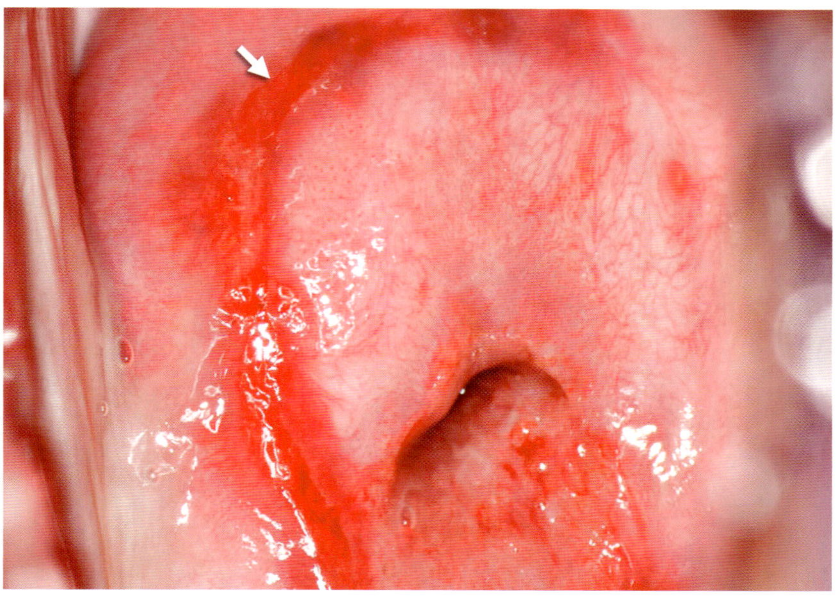

Figure 306 - Semicircular hemorrhagic effusion (arrow), due to a previous diathermy.

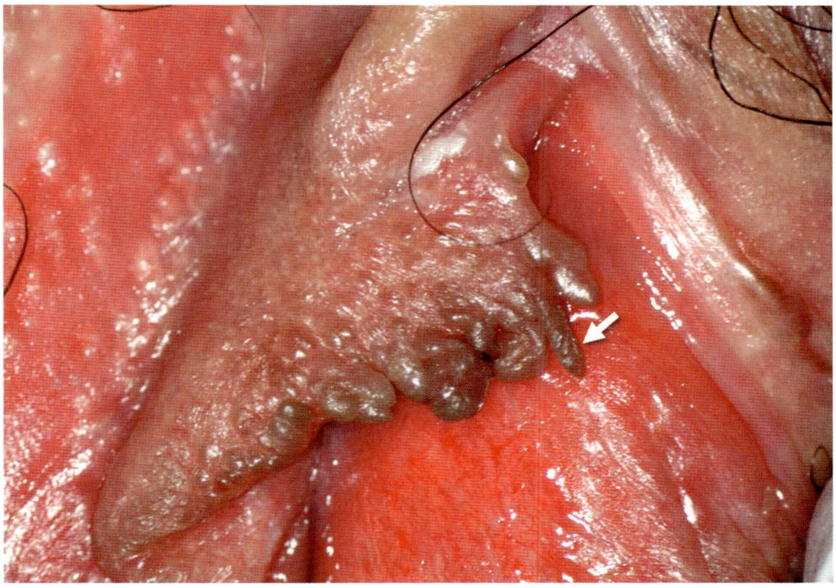

Figure 307 - The margin of the right labium minor appears fimbriated (arrow).

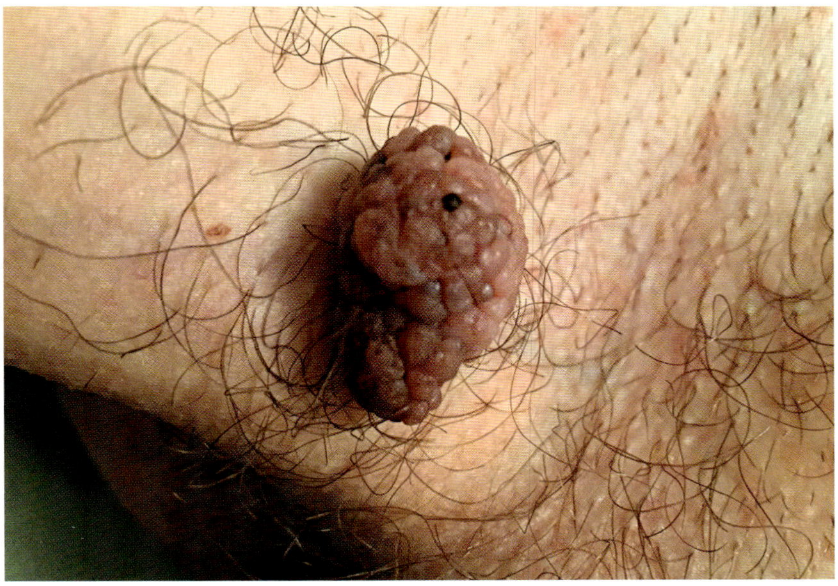

Figure 308 - Crural seborrheic keratosis.

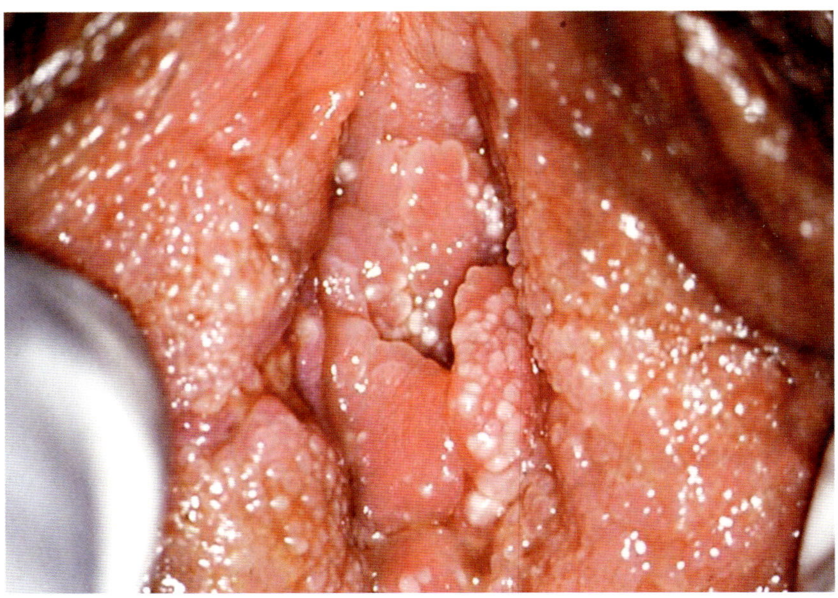

Figure 309 - Scattered vulvar flat condylomas.

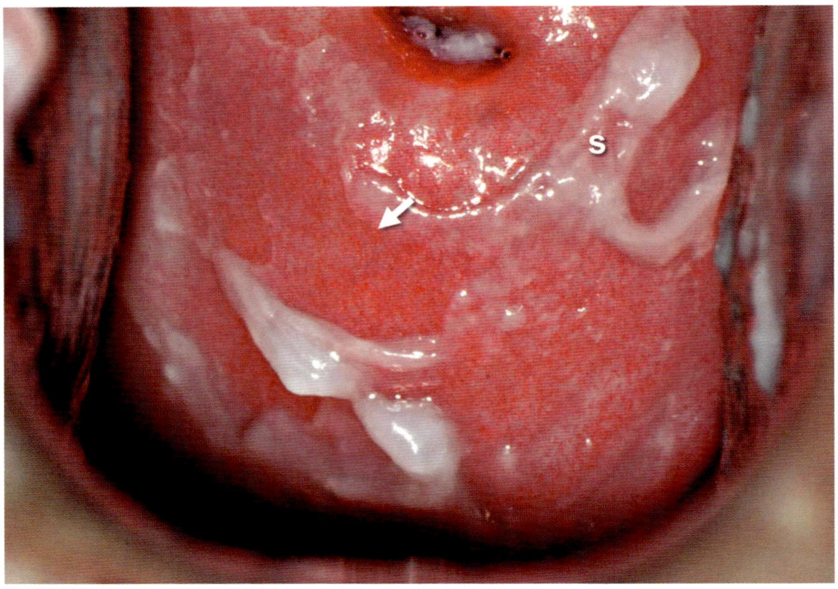

Figure 310 - Epithelial sheet (s), shed from the underlying stroma is responsible for a red area (arrow).

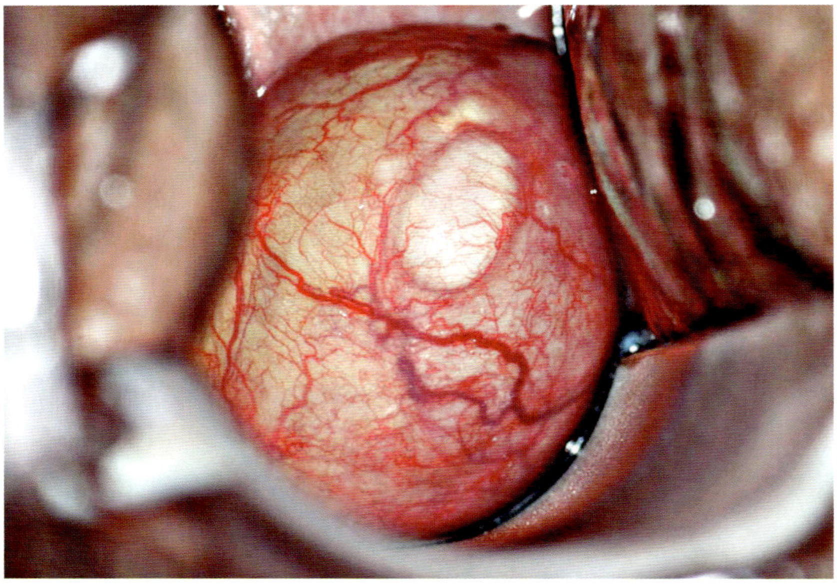

Figure 311 - A voluminous cystic polyp of the endocervical canal protrudes into the vagina.

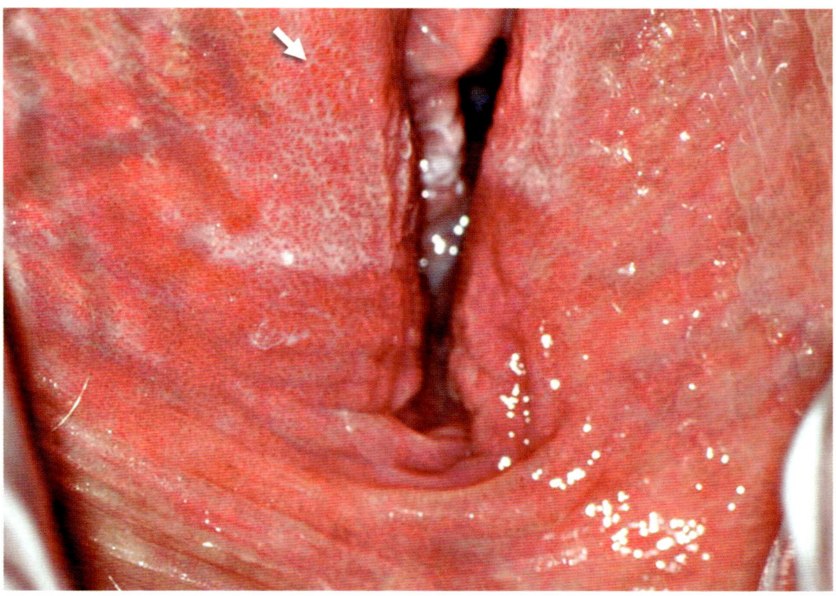

Figure 312 - Acetowhite area with coarse red punctation (arrow). Punch biopsy disclosed a vulvar L-SIL.

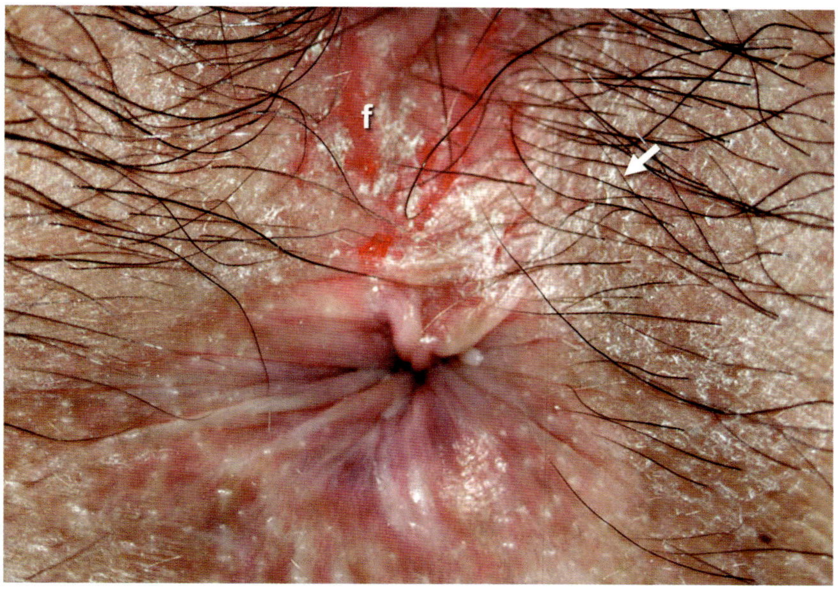

Figure 313 - Vulvar psoriasis. Perineal fissures (f) may resemble fungal infection, but typical silver scaly crusts (arrow) can provide helpful diagnostic hints.

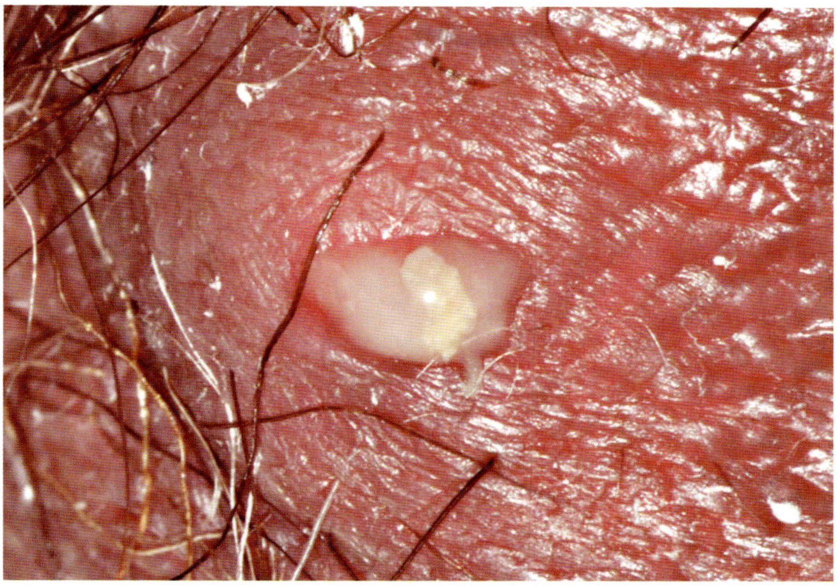

Figure 314 - A spontaneous opening in the weakest part of the wall of the vulvar abscess allows the pus to drain through it.

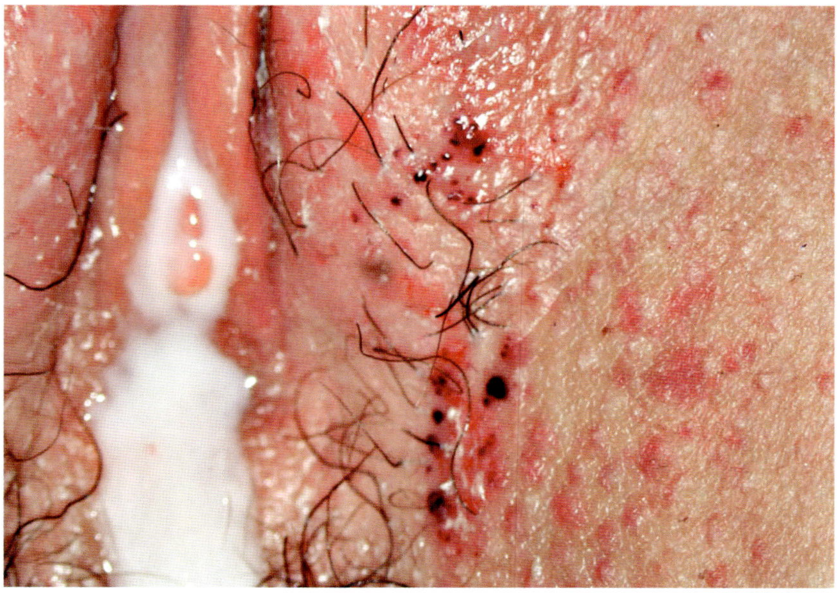

Figure 315 - Cutaneous lesions following waxing for hair removal.

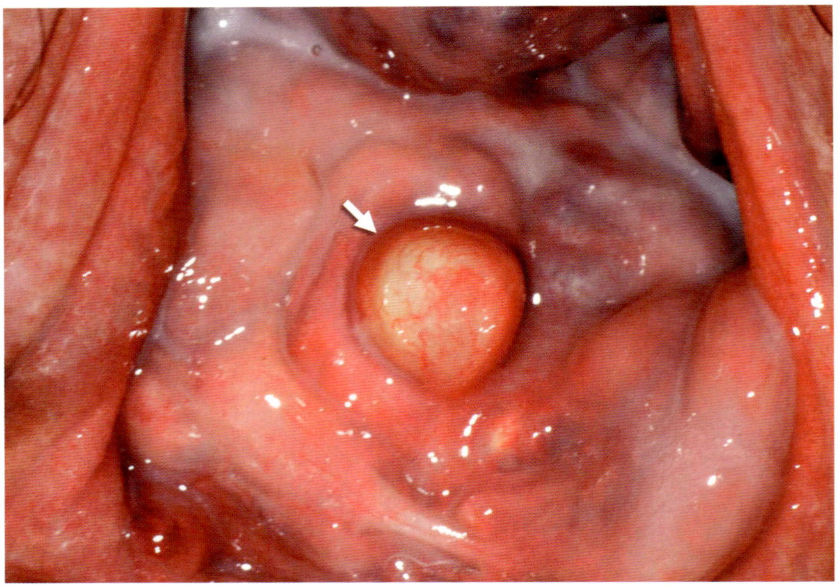

Figure 316 - Cyst (arrow) at the vulvar fourchette.

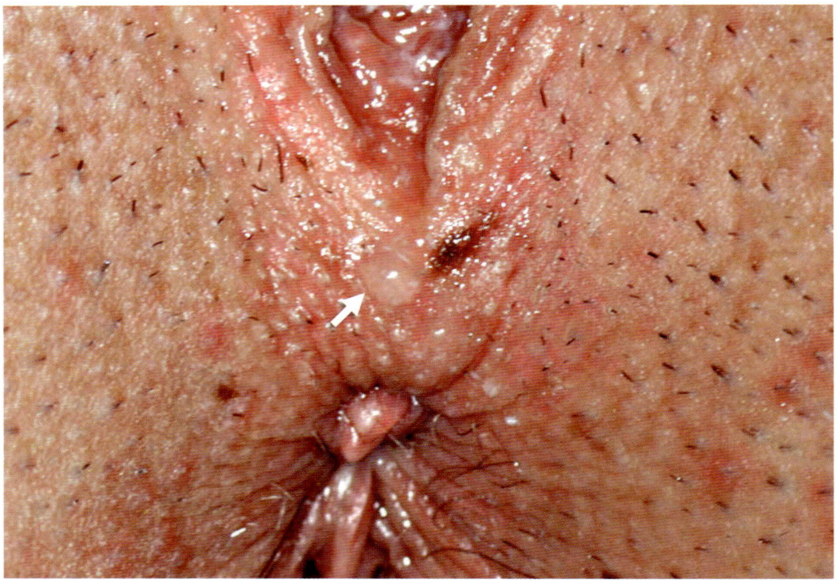

Figure 317 - Single perineal herpetic blister (arrow).

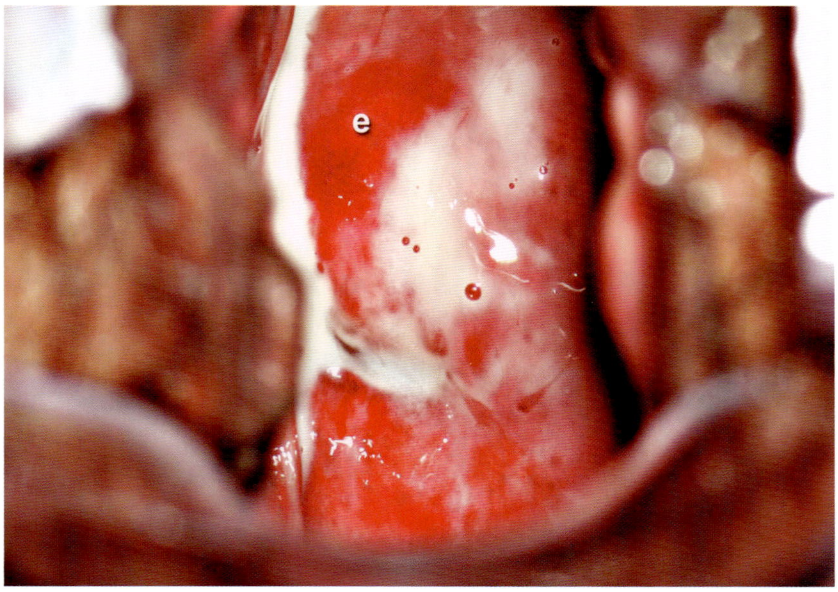

Figure 318 - Exposed columnar epithelium (e) is associated with a white frothy discharge (bacterial vaginosis).

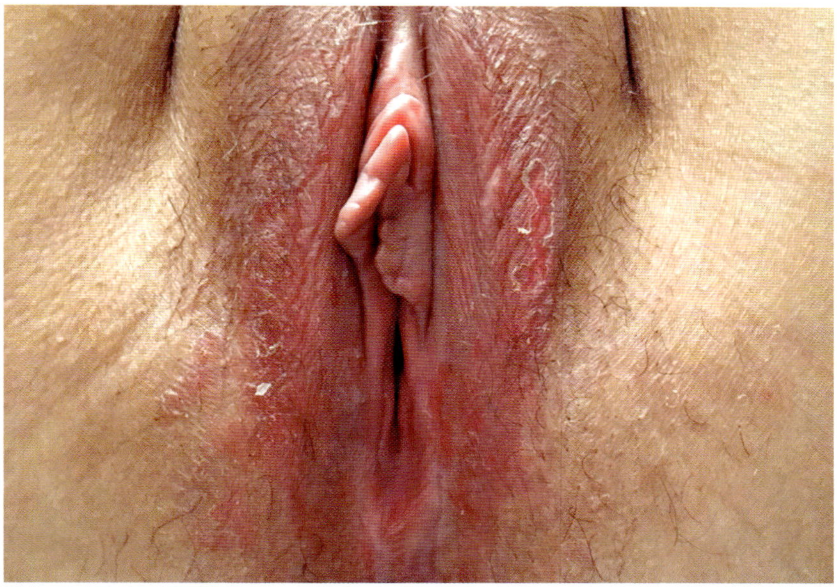

Figure 319 - Vulvar psoriasis.

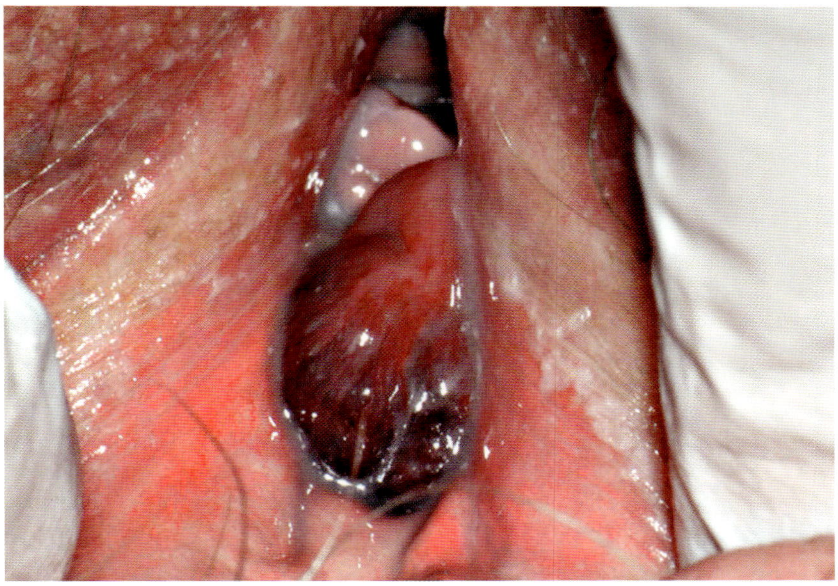

Figure 320 - Congested polyp at the vaginal introitus.

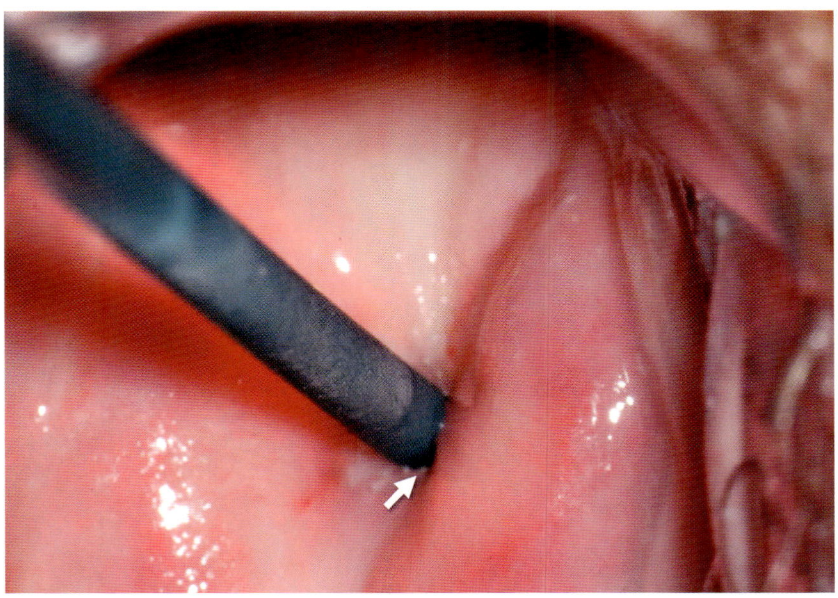

Figure 321 - The extremity of the cytobrush passes through a small hole of the vaginal wall (arrow). Computed tomography urogram with and without iv contrast, revealed a coarse left paraureteral tubular formation, 35 cm long, originating from the parenchyma of the upper pole of the left kidney and opening into the vagina.

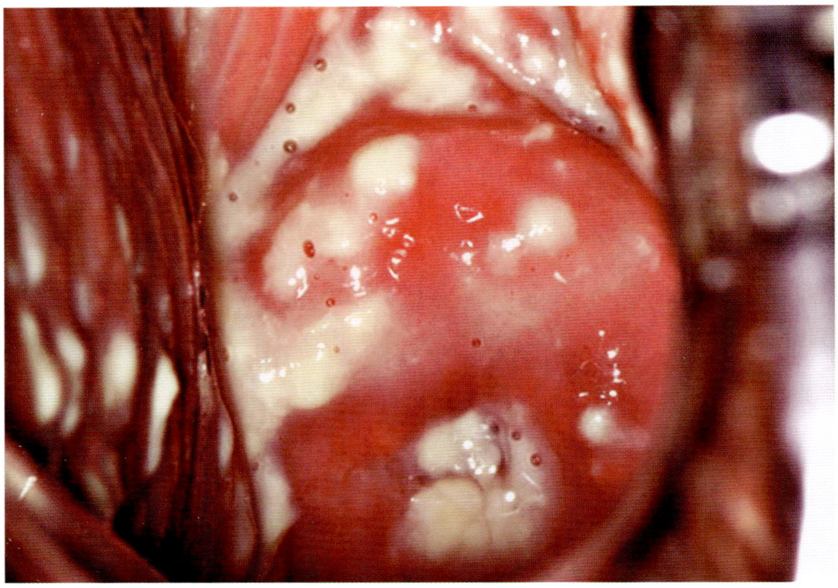

Figure 322 - Creamy and frothy discharge produced by Candida infection and bacterial vaginosis.

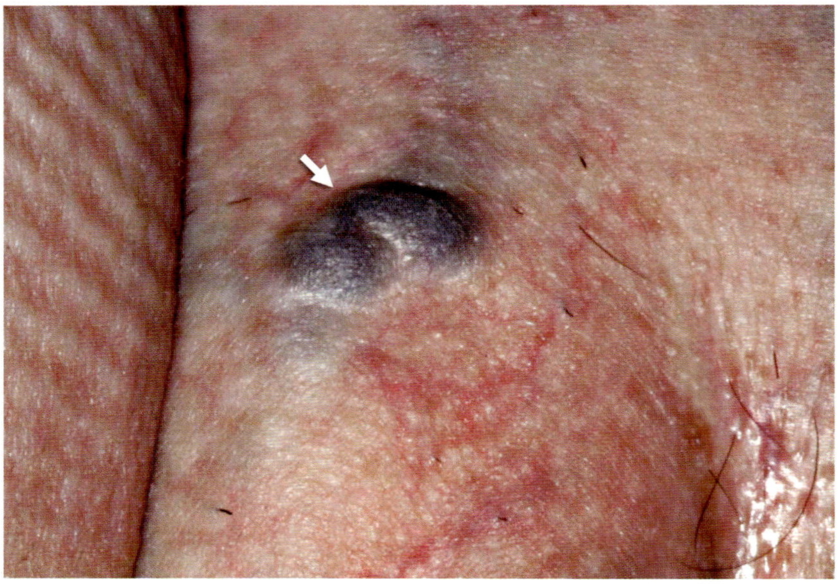

Figure 323 - Pubic varices (arrow).

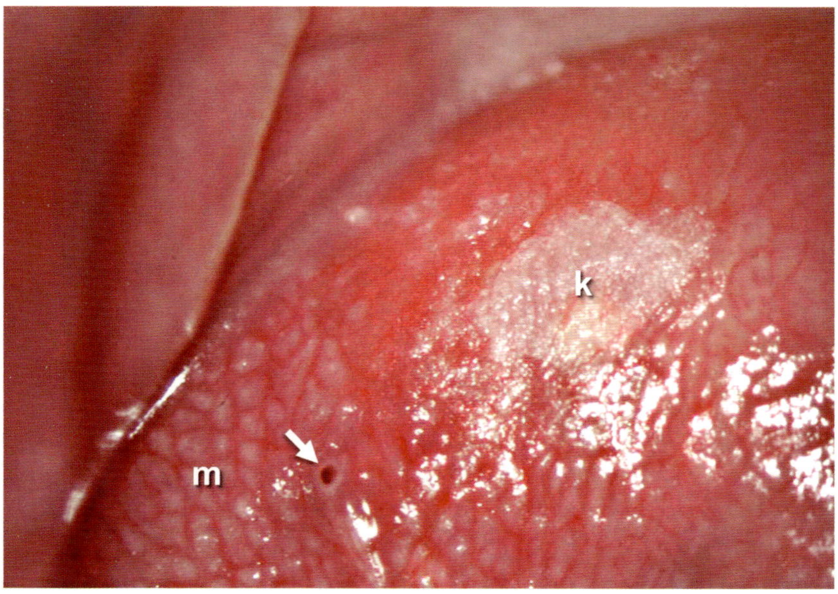

Figure 324 - The colpophotograph shows thick keratosis (k), a mosaic pattern (m) and a grade II gland opening (arrow).

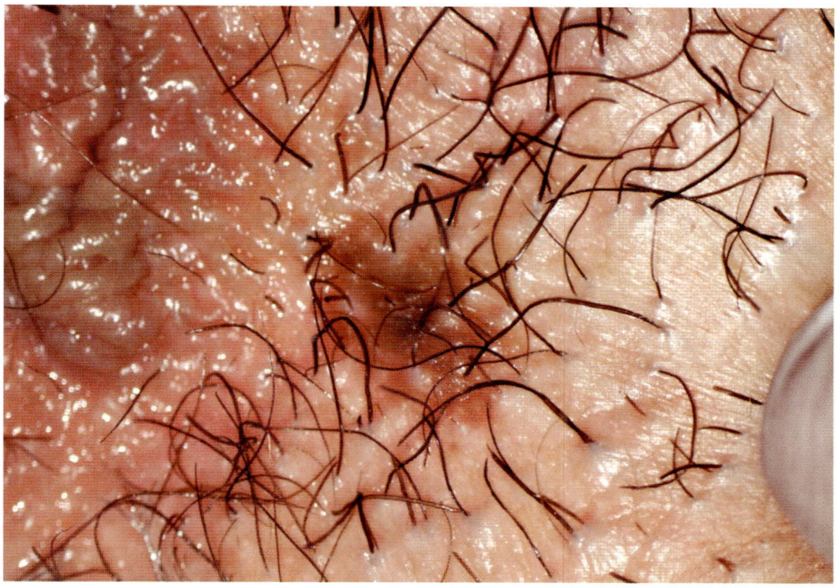

Figure 325 - Vulvar supernumerary nipple. Note an areola around the nipple area, but instead of breast tissue underneath, fat tissue is found (category 5, known as pseudo mamma).

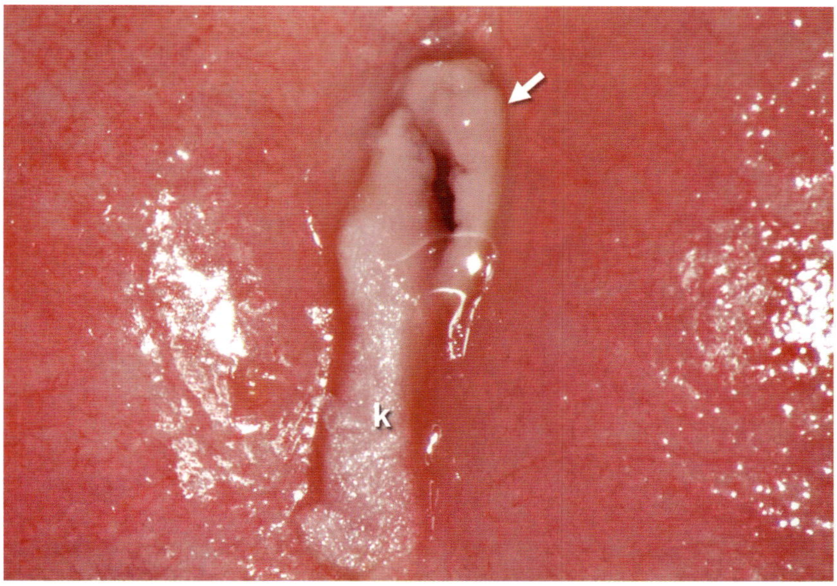

Figure 326 - A thick rim of acetowhite epithelium (arrow) surrounds the squamocolumnar junction and gradually passes into a ridge of thick keratosis (k). Excision biopsy of the acetowhite area confirmed a high-grade HPV-CIN lesion.

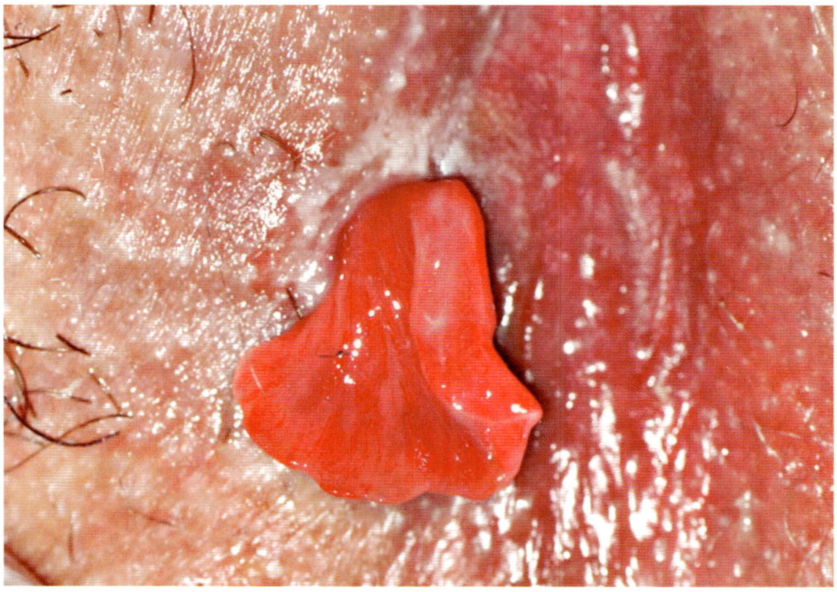

Figure 327 - Polypoid granulation tissue comes out of a scarred episiorrhaphy.

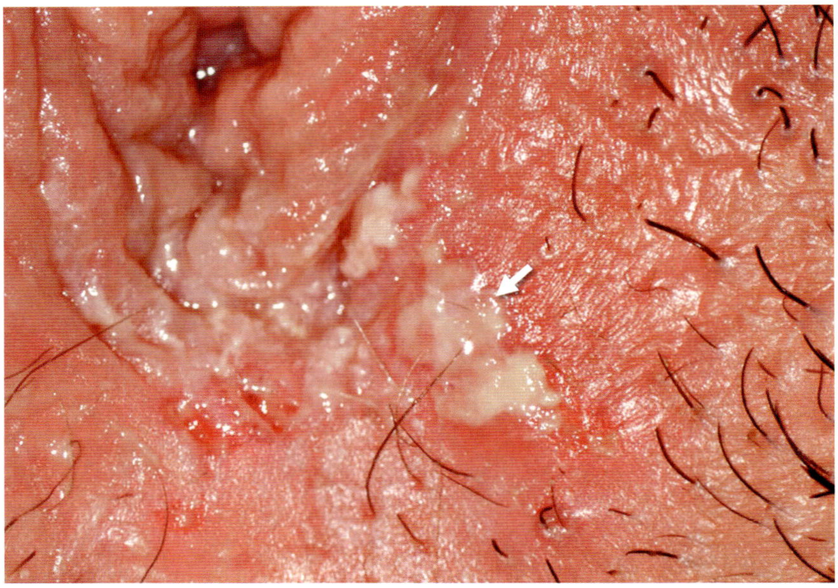

Figure 328 - Herpetic ulcers are covered with fibrin (arrow).

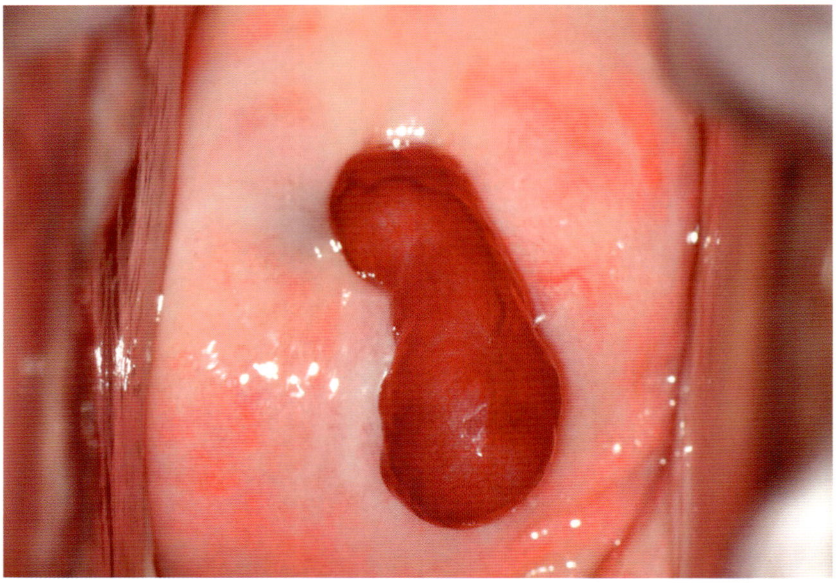

Figure 329 - A congested polyp protrudes out of the cervical canal.

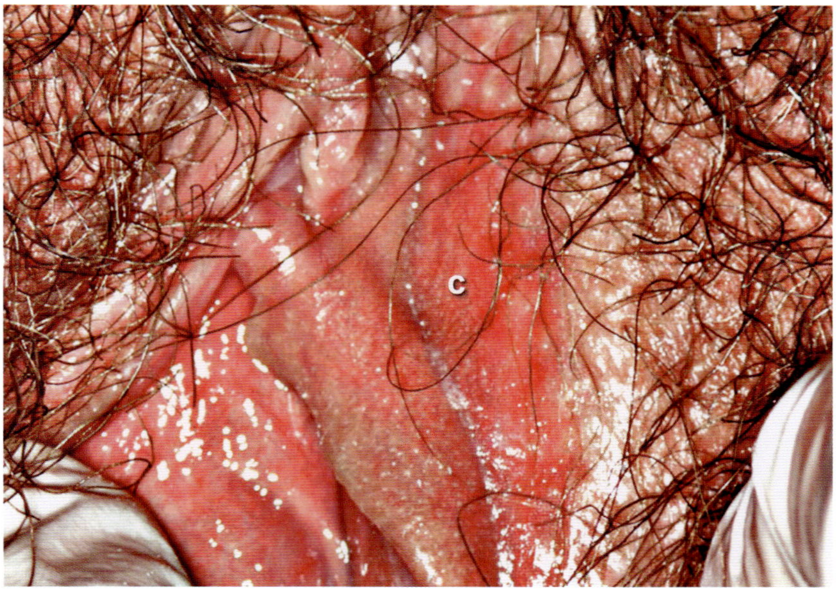

Figure 330 - Cellulitis of the left labium majus (c) appears as a red, swollen area that feels hot and tender to the touch. The borders of inflammation are much less defined than in abnormalities as the stroma is more affected than epithelium.

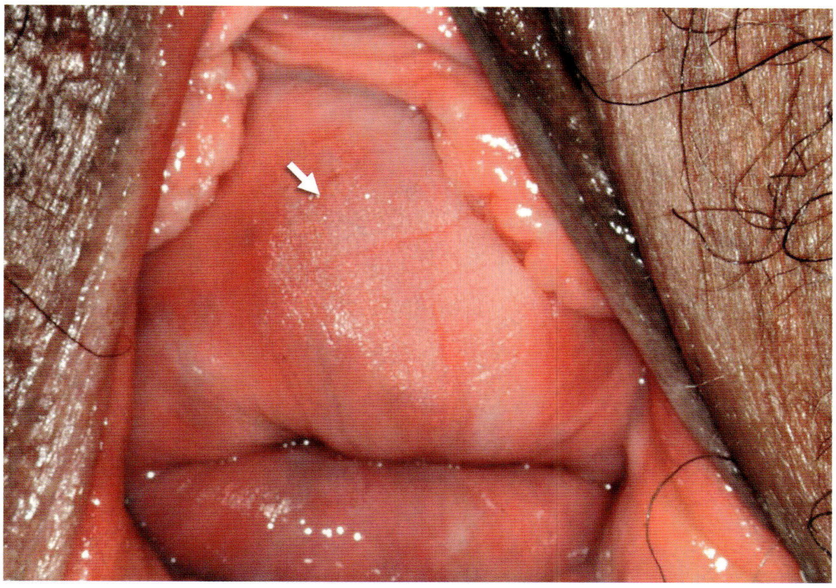

Figure 331 - Epidermization (arrow) of the prolapsed cervix. Due to constant scratching and rubbing, the nonkeratinized cervical squamous epithelium becomes wrinkled and skin-like, characterized by acanthosis and hyperkeratosis.

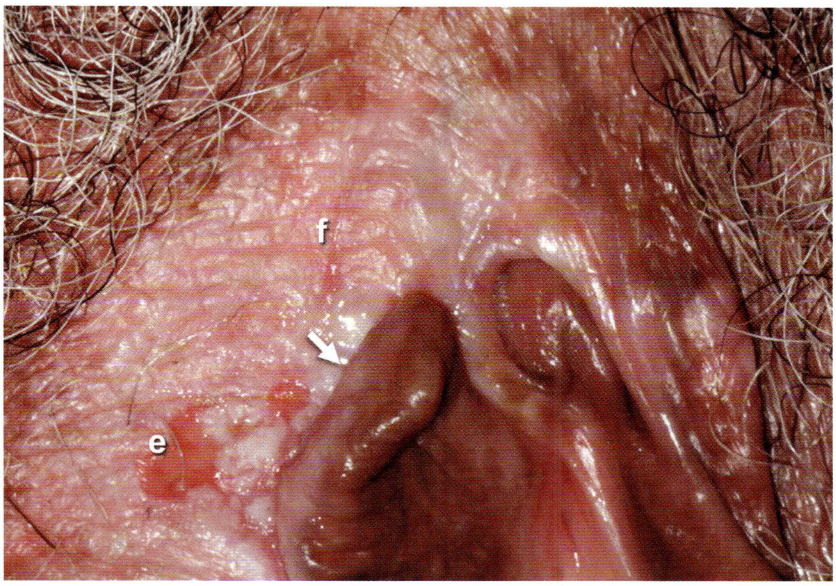

Figure 332 - Lichen sclerosus. Erosions (e) and a fissure (f) are scattered in a plaque of sclerosis and hyperkeratosis. The arrow indicates the site of labial fusion.

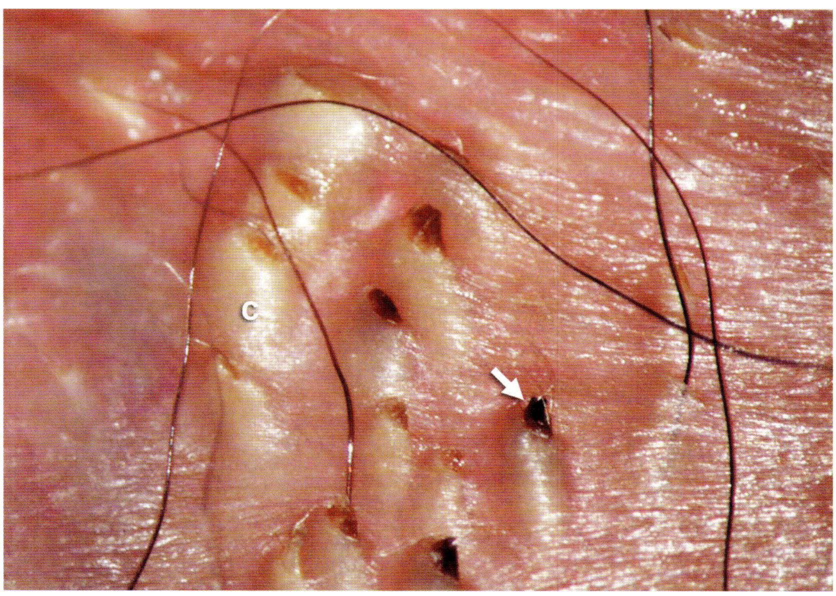

Figure 333 - Perianal sebaceous cysts (c). Hardened sebum can form quills (arrow).

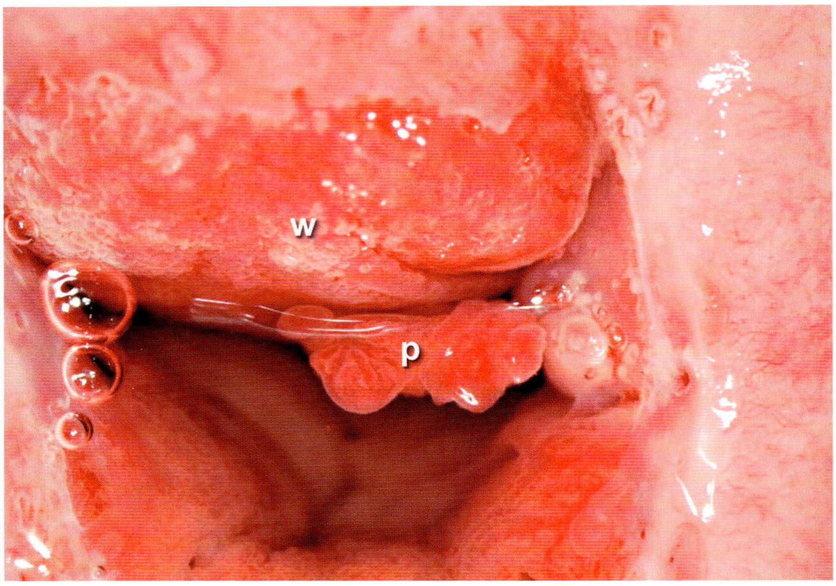

Figure 334 - Endocervical polyp (p) and faint whitening (w) of villi for the development of an immature metaplastic epithelium.

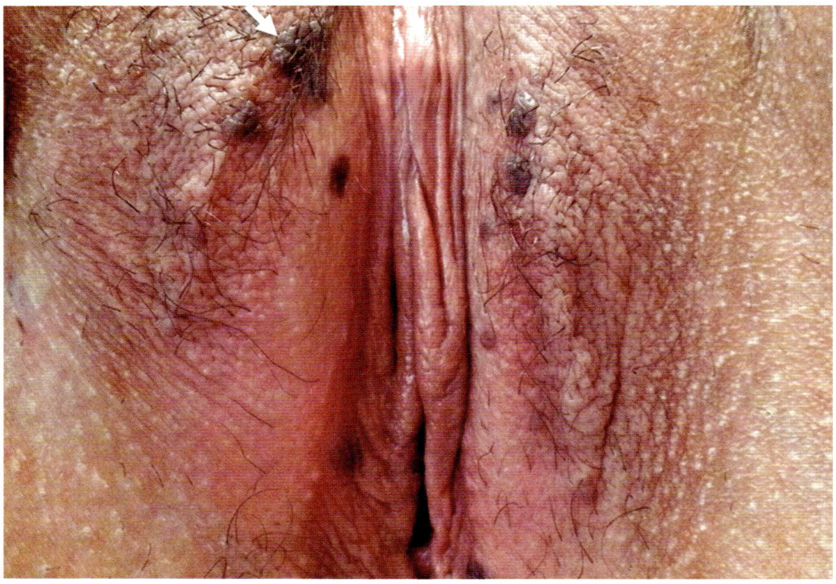

Figure 335 - Multicentric, pigmented verrucous papules (arrow) on labia majora. Excision biopsy and the resultant histology disclosed VIN usual type, warty subtype.

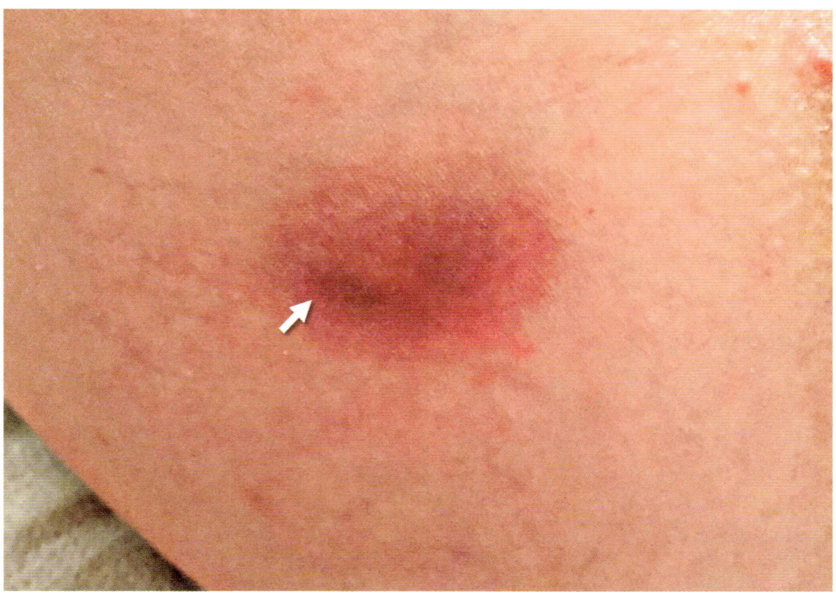

Figure 336 - A painful firm subcutaneous nodule (arrow), surrounded by a purple effusion with faded margins, involves the right crural region. The lesion was associated with cyclical pain during menses. Biopsy revealed an unusual cutaneous endometriosis.

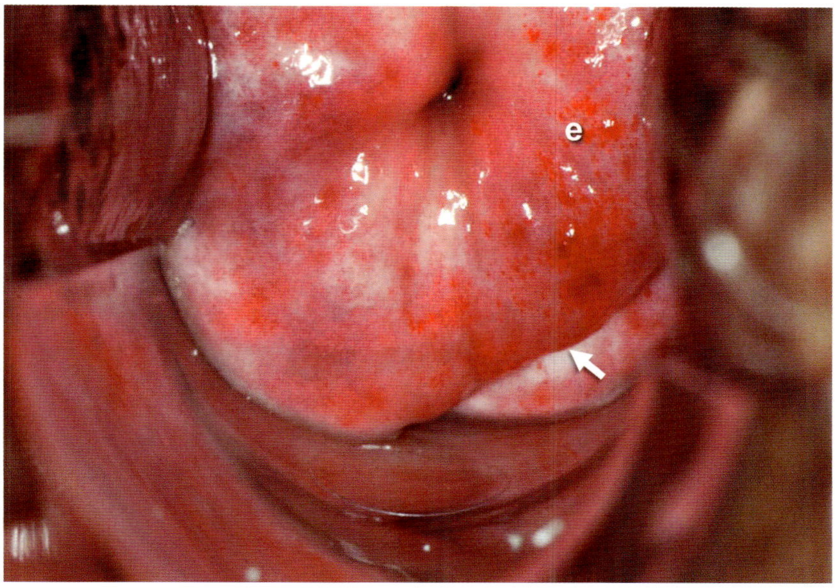

Figure 337 - The dystrophic cervix exhibits capillary effusions (e). The arrowed deep sulcus is the outcome of a previous cervical cerclage.

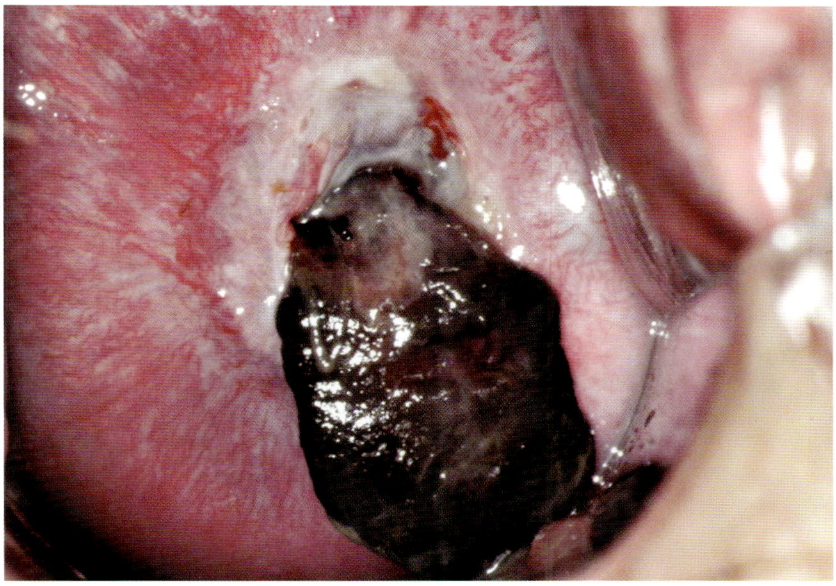

Figure 338 - Infarcted cervical polyp.

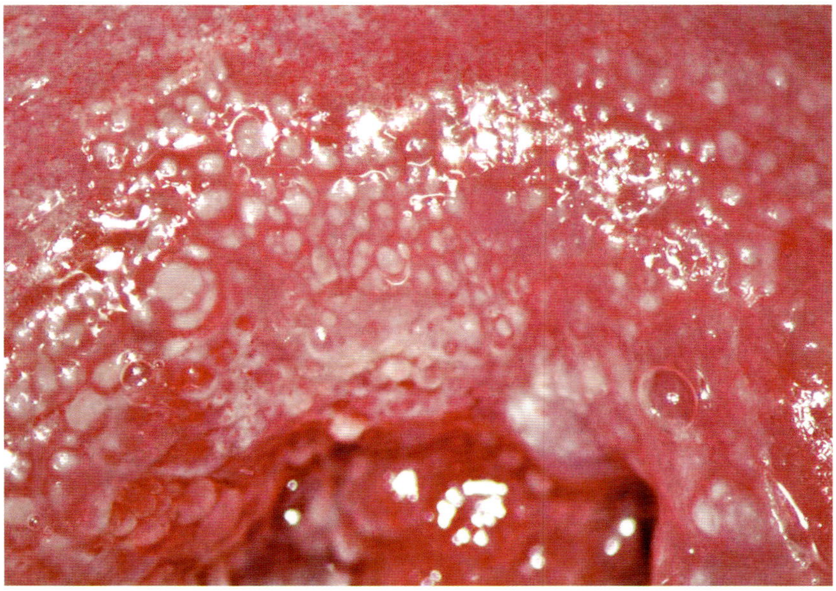

Figure 339 - Coarse mosaic. Histology disclosed a CIN 3 lesion.

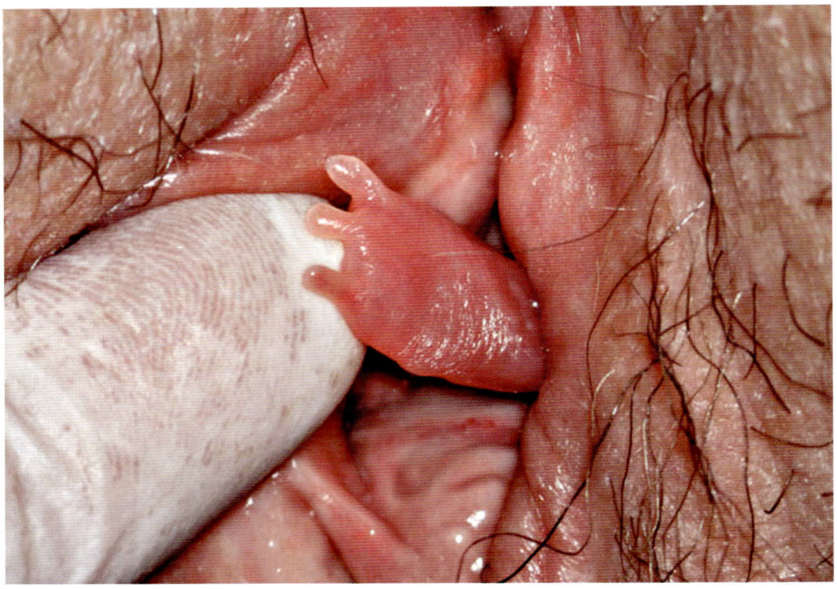

Figure 340 - Hand-shaped hypertrophic hymenal caruncle.

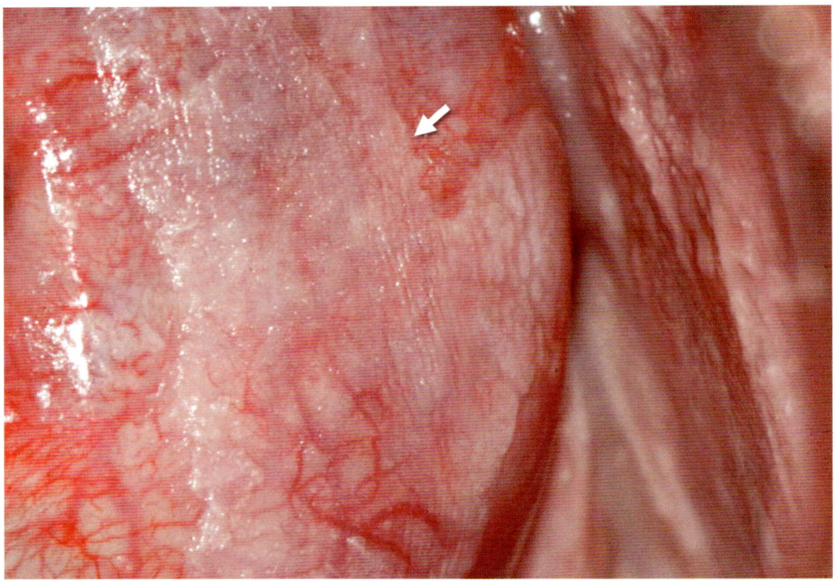

Figure 341 - Extensive sheet of thin keratosis (arrow).

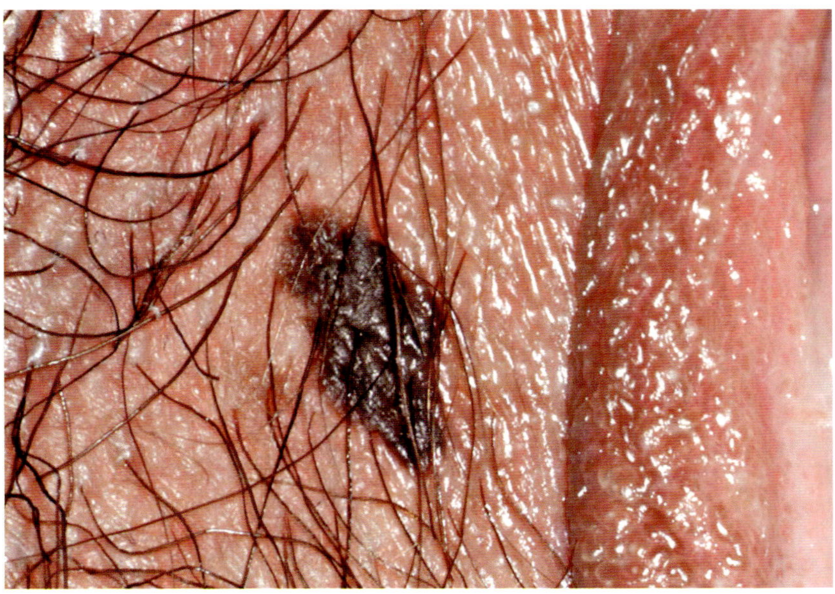

Figure 342 - Vulvar melanocytic nevus.

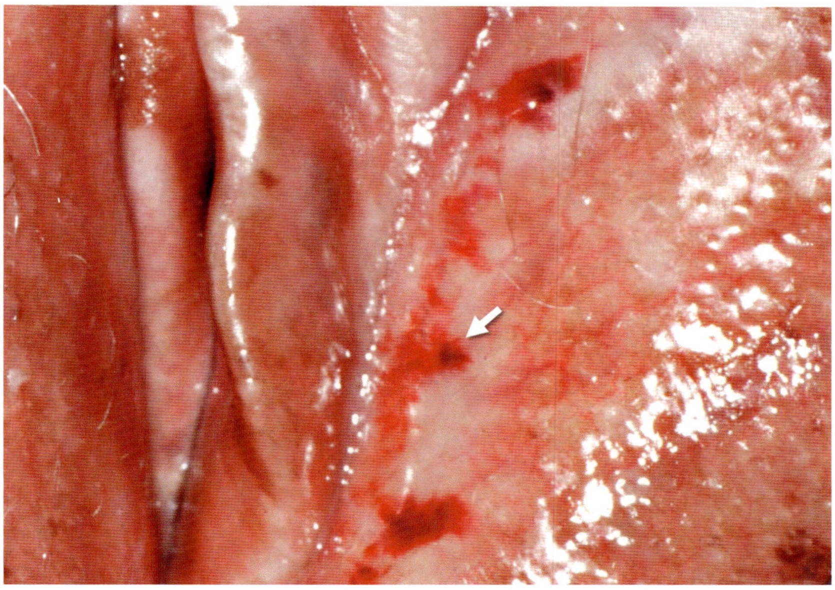

Figure 343 - Vulvar dystrophic hemorrhagic effusions (arrow).

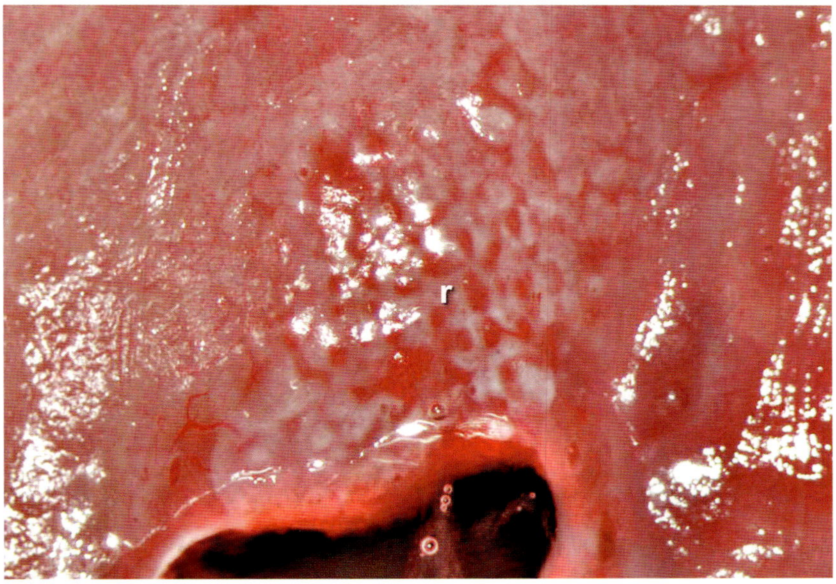

Figure 344 - Reverse mosaic (r).

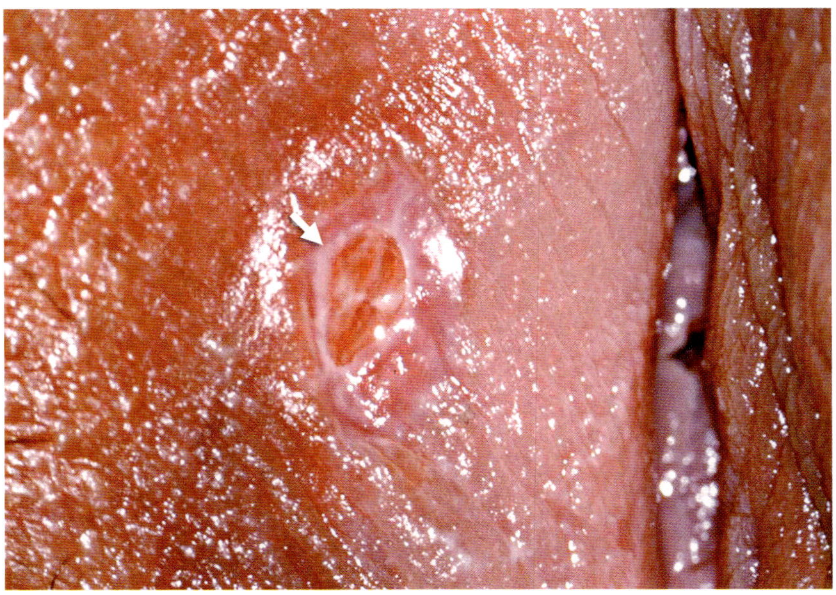

Figure 345 - Hard ulcer (arrow) with an eroded center (chancre).

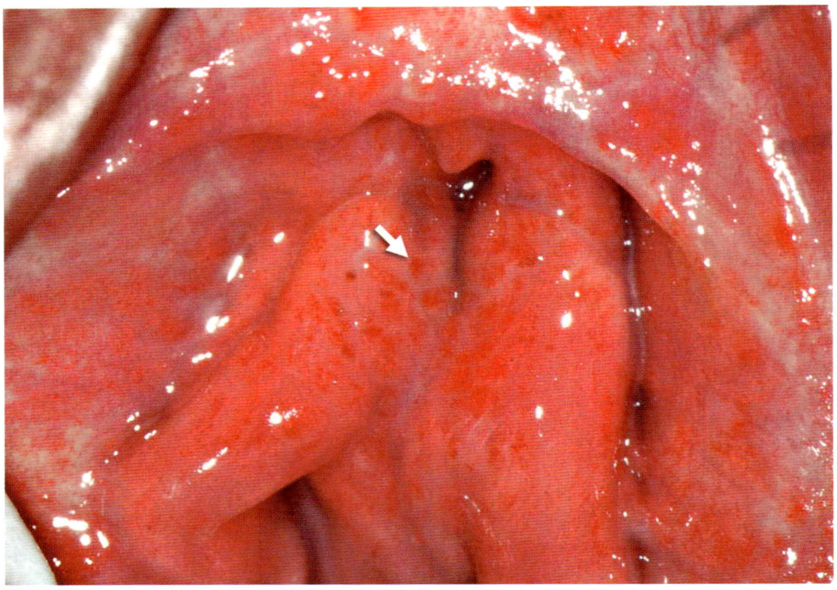

Figure 346 - Patched dilated capillaries (arrow) in fungal candidiasis, involve the paraurethral region.

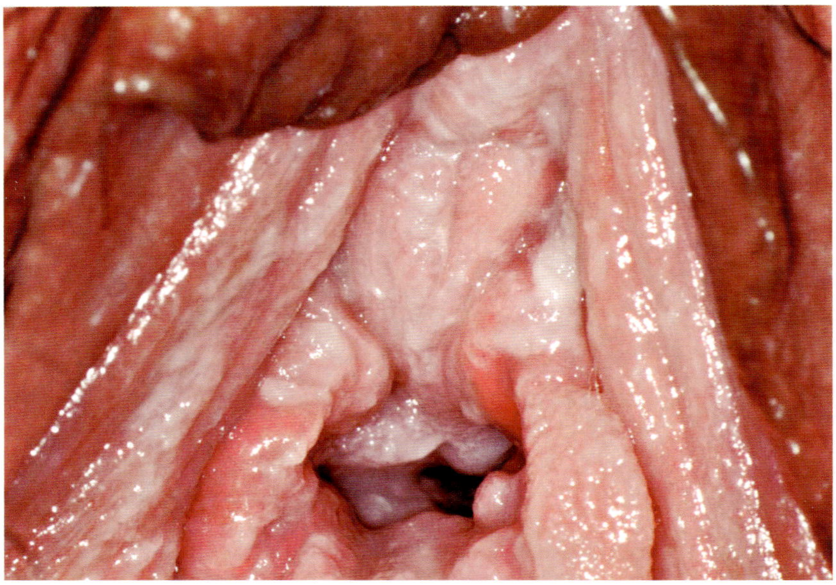

Figure 347 - Diffuse vulvar acetowhitening due to poorly glycogenated epithelium.

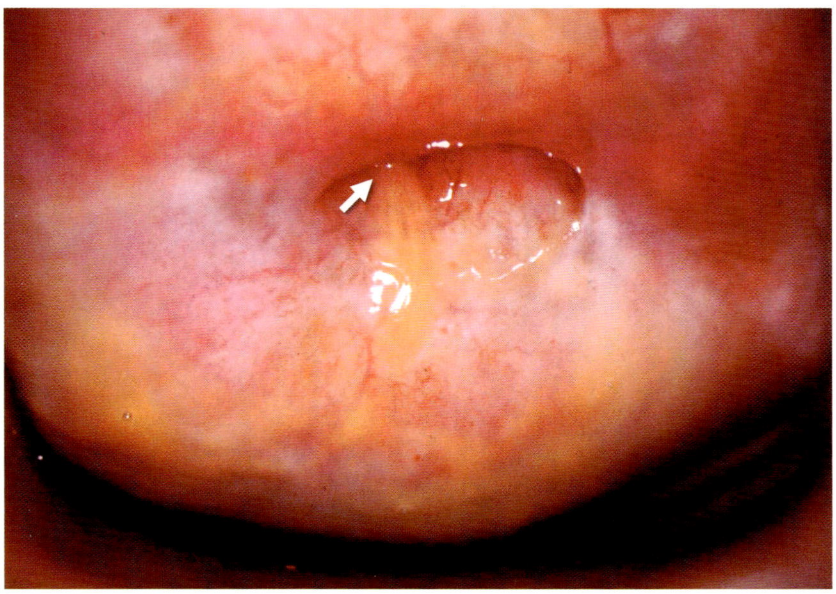

Figure 348 - Yellowish discharge comes out of the endocervical canal (arrow) in Chlamydia trachomatis infection.

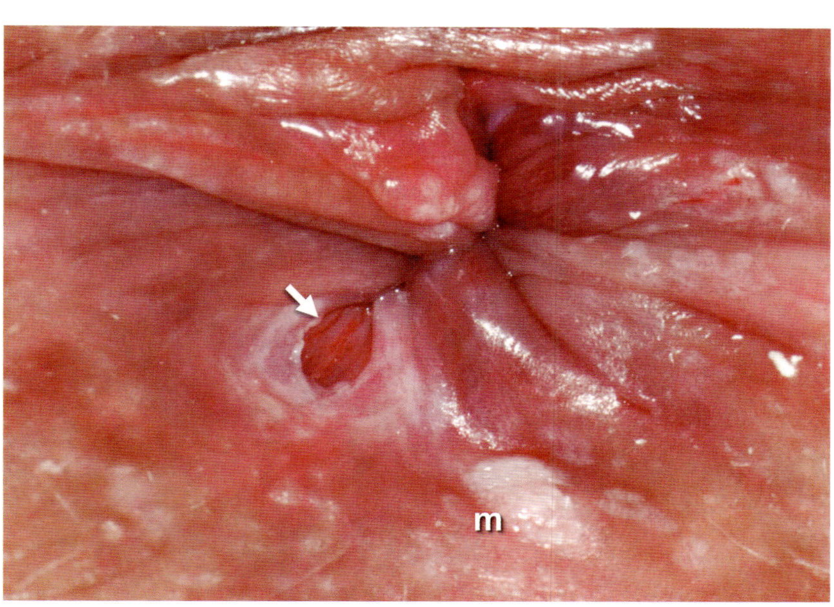

Figure 349 - A perianal healing fissure (arrow) is associated with an HPV micropapillary lesion (m).

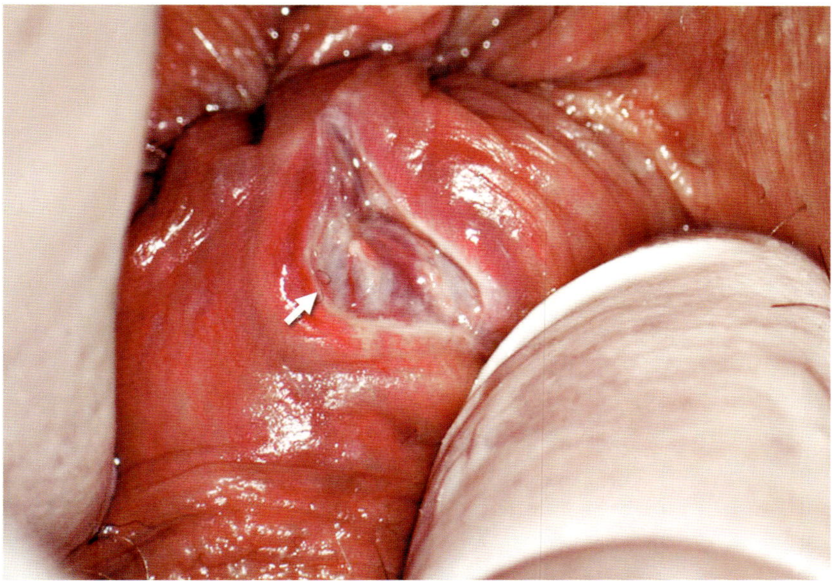

Figure 350 - The arrowed syphilitic anal ulcer can be misdiagnosed as perianal fissures.

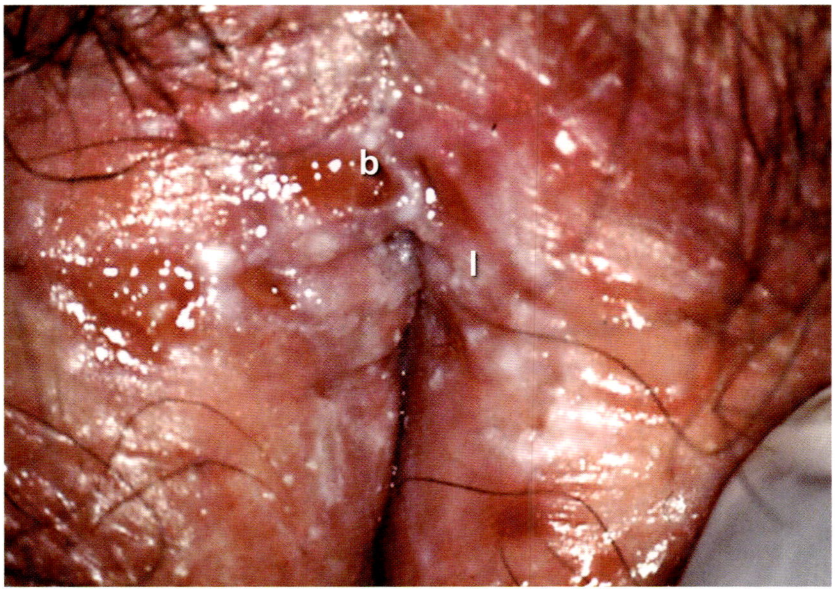

Figure 351 - Widespread herpetic blisters (b) surmount lichen sclerosus (l).

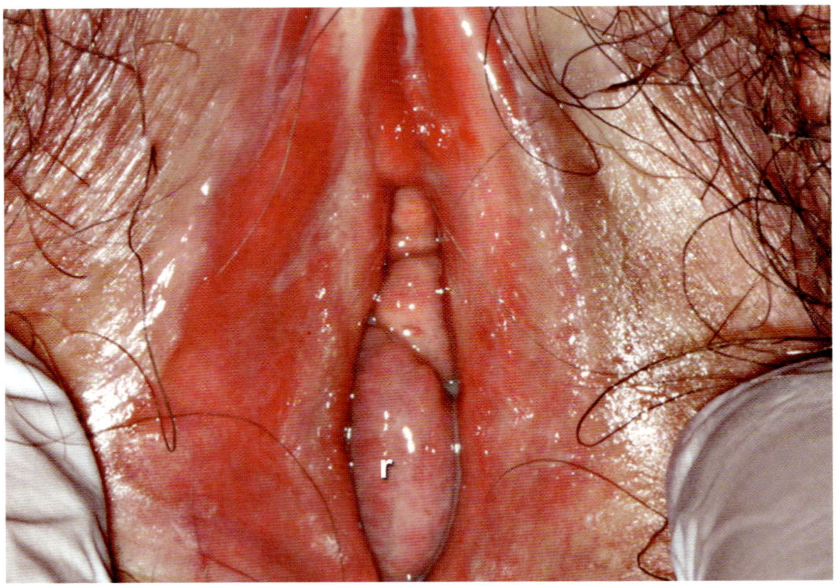

Figure 352 - Red vestibule in desquamative inflammatory vaginitis (DIV). Rectocele (r).

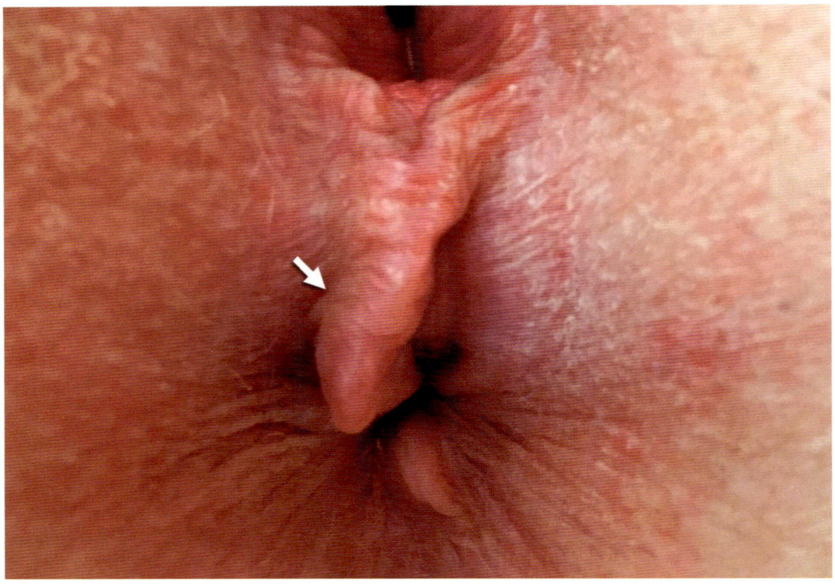

Figure 353 - Perianal skin tag (arrow) of Crohn's disease may resemble a swollen hemorrhoid.

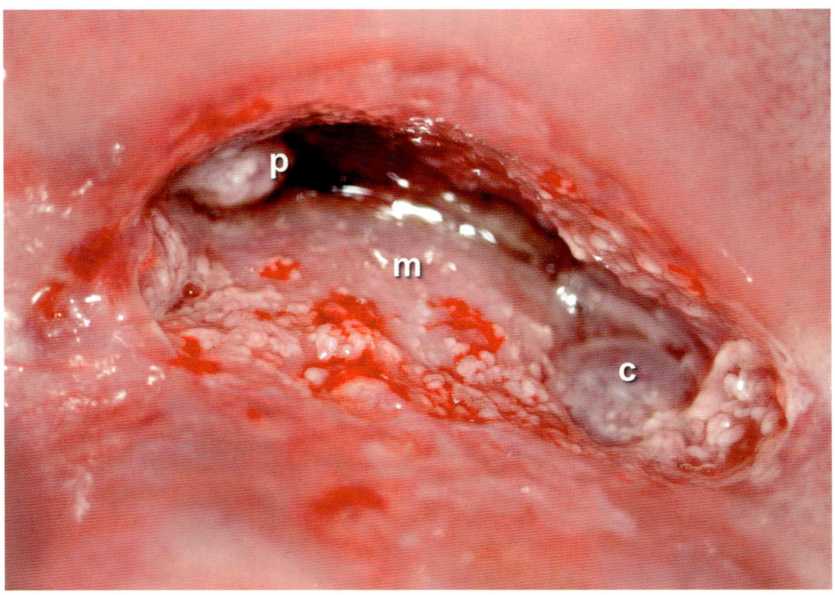

Figure 354 - The cervical canal, lined with a faint acetowhite metaplastic epithelium (m), shows a polyp (p) and a glandular cyst (c).

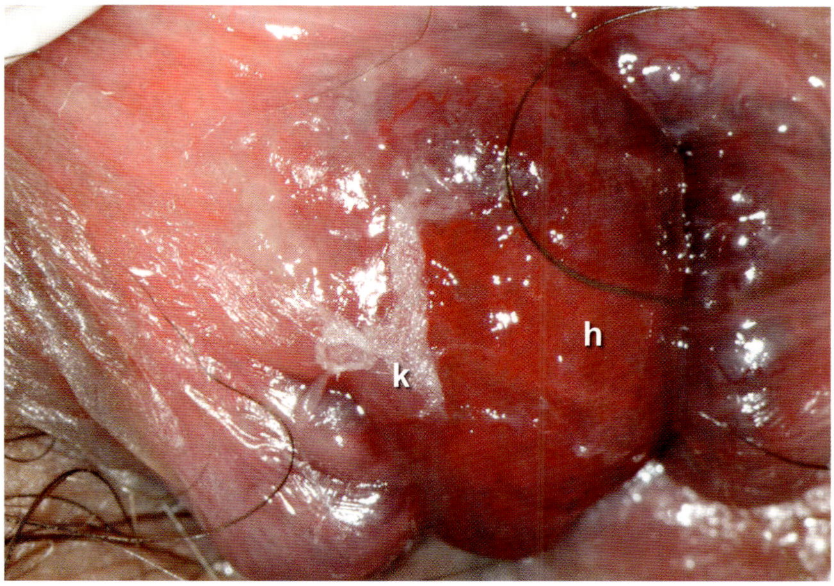

Figure 355 - A thrombosed hemorrhoid (h), protruding from the anus, appears as a lump at the anal verge. The dark reddish color is due to the blood clot contained inside the swollen blood vessel. Thin keratosis (k).

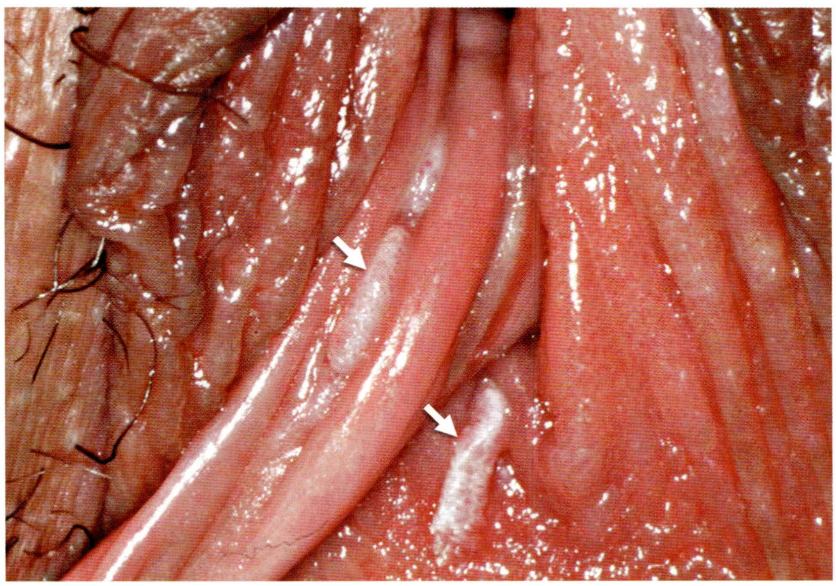

Figure 356 - Vulvar flat condylomas (arrows).

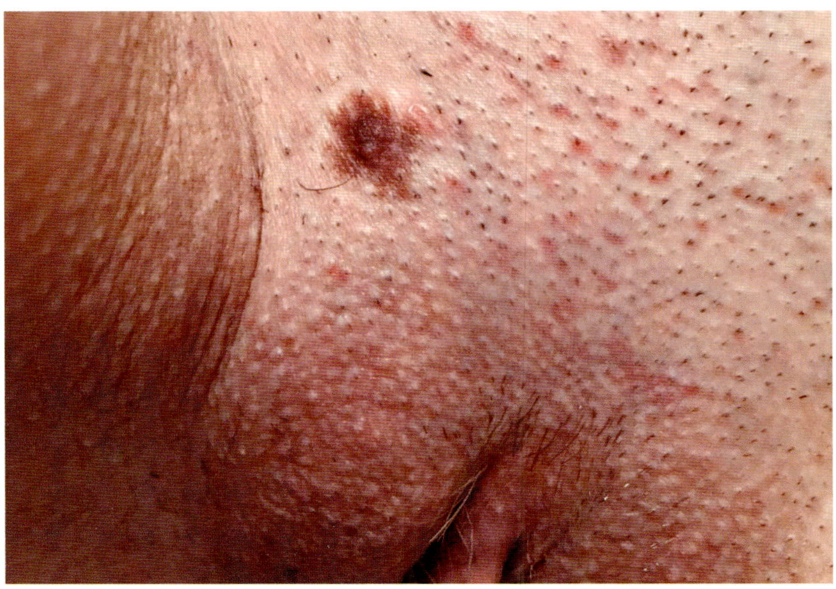

Figure 357 - Pubic supernumerary nipple.

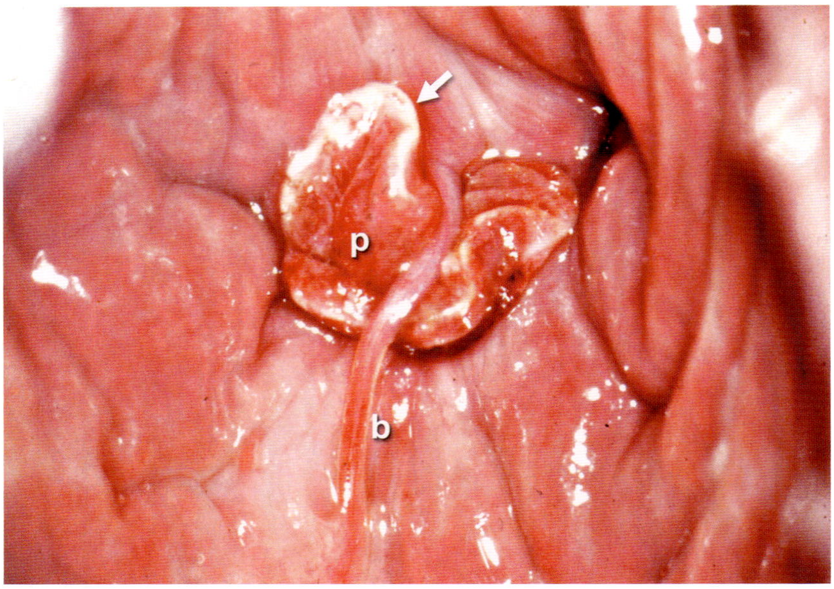

Figure 358 - A tissue bridle (b) passes over a polyp (p) of the vaginal vault, following hysterectomy. The polyp shows a dense acetowhite epithelium on its tip (arrow).

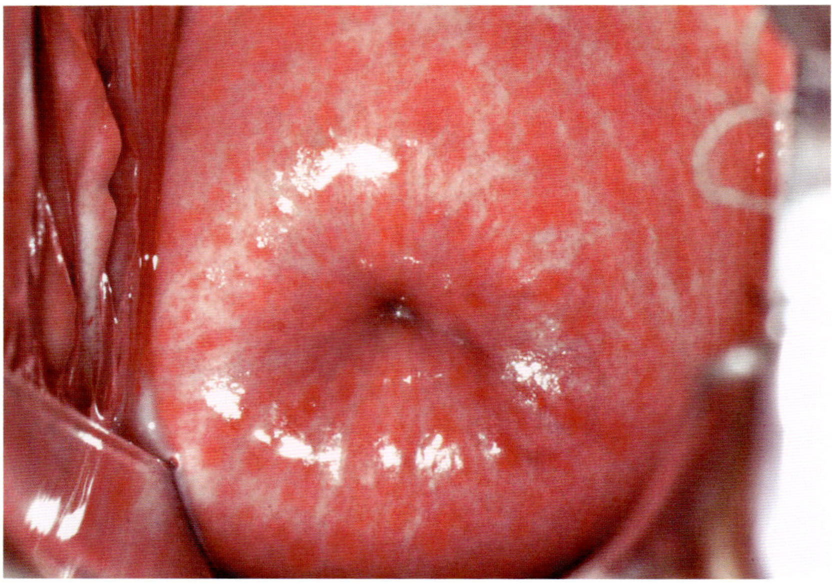

Figure 359 - Widespread dystrophic petechiae in menopause.

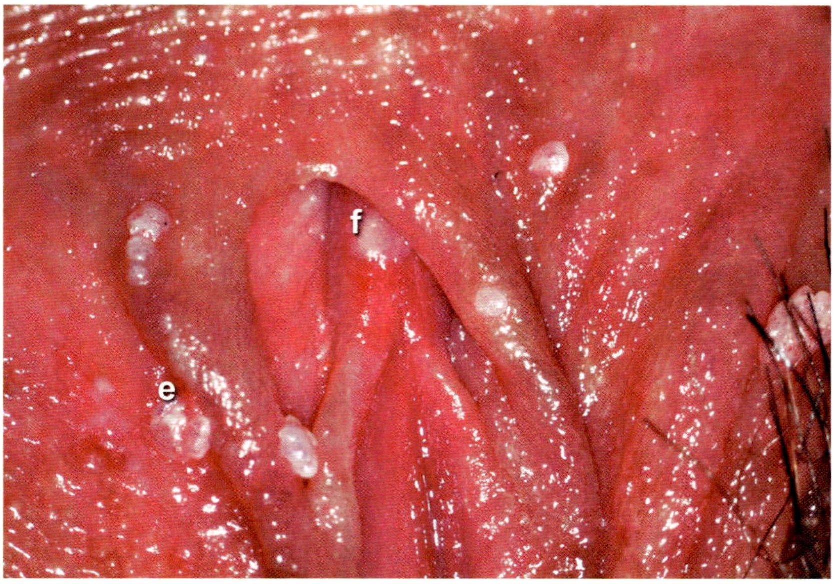

Figure 360 - Para-clitoral flat condyloma (f) and vulvar exophytic condylomas (e).

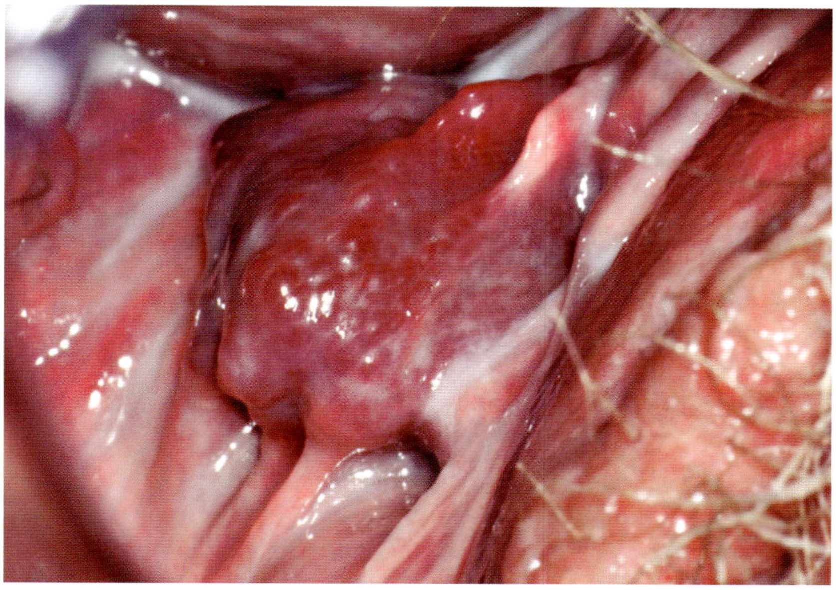

Figure 361 - Vaginal hemangioma.

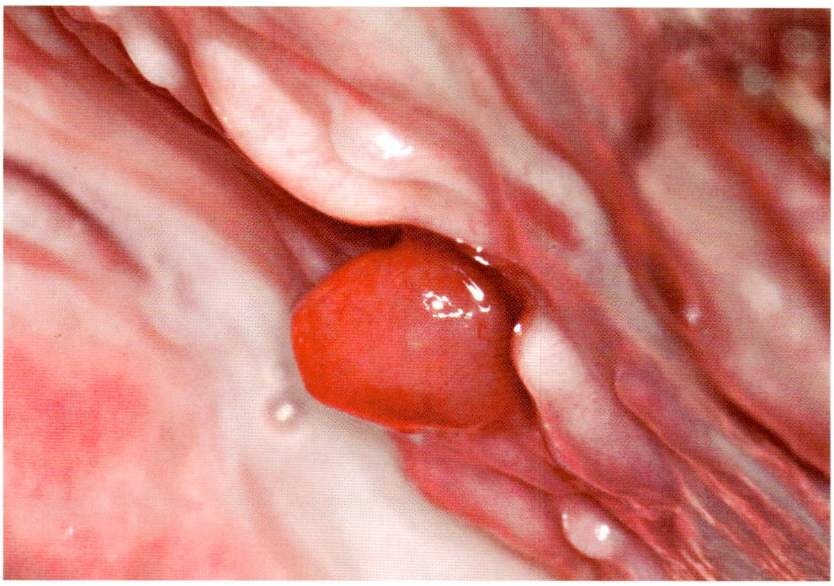

Figure 362 - Congested fibroid of the left lateral wall of vagina.

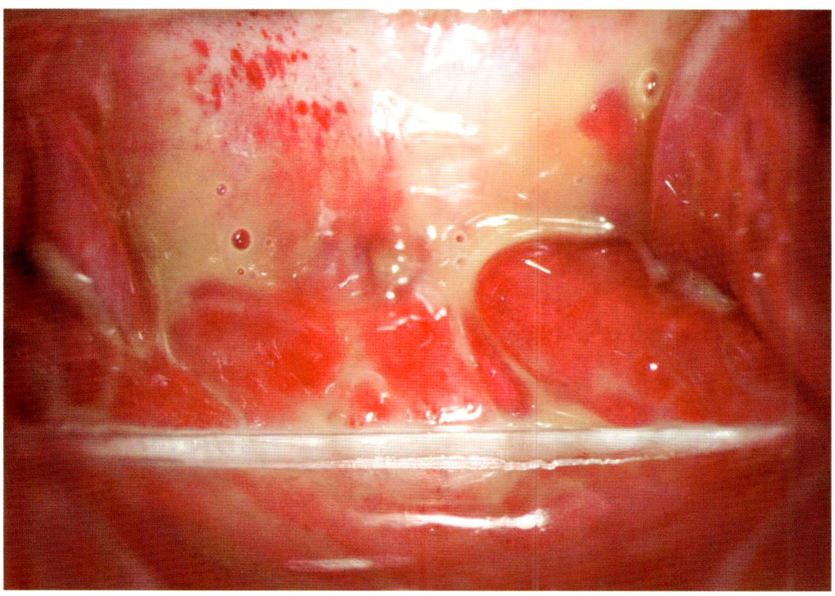

Figure 363 - Vaginal vault following hysterectomy exhibits a yellowish discharge due to aerobic vaginitis.

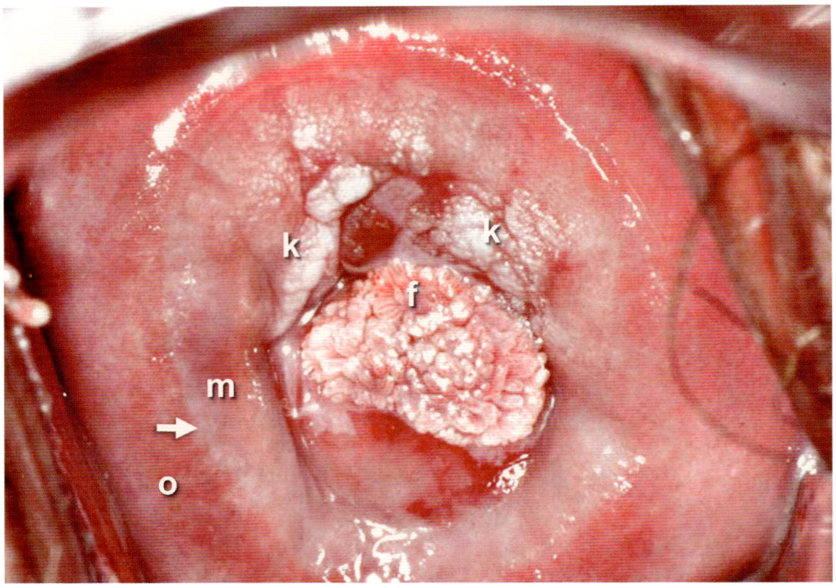

Figure 364 - Endocervical florid condyloma (f) and thick keratosis (k). The arrow indicates the border between the light pink mature metaplastic epithelium (m) and the darker pink original squamous epithelium (o).

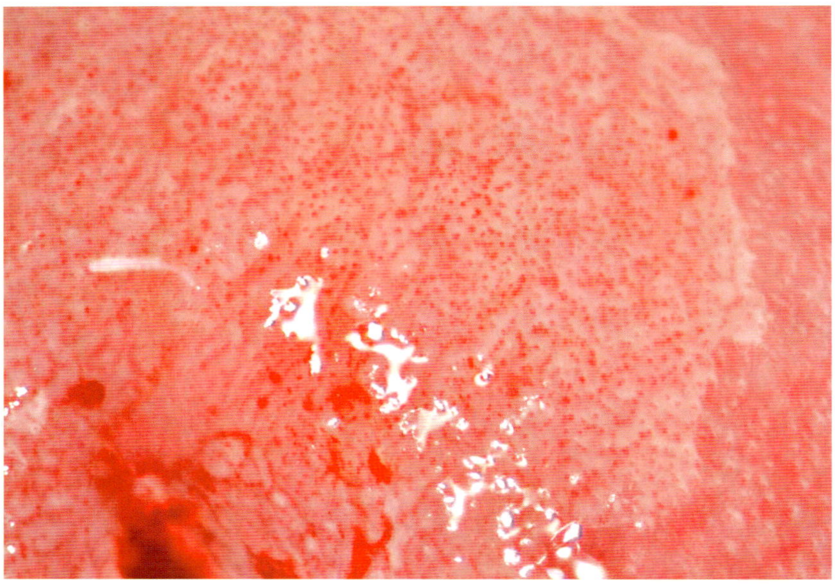

Figure 365 - Fine punctation.

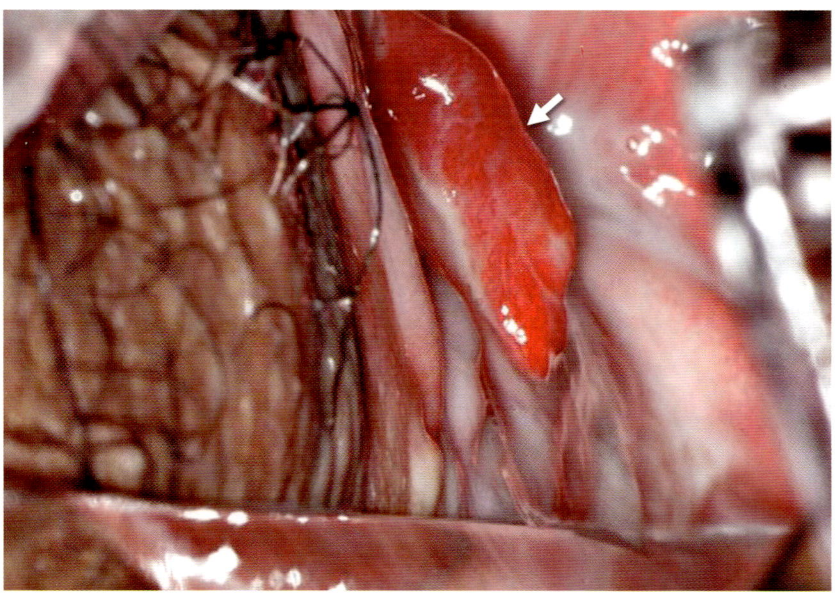

Figure 366 - A polypoid granulation tissue (arrow), protrudes from the right lateral wall, following vaginorrhaphy.

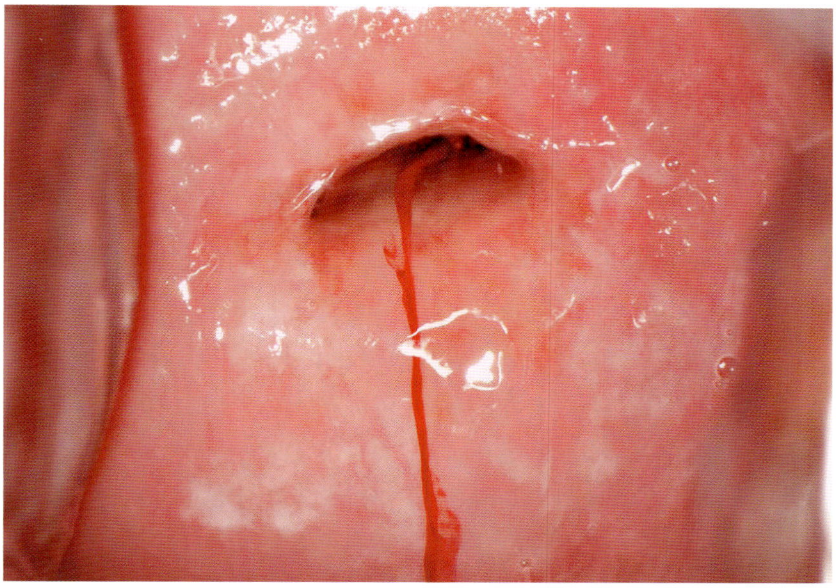

Figure 367 - The midcycle bleeding is a result of an occasionally precipitant drop in estrogen level between the functional peak of the mature follicle and that of the fully developed corpus luteum (minimum "estrogen withdrawal" menstruation).

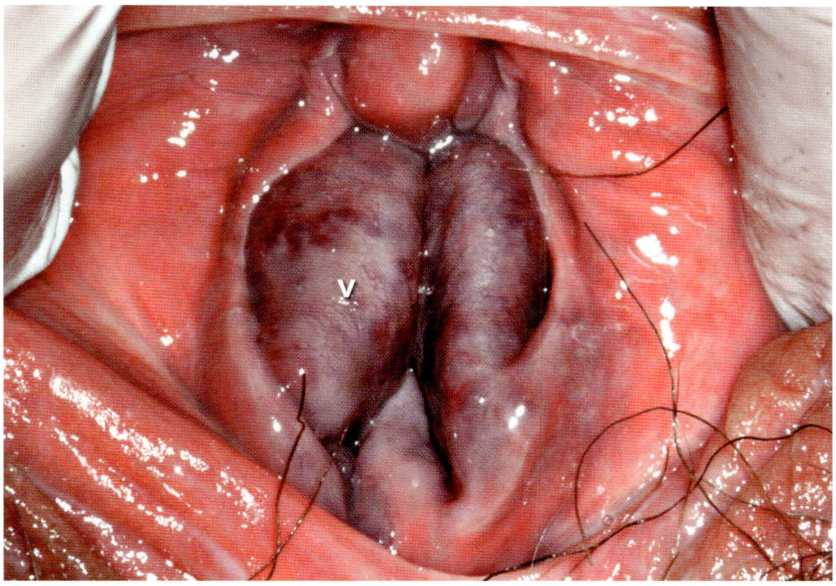

Figure 368 - Vestibular varices (v) at 18th week of gestation.

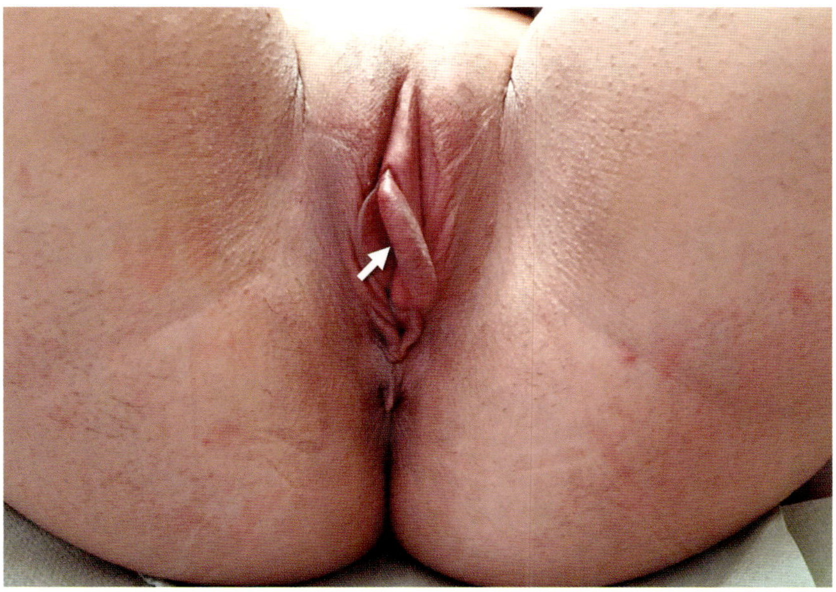

Figure 369 - Edema of the left inner labium (arrow) due to lymphorrhagia following sexual intercourse.

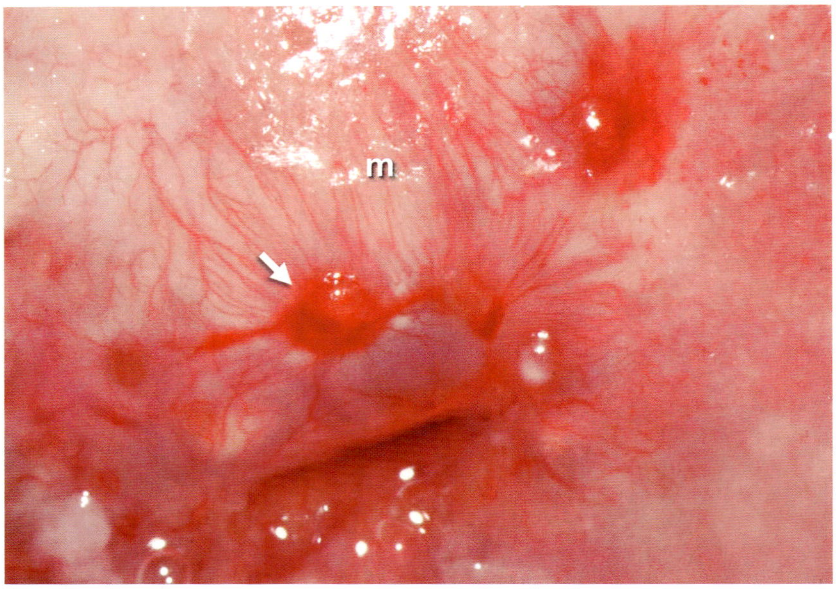

Figure 370 - Mature metaplastic epithelium (m) and hemorrhagic effusions (arrow) following diathermy.

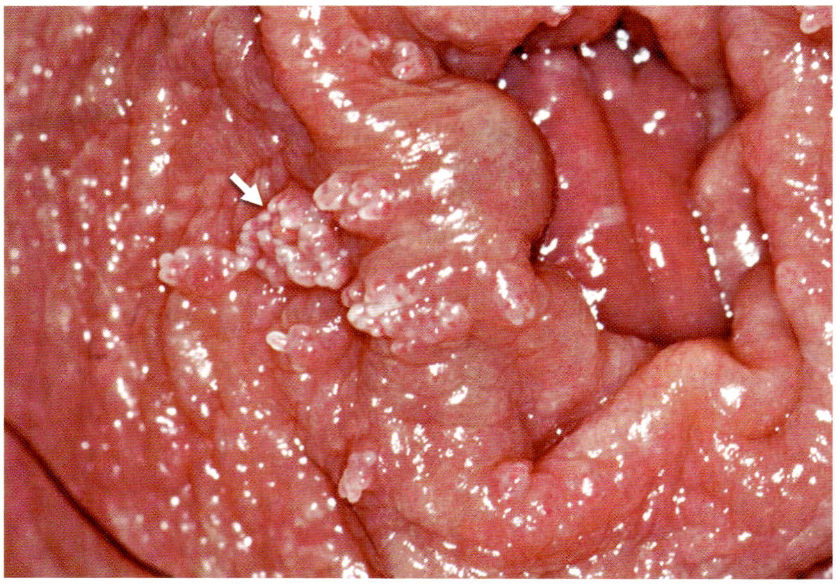

Figure 371 - Vulvar warts (arrow).

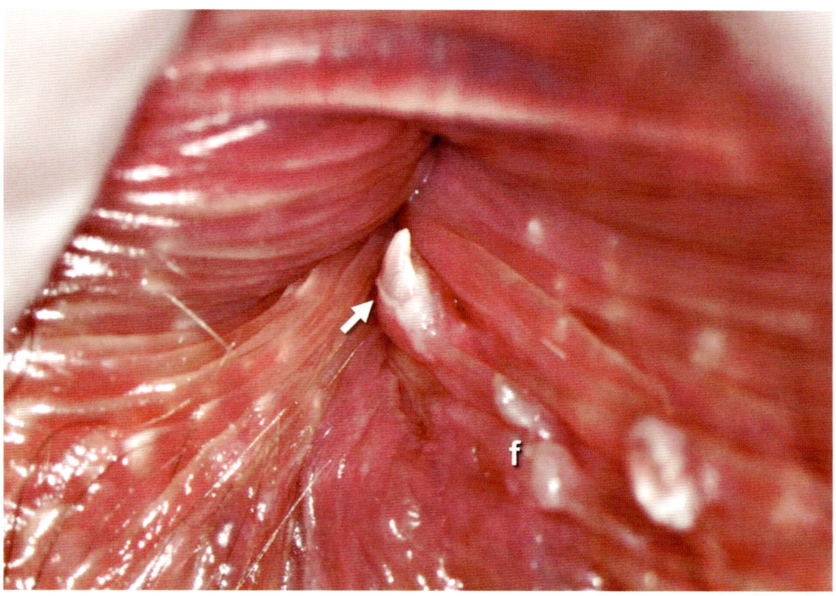

Figure 372 - Perianal HPV flat condyloma (f) and horn-like exophytic condyloma (arrow).

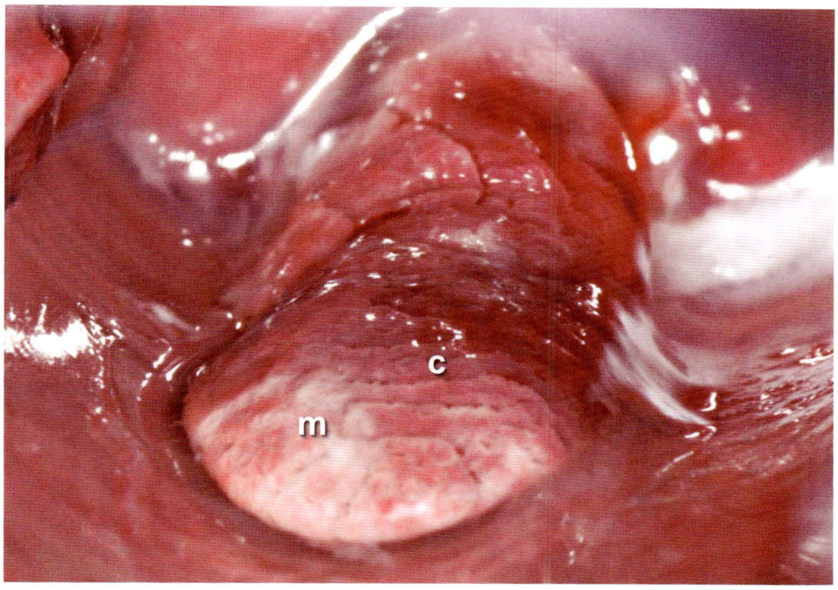

Figure 373 - Vaginal adenosis on the posterior wall. Ectopic glandular tissue in the vagina is termed vaginal adenosis. Colposcopy of this uncommon case exhibits both pure columnar epithelium (c) with crypt openings secreting mucus, and a mix of columnar and metaplastic epithelial tissue (m). Biopsy of this vaginal abnormality is indicated because it may be difficult to differentiate vaginal adenosis from primary vaginal carcinoma.

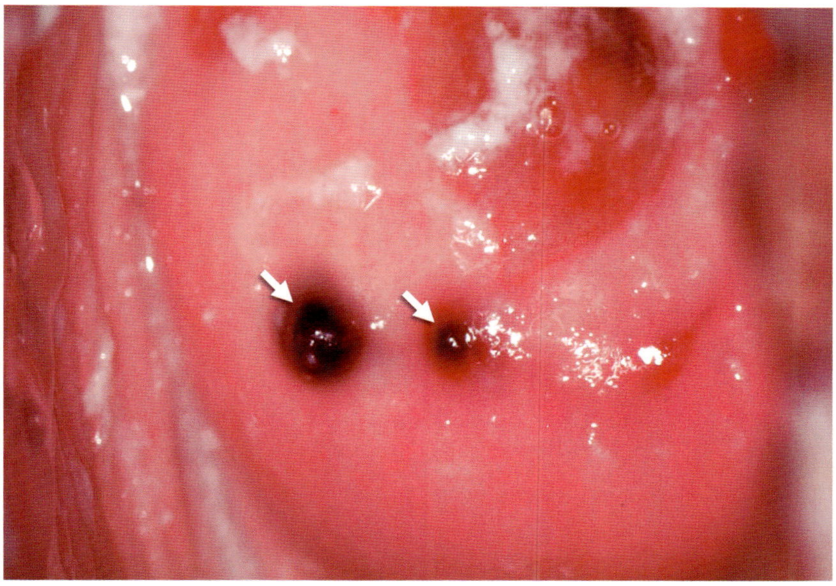

Figure 374 - Newly developed bluish Nabothian follicles (arrows) can mimic endometrial cysts.

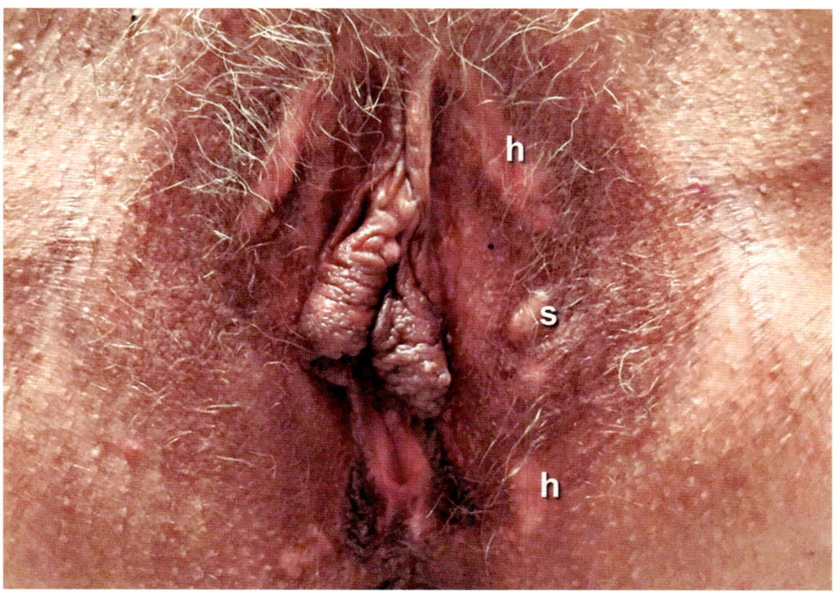

Figure 375 - Hypopigmented macules (h) and sclerosis (s) of the dermis, following laser vaporization.

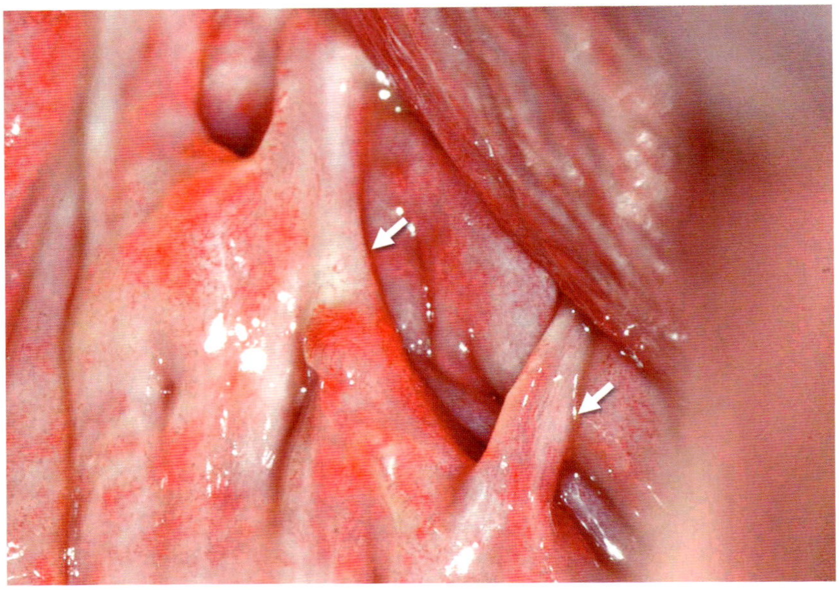

Figure 376 - The vaginal vault following hysterectomy shows irregular ravines, due to cicatricial bridges (arrows), thus making the follow-up more difficult.

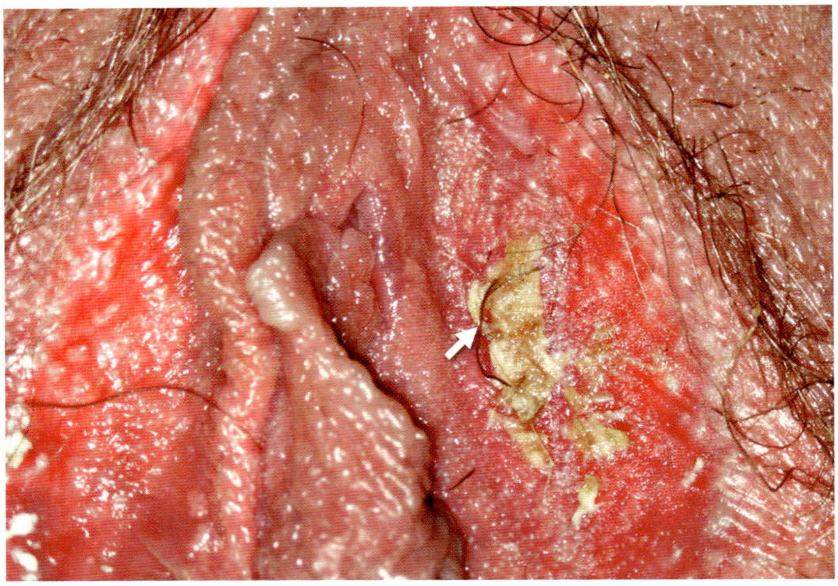

Figure 377 - Vulvar erythema and yellowish smegma (arrow).

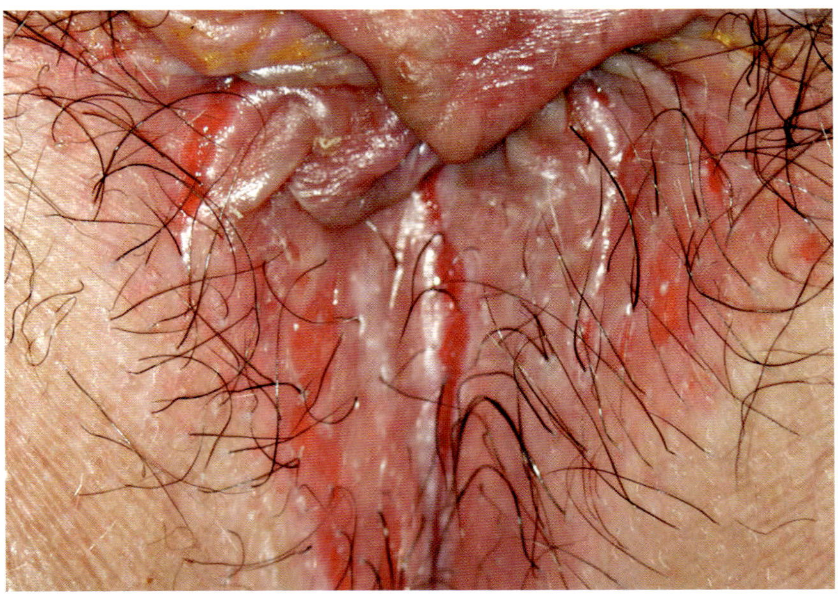

Figure 378 - Perianal fissures due to psoriasis.

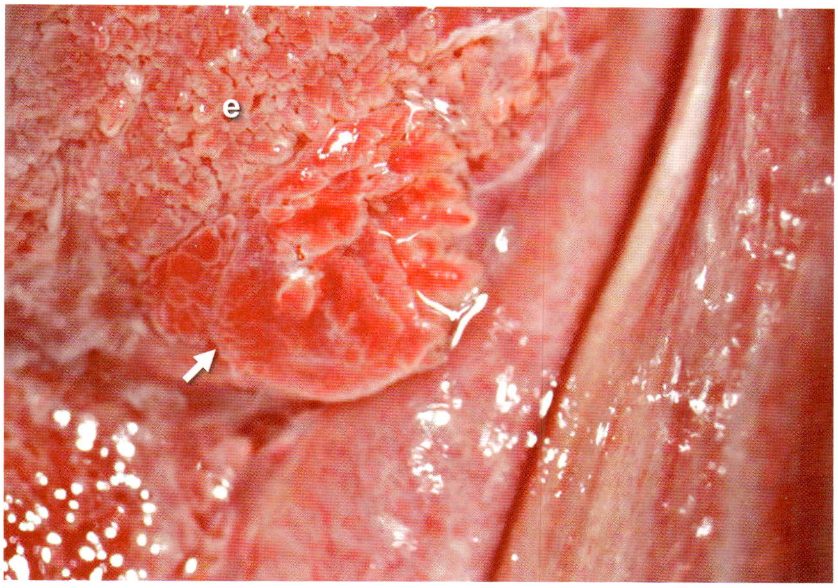

Figure 379 - A florid condyloma (arrow) rises from an area of exposed columnar epithelium (e).

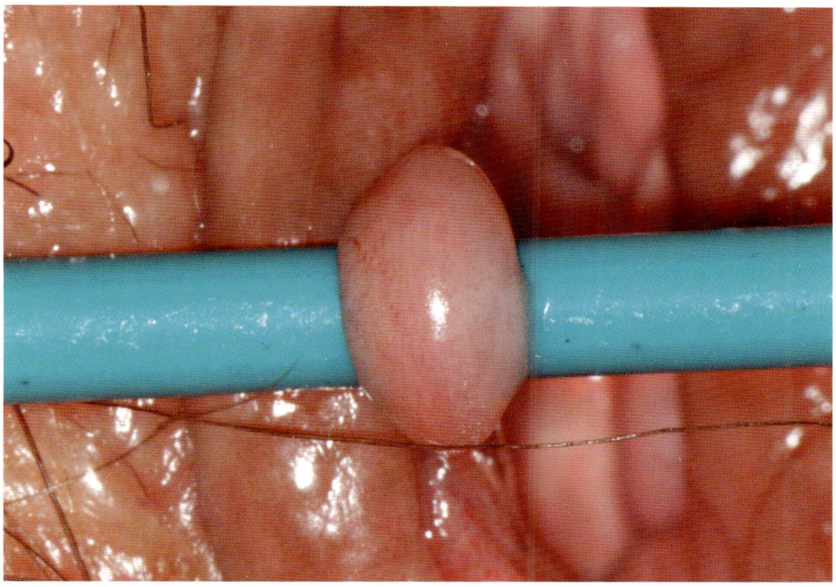

Figure 380 - A tissue ring is anchored to the lateral wall of the vagina.

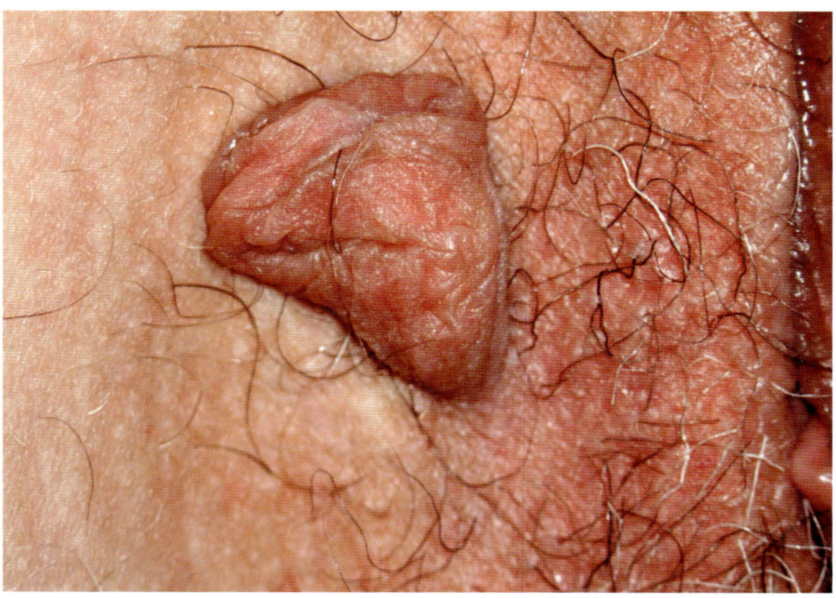

Figure 381 - Vulvar pedunculated fibroid.

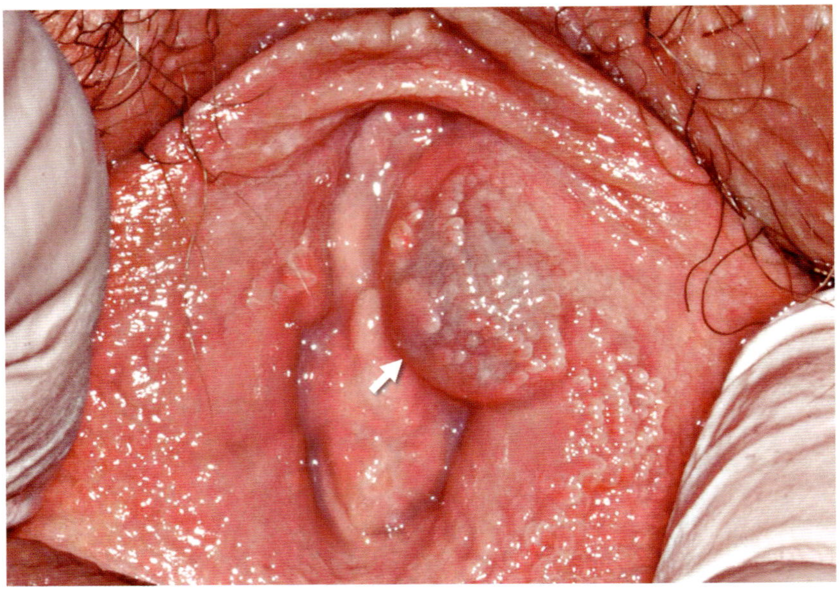

Figure 382 - Mesonephric cyst of the vulva (arrow). Mesonephric cyst is a vestigial remnant of the Wolffian duct.

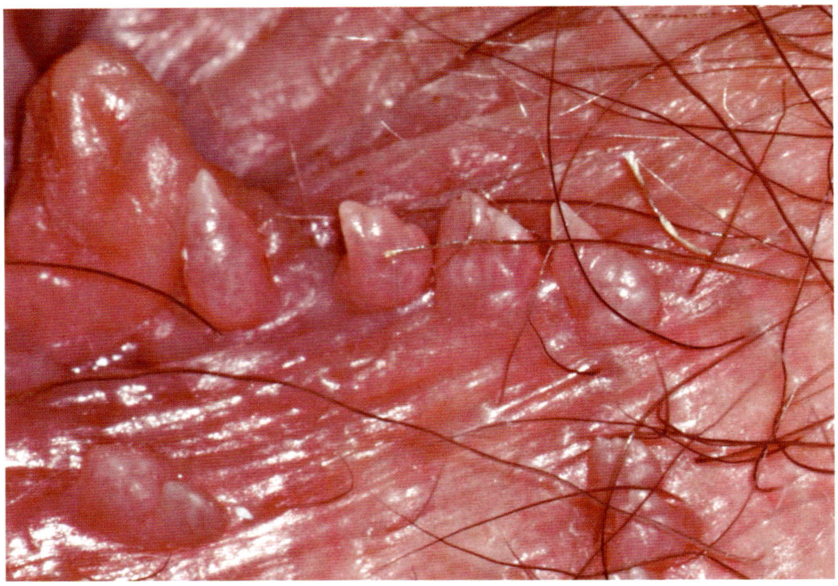

Figure 383 - Perianal HPV exophytic condylomas.

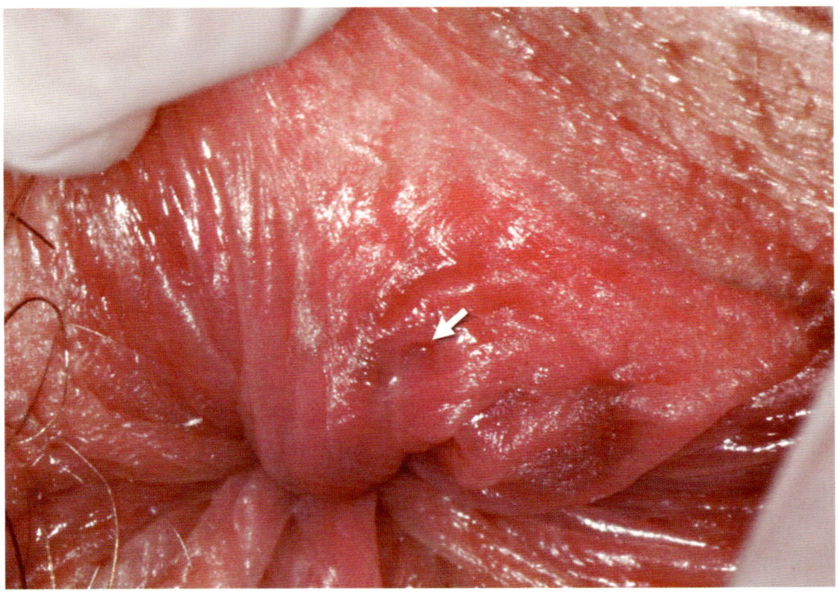

Figure 384 - The arrow indicates the external opening of an intersphincteric anal fistula.

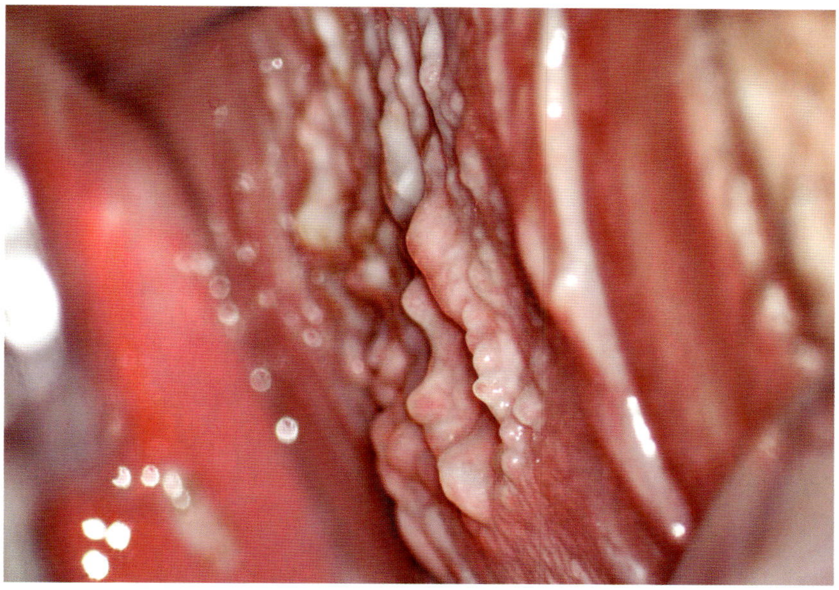

Figure 385 - Normal mucosal wrinkling of the vaginal wall.

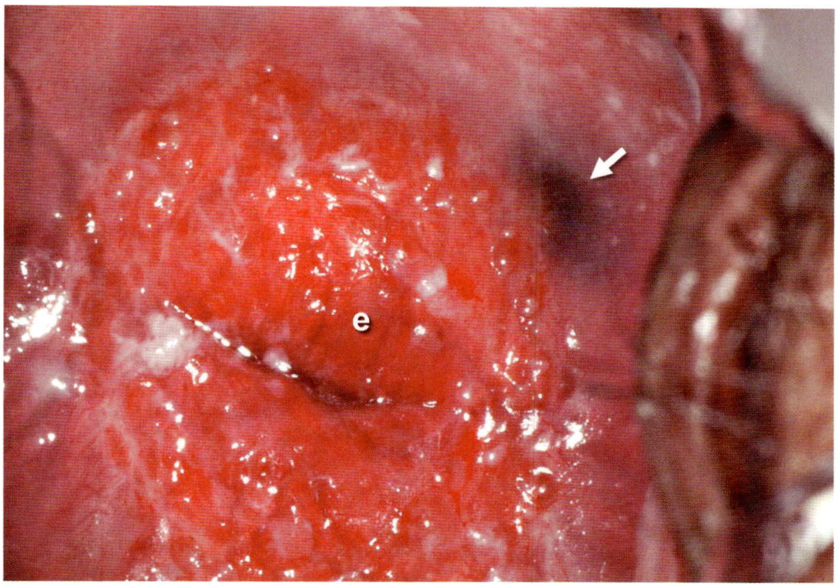

Figure 386 - The arrowed endometrial focus shows a circumscribed, bluish area beneath squamous epithelium. Exposed columnar epithelium (e).

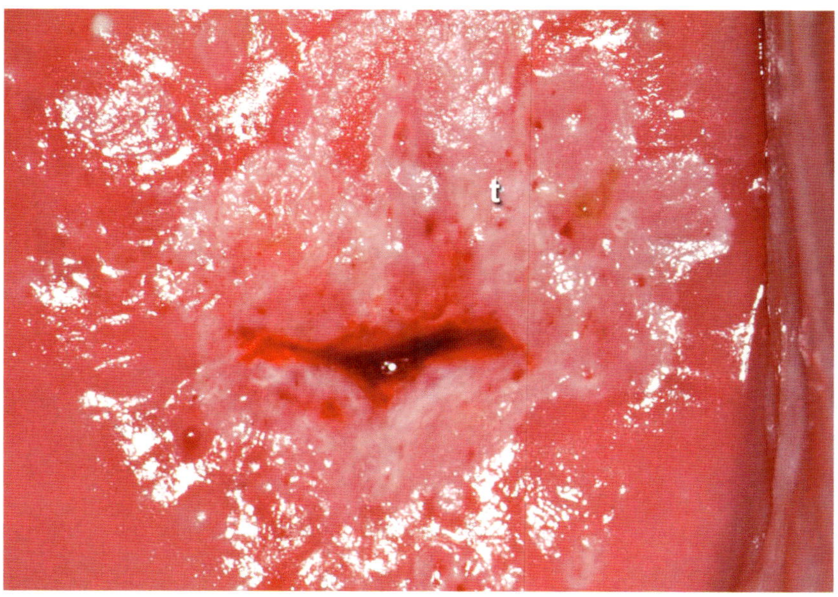

Figure 387 - Thick acetowhite epithelium (t). Excision biopsy and the resultant histology confirmed a high-grade HPV lesion.

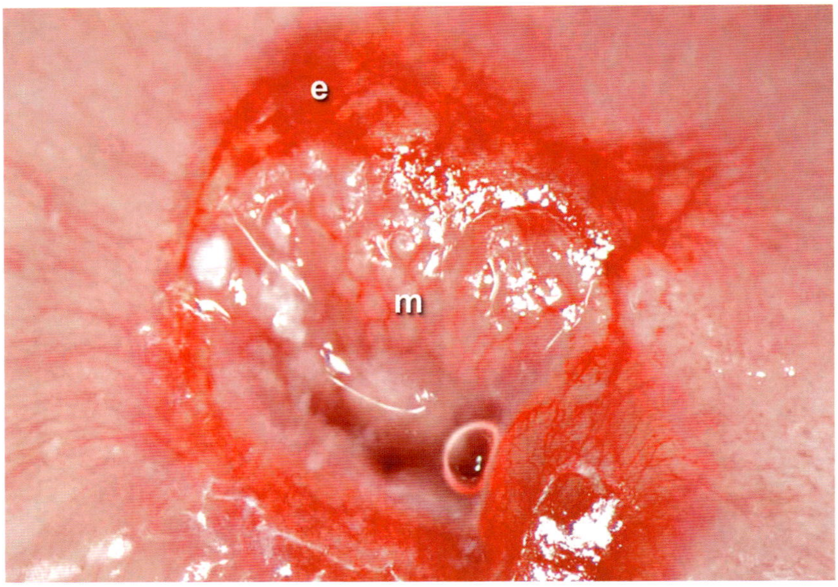

Figure 388 - A fine mosaic (m) is surrounded by a circular hemorrhagic effusion (e), due to a previous diathermy.

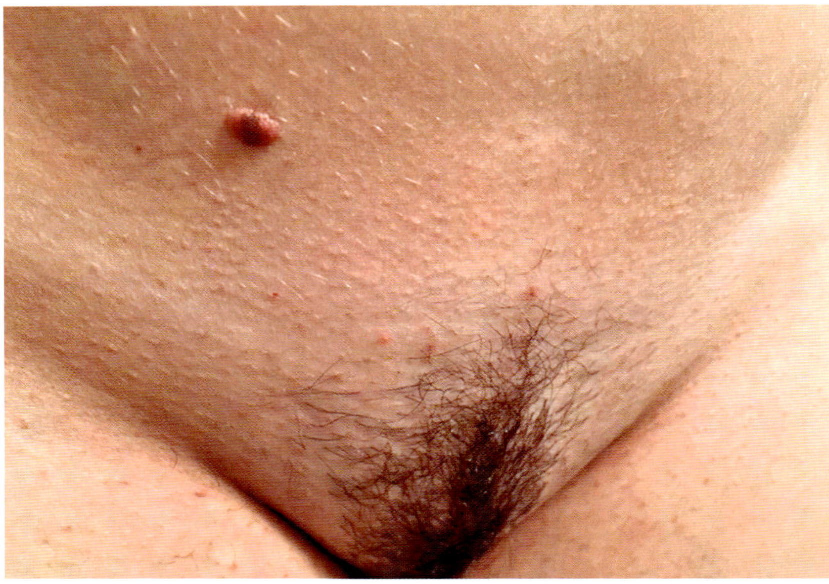

Figure 389 - Abdominal supernumerary nipple.

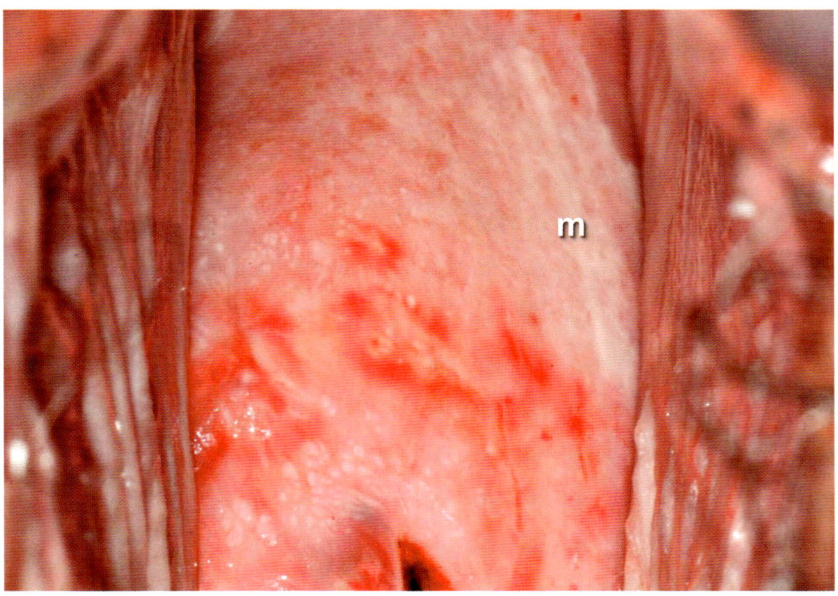

Figure 390 - A faint acetowhite epithelium (m) involves the anterior vaginal wall (congenital metaplasia).

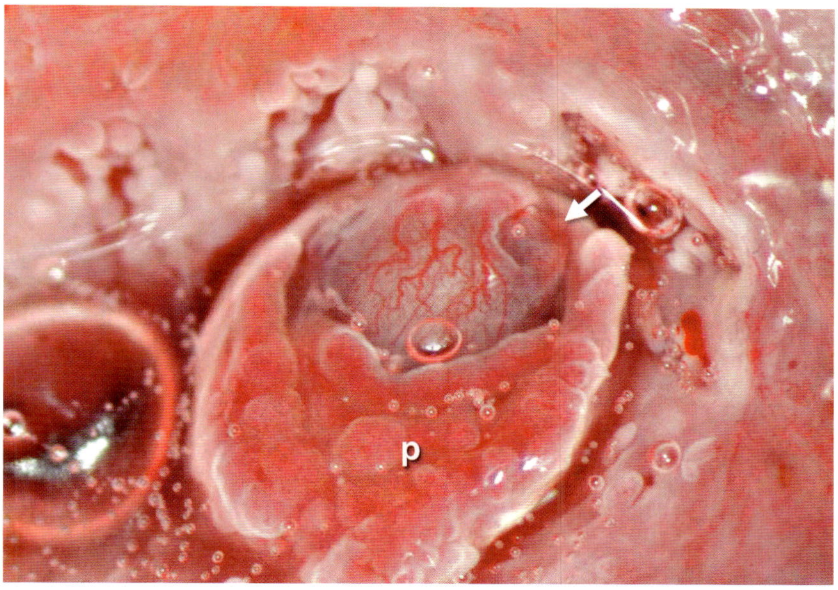

Figure 391 - A serous cyst (arrow) has developed inside the endocervical polyp (p).

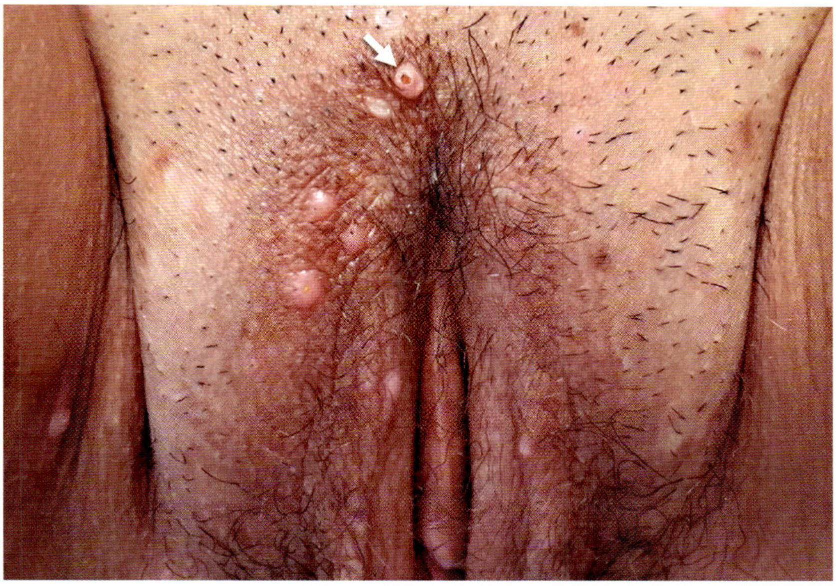

Figure 392 - Scattered pink, shiny and smooth bumps with a dimple in the center (arrow) (molluscum contagiosum).

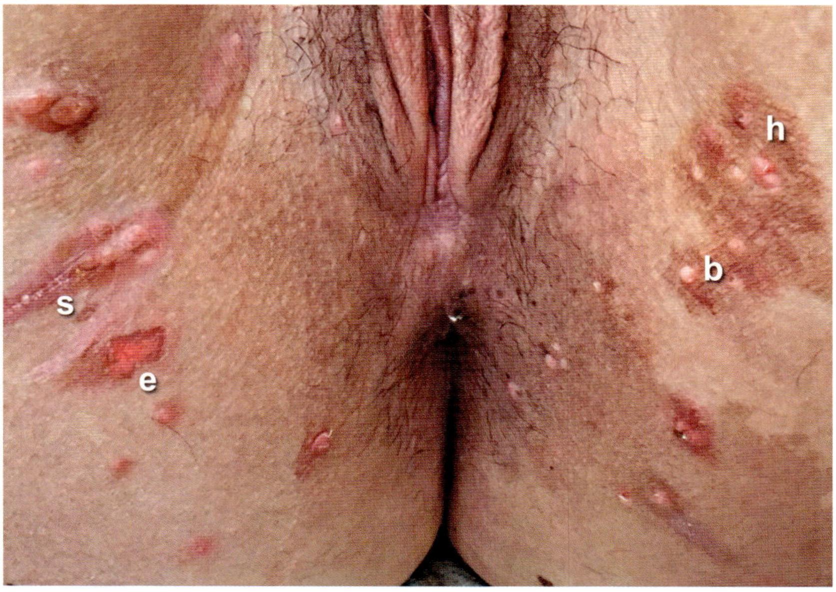

Figure 393 - The same patient of the previous image underwent cryotherapy. This picture shows the disadvantages of this treatment, such as the possibility of erosions (e), blistering (b), scarring (s), and post-inflammatory hyperpigmentation (h).

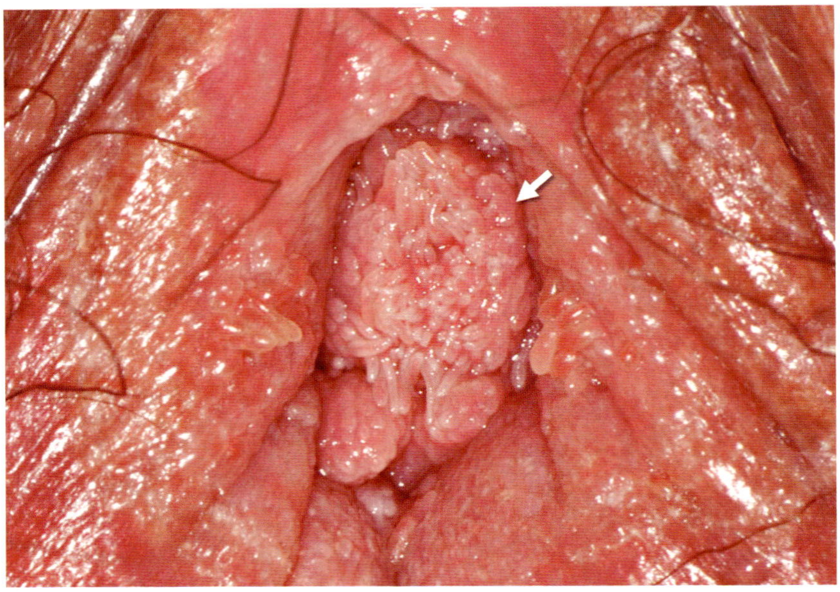

Figure 394 - Periurethral hypertrophic papillae (arrow).

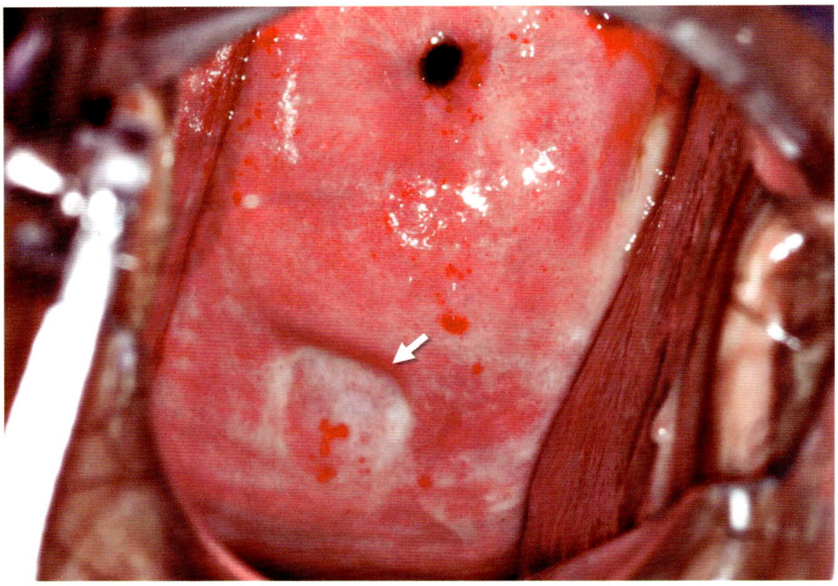

Figure 395 - The arrowed dimple is the outcome of a previous cervical cerclage.

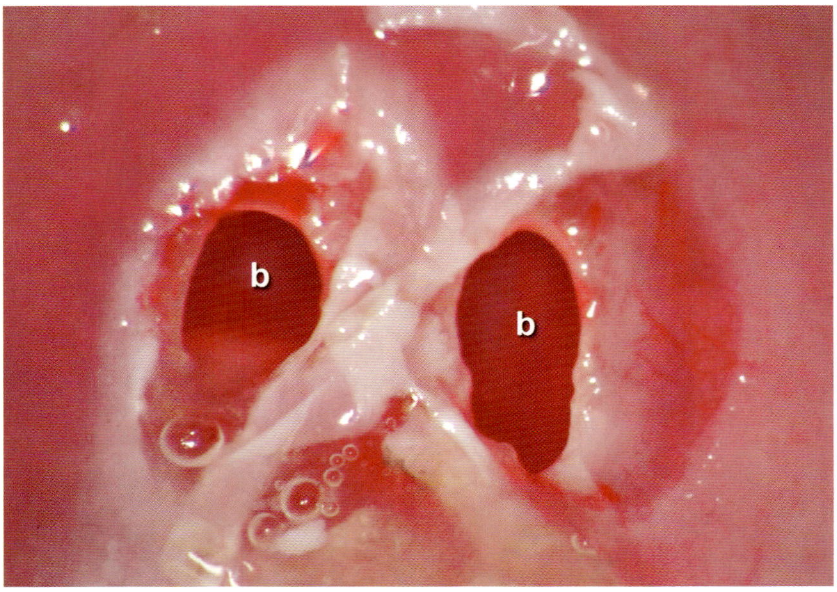

Figure 396 - Beds (b) of spontaneously opened retention cysts.

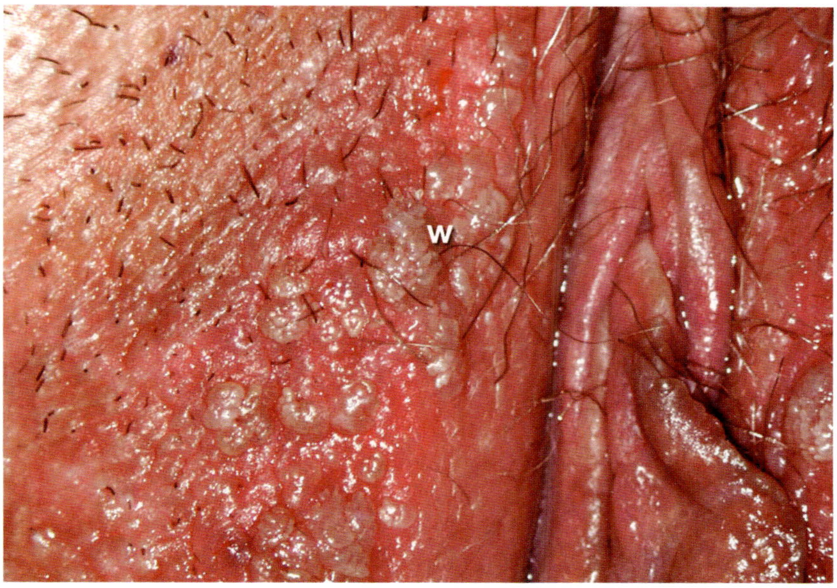

Figure 397 - Vulvar warts (w).

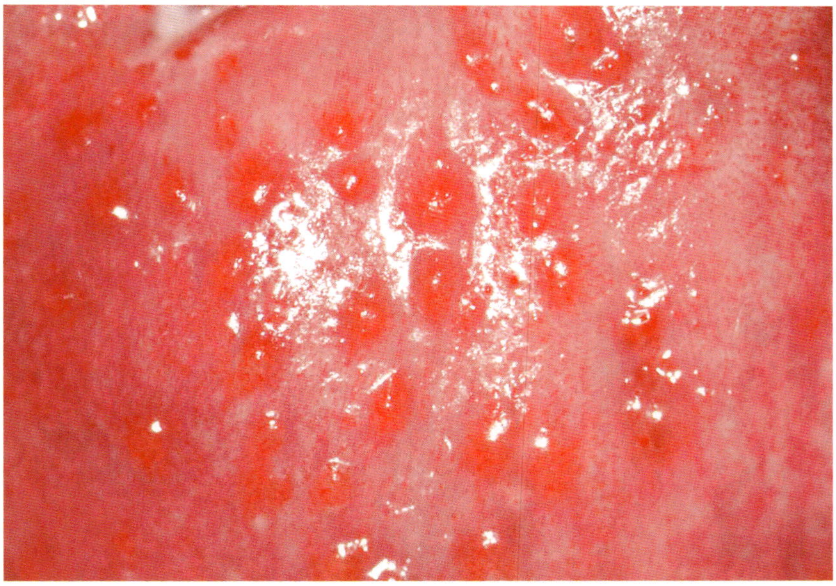

Figure 398 - Erythematous papules induced by Candida infection.

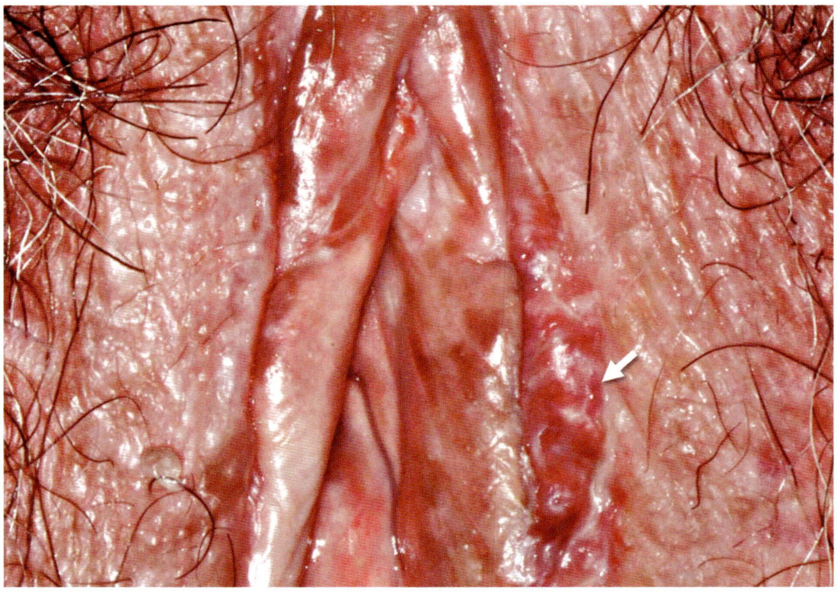

Figure 399 - Extensive angiokeratoma (arrow) of the left interlabial sulcus.

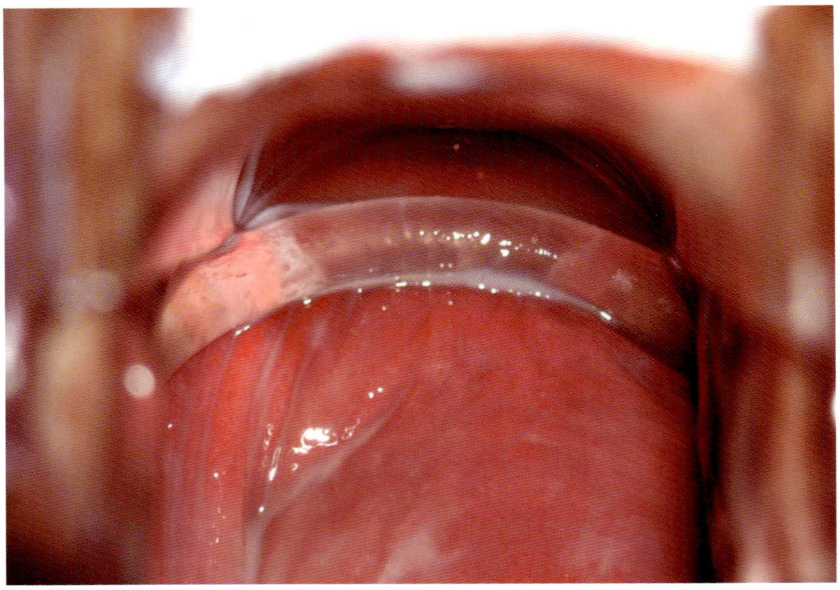

Figure 400 - Contraceptive ring.

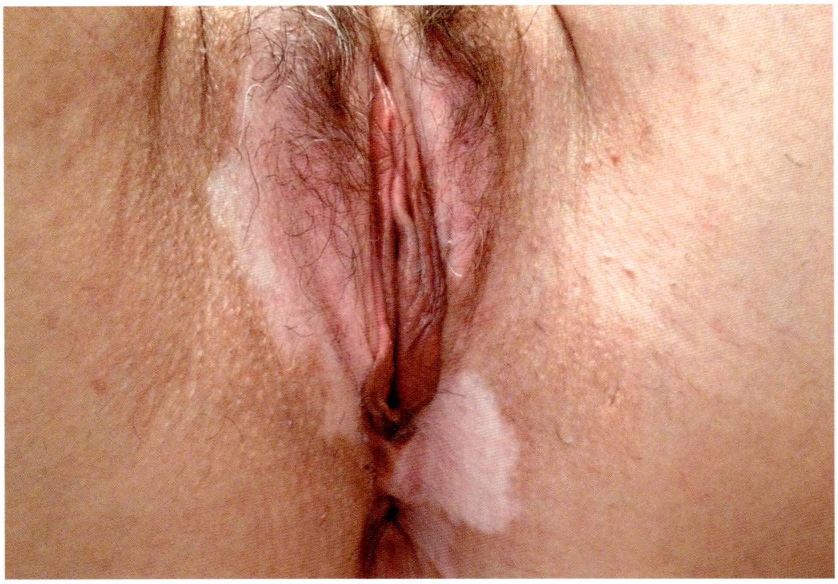

Figure 401 - Vulvar vitiligo.

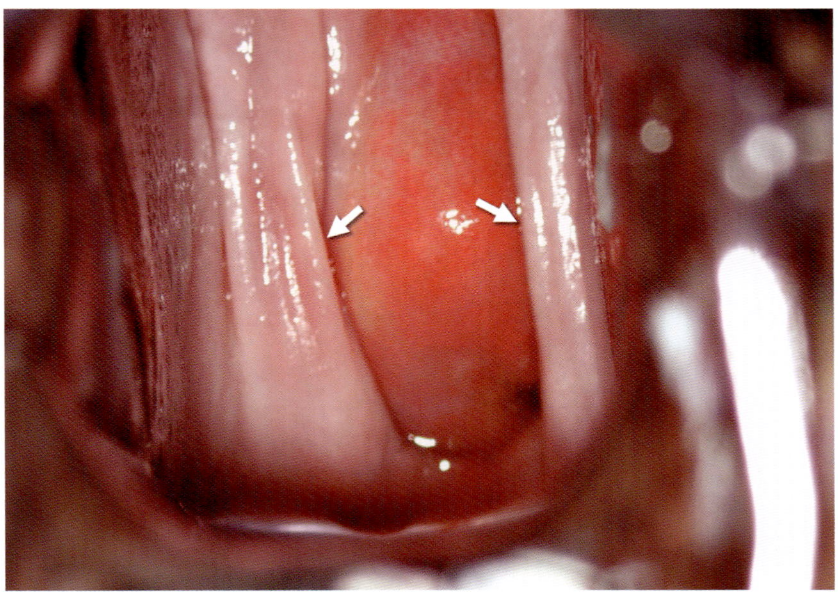

Figure 402 - Two congenital bridles (arrows) cause a stenosis of the proximal tract of vagina.

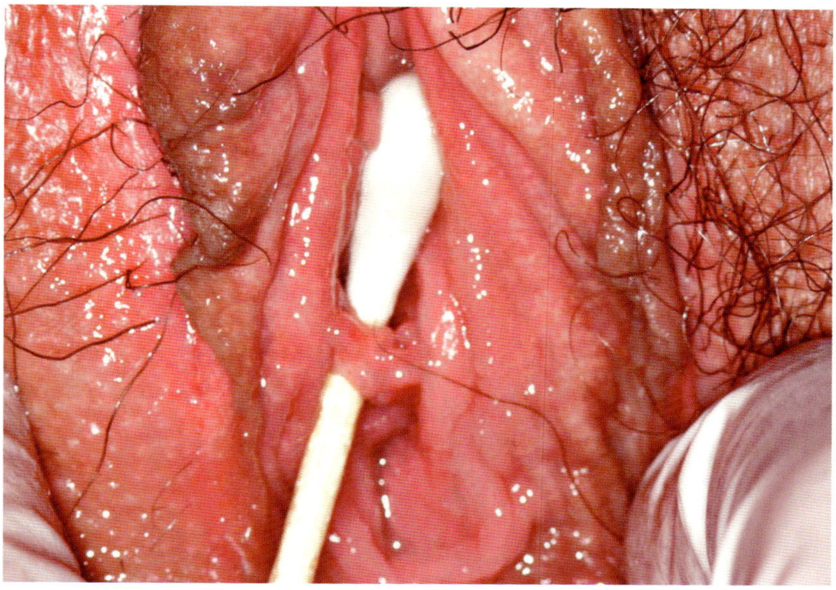

Figure 403 - The cotton-tipped applicator reveals a transverse introital septum.

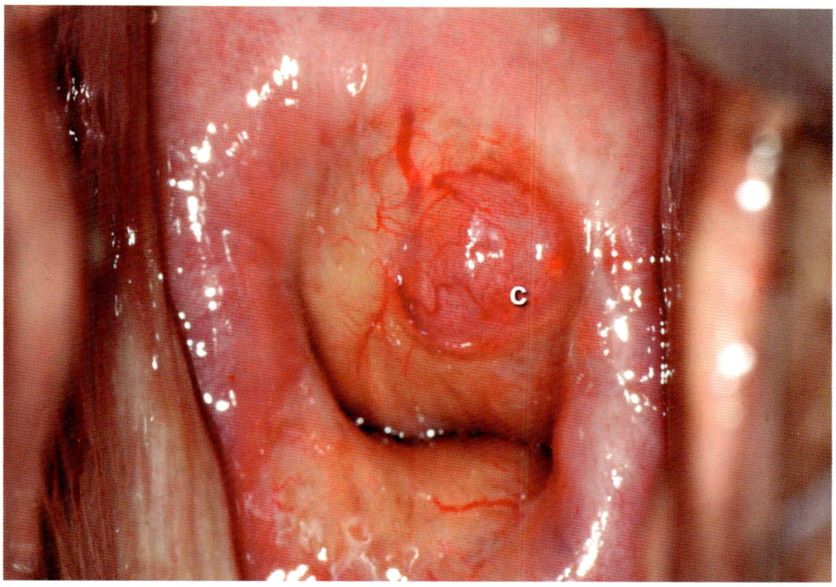

Figure 404 - Voluminous endocervical serous cyst (c) and yellowish discharge coming from the cervical canal caused by gonorrhea.

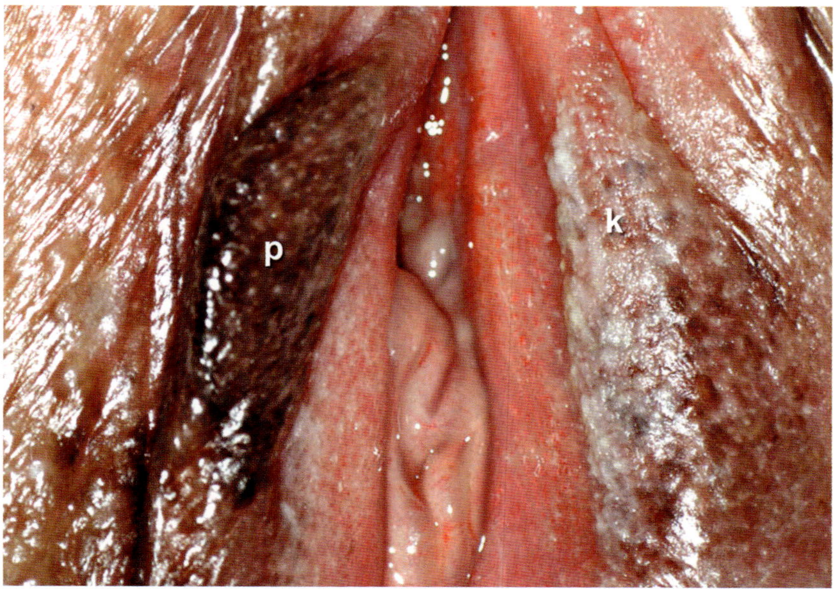

Figure 405 - Pigmented right labium minus (p) and thin keratosis (k) at the left labium minus.

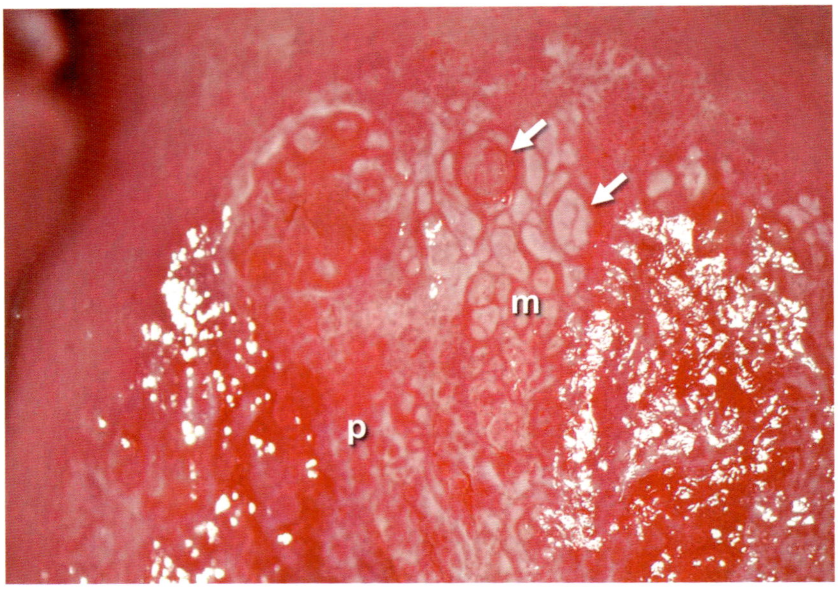

Figure 406 - Combination of coarse mosaic (m) and coarse punctation (p). The arrows indicate convoluted blood vessels defining oval tiles.

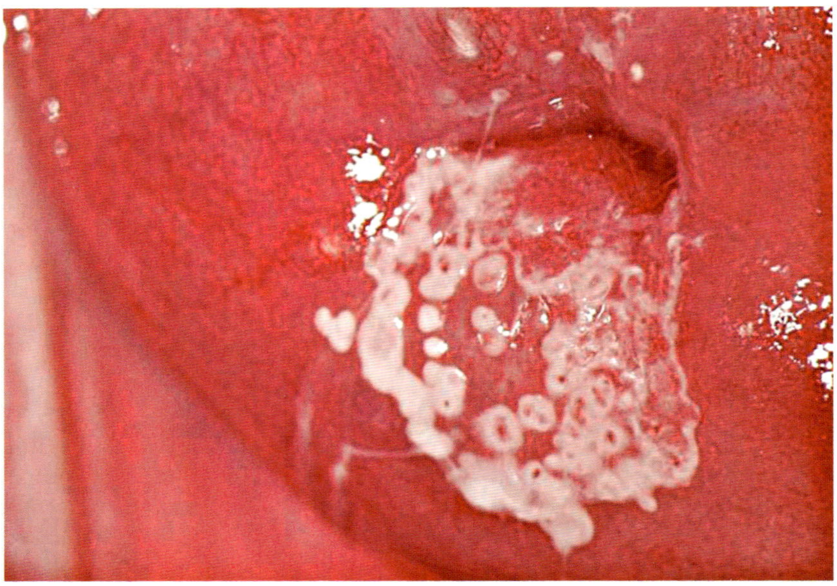

Figure 407 - Scattered grade IV gland openings, characterized by a dense acetowhite rim, raised from the surface like a doughnut. Biopsy disclosed a high-grade CIN lesion.

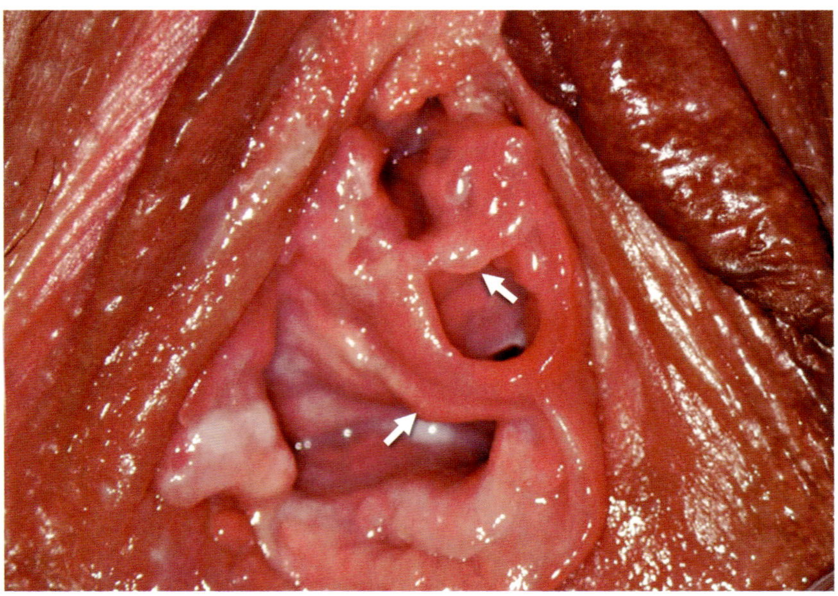

Figure 408 - Congenital vulvar annular bridles (arrows).

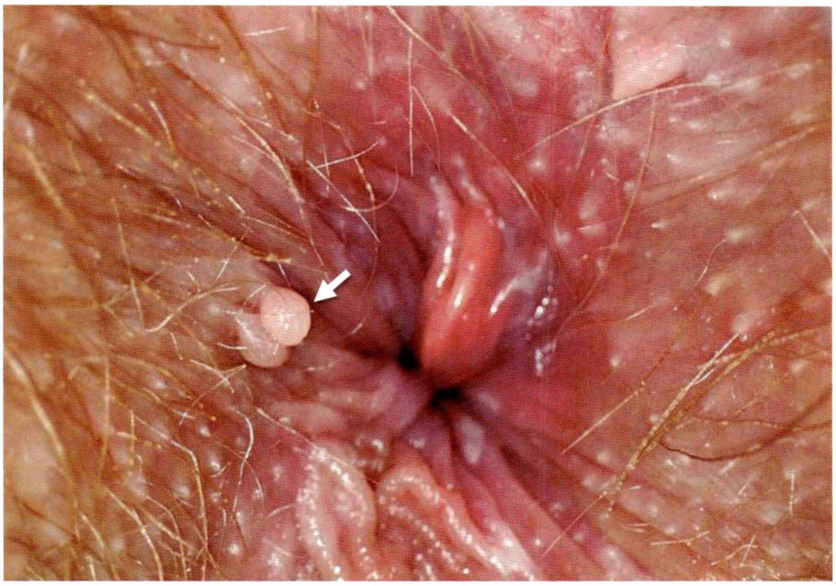

Figure 409 - Pedunculated condylomas (arrow).

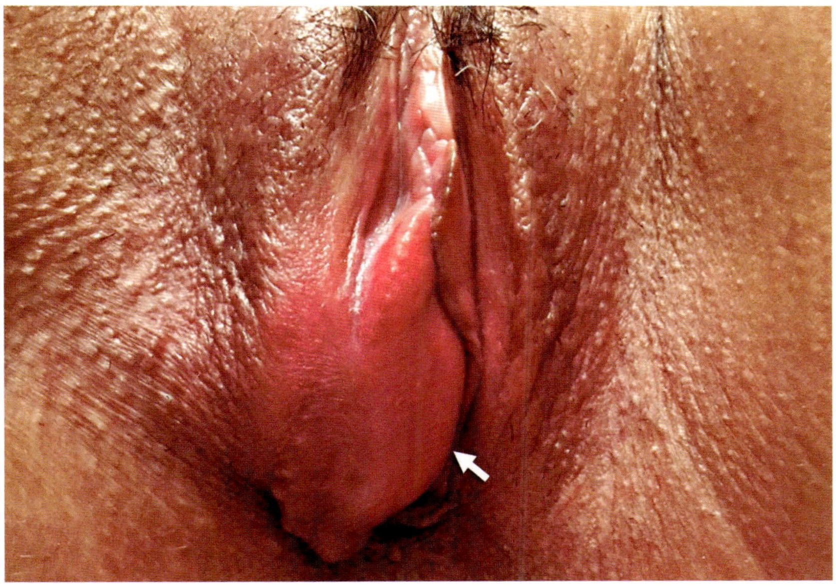

Figure 410 - Bartholin's gland abscess (arrow).

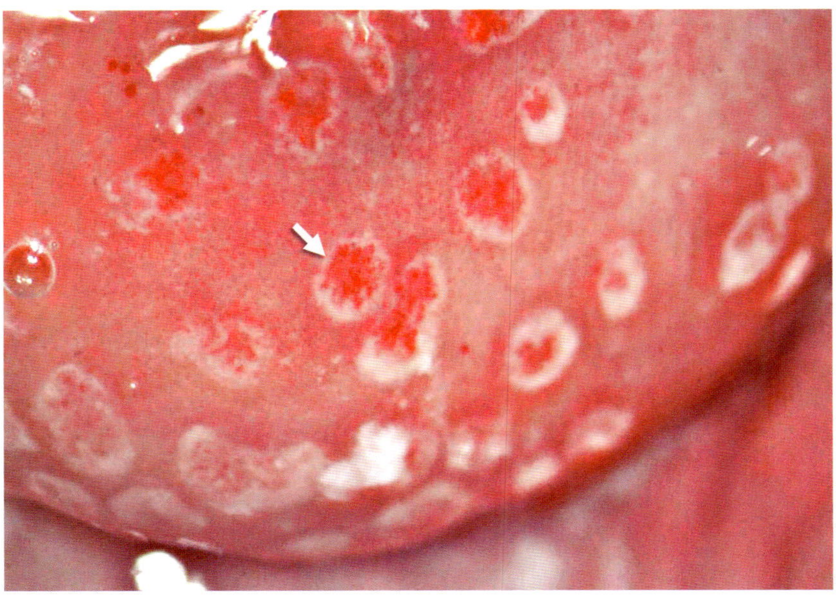

Figure 411 - These scattered lesions characterized by white acetowhite spots centered by dilated capillaries (arrow) are due to Candida infection.

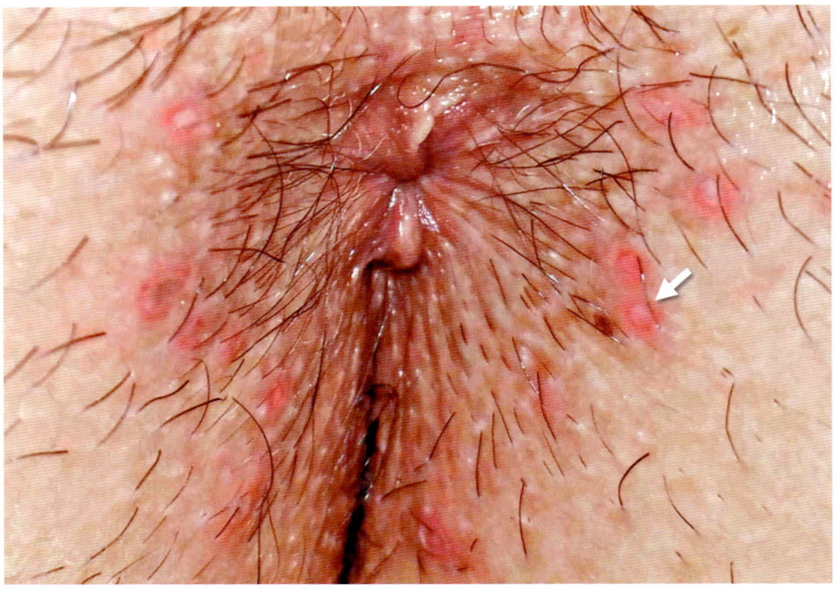

Figure 412 - Perianal herpetic blisters (arrow).

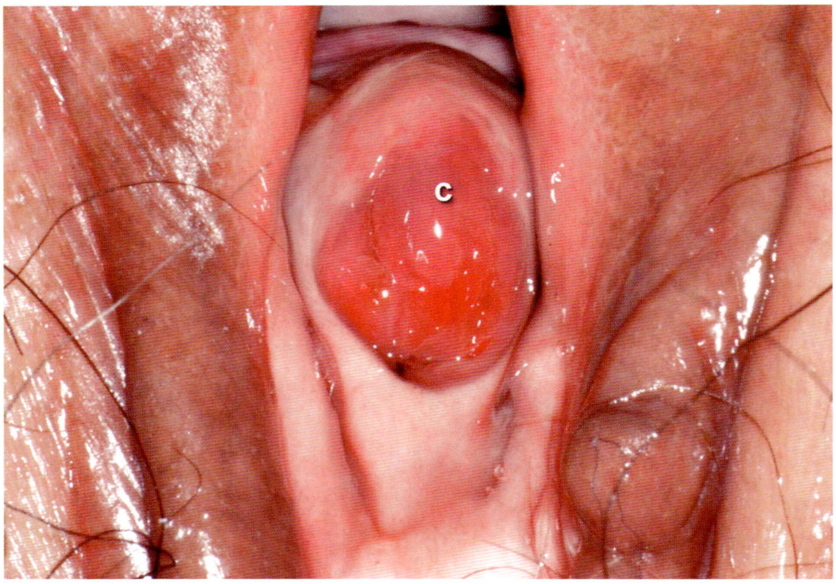

Figure 413 - The urethral caruncle (c) is lined with a thin immature metaplastic tissue.

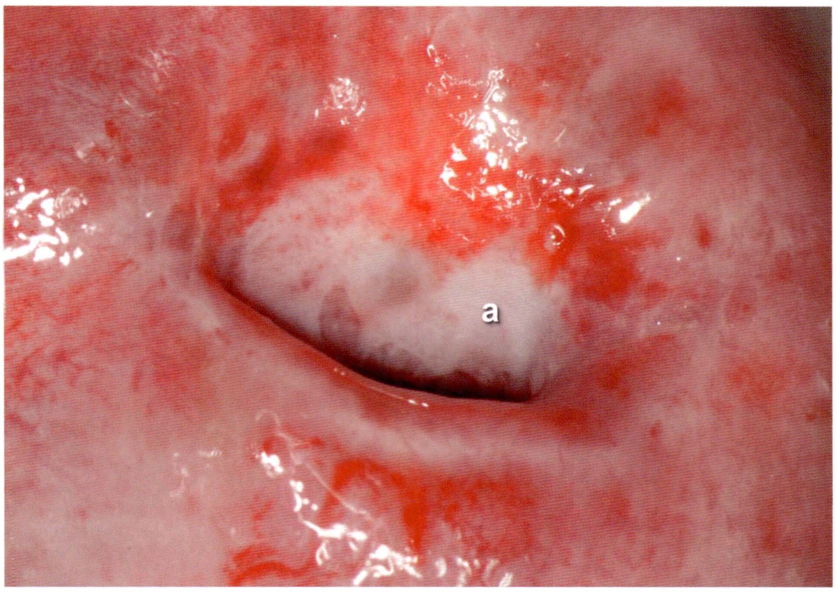

Figure 414 - Dystrophic cervix in menopause. Biopsy of the acetowhite area (a) disclosed a low-grade HPV-CIN lesion.

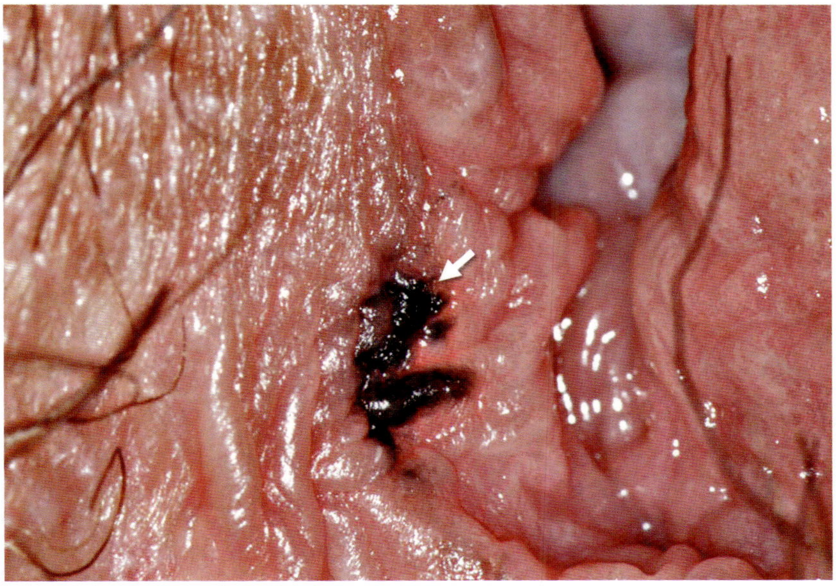

Figure 415 - Vulvar melanoma (arrow).

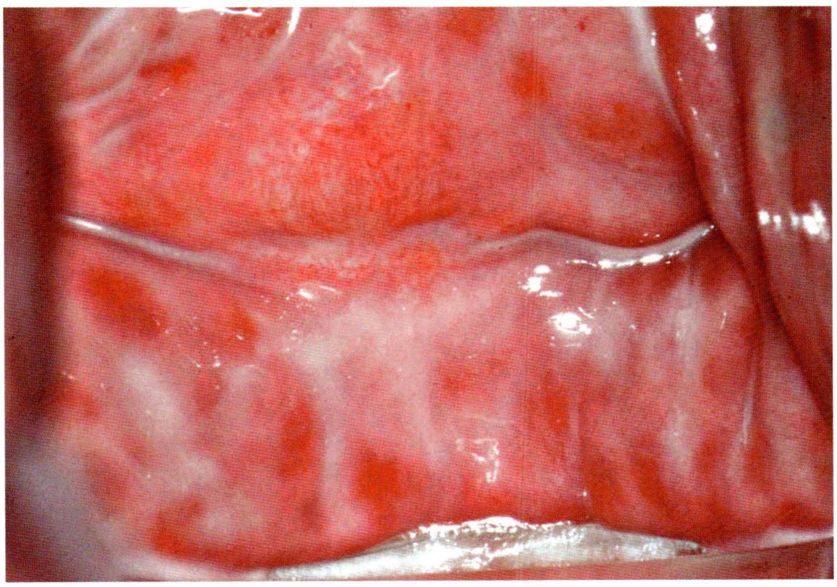

Figure 416 - Vaginal vault following hysterectomy shows dystrophic dilated capillaries clustered in patches.

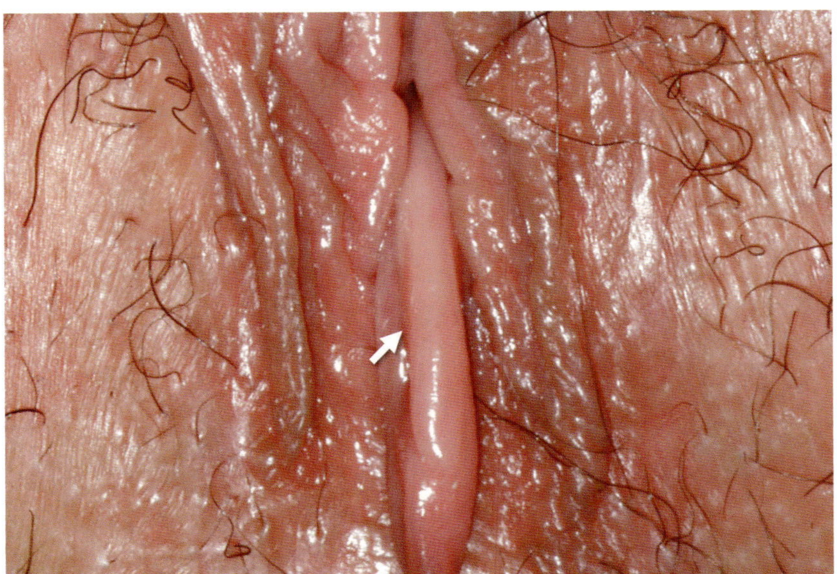

Figure 417 - Hypertrophic hymenal caruncle (arrow).

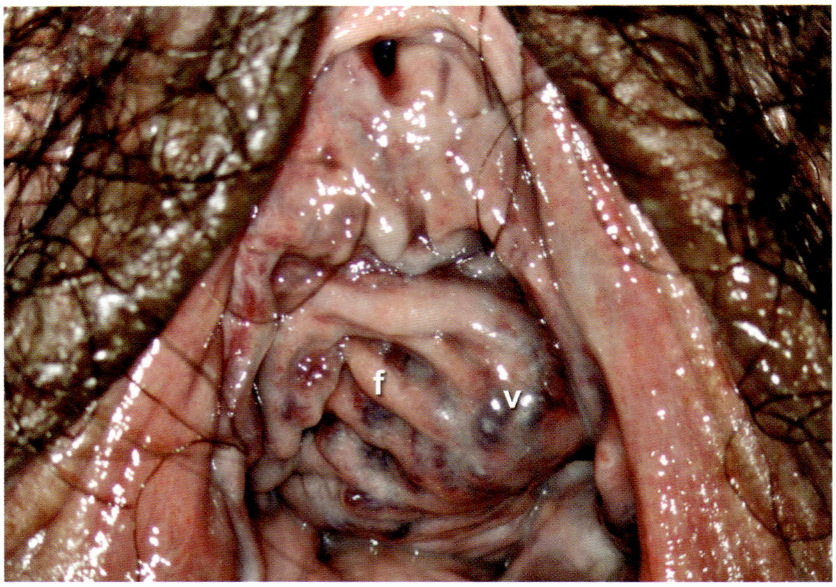

Figure 418 - Mucosal folds (f) of the anterior vaginal wall are associated with vaginal varices (v).

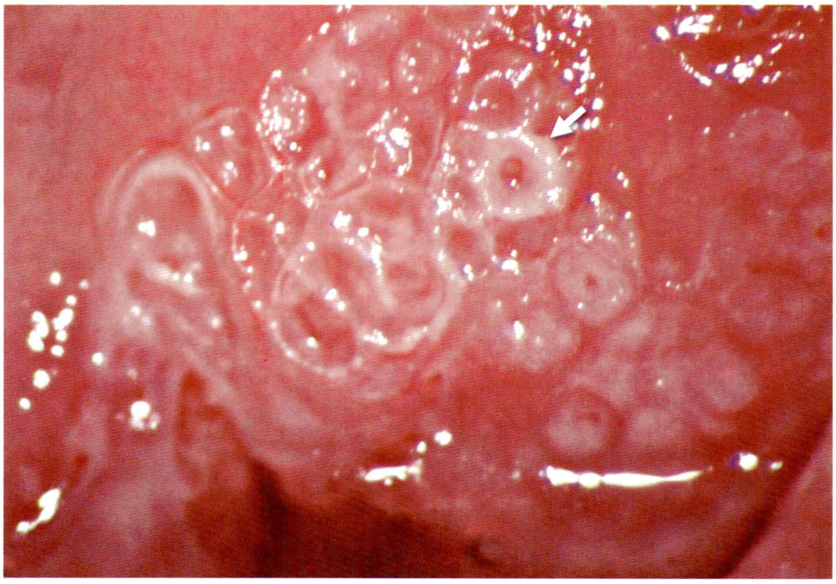

Figure 419 - The arrow indicates a grade IV gland opening, characterized by a distinct and elevated dense acetowhite ring (cuffed gland openings). Histology showed CIN III.

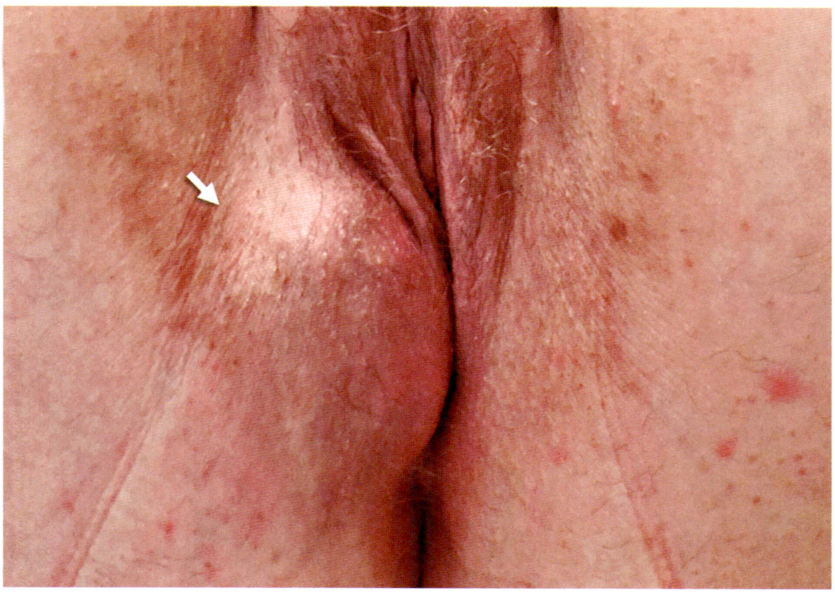

Figure 420 - The voluminous vulvar bulge mimics a Bartholin's cyst but its particular hardness on palpation and extension up to the crural region (arrow), were suspicious. Surgical excision and the resultant pathology disclosed an alveolar rhabdomyosarcoma, involving the pelvis.

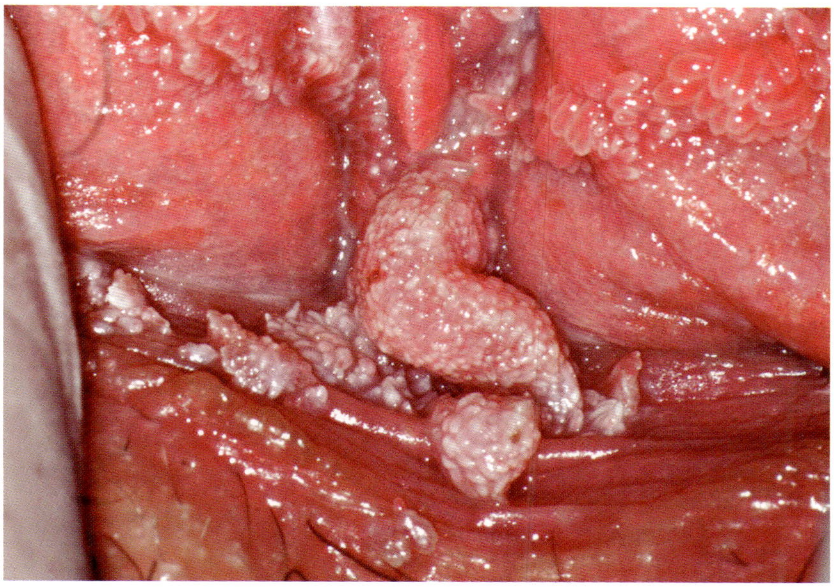

Figure 421 - Florid condylomas at the fourchette.

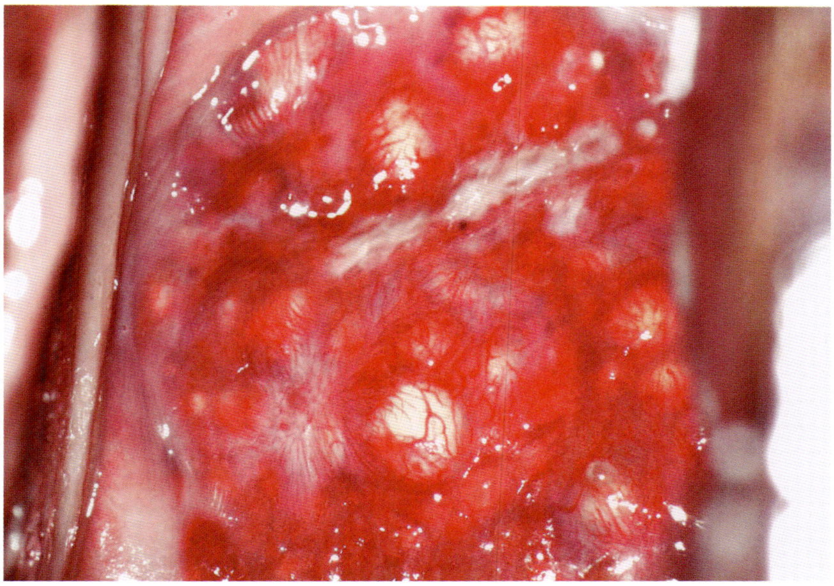

Figure 422 - The cervix is studded with inflamed glandular cysts.

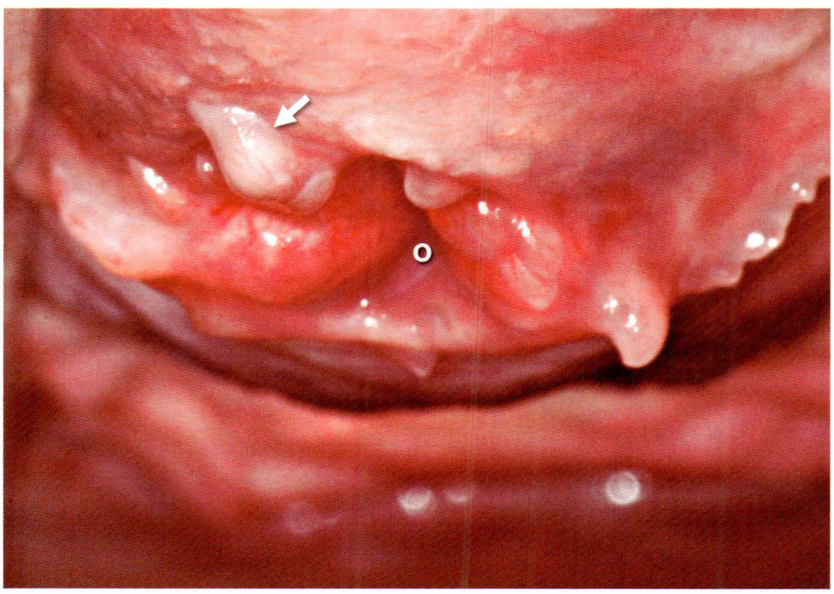

Figure 423 - A flat condyloma (arrow) rises close to the external urethral orifice (o).

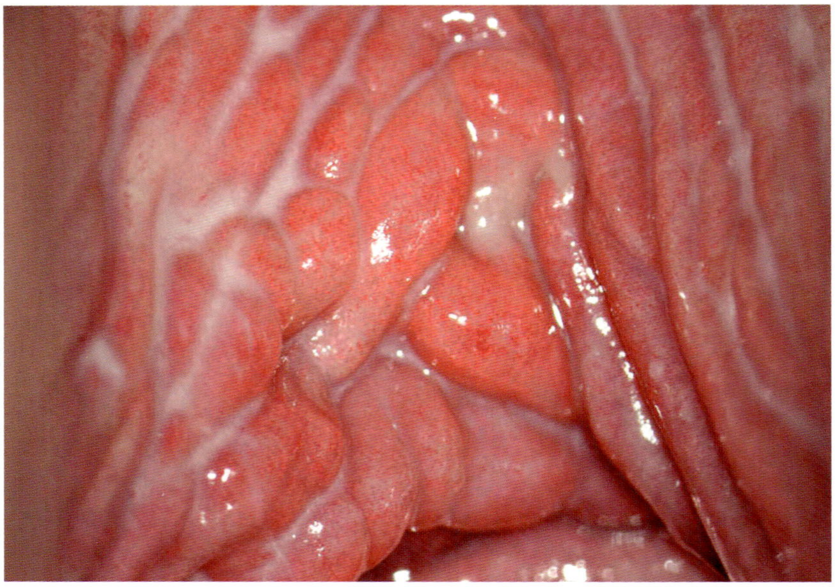

Figure 424 - Normal mucosal bumps of the vaginal wall.

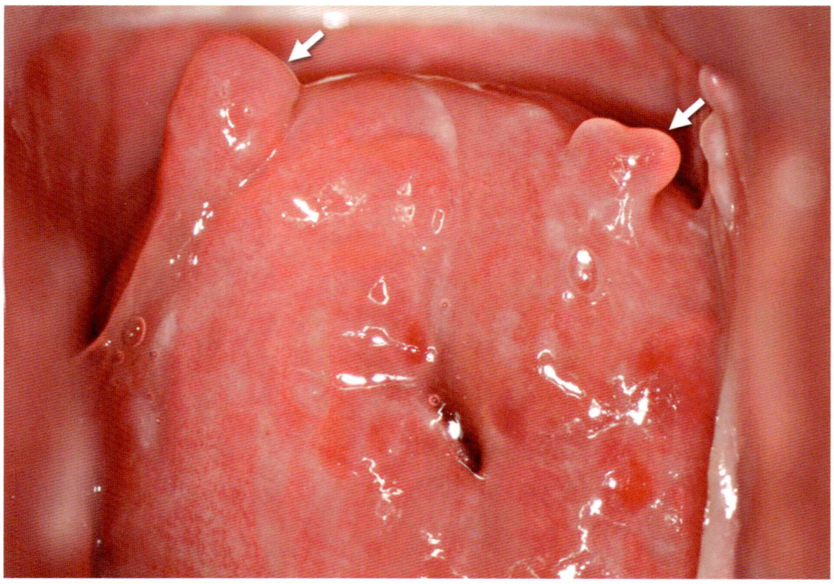

Figure 425 - "Piggy bank" localized cervical hypertrophies (arrows).

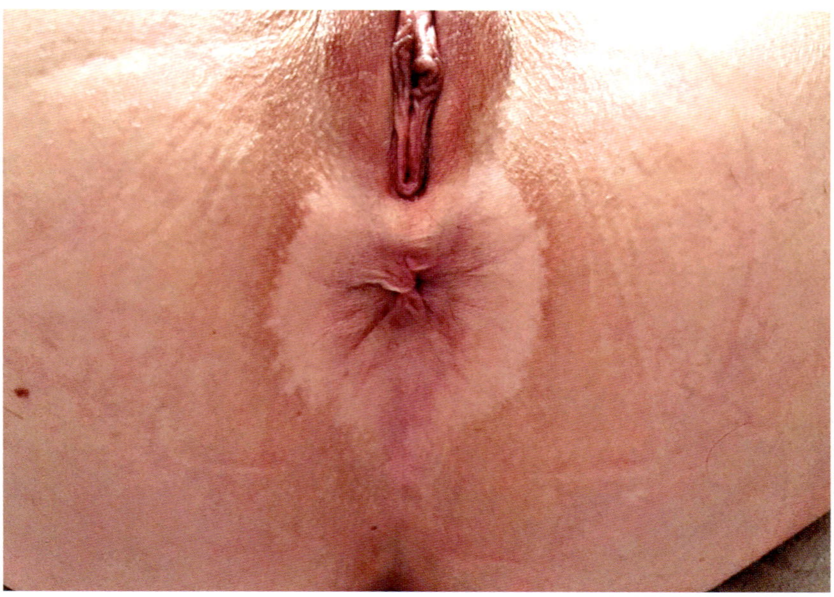

Figure 426 - Perianal hypopigmentation following healed psoriasis.

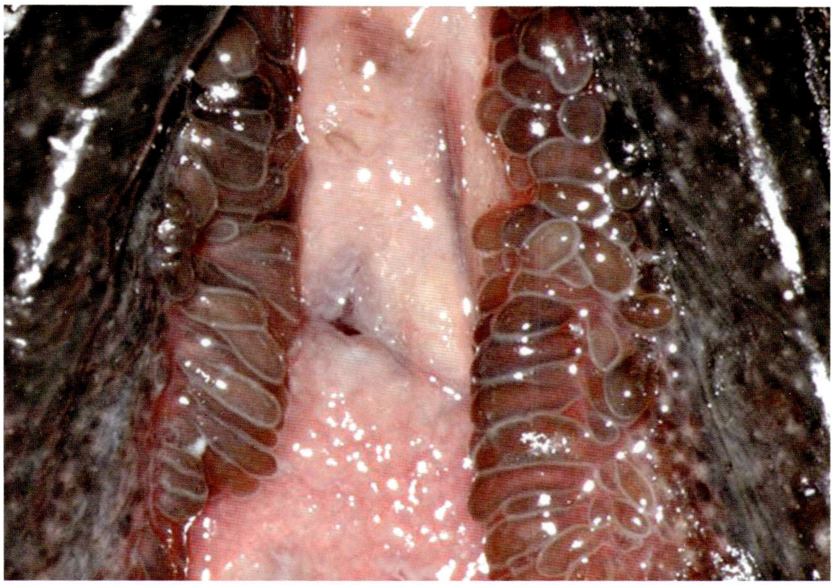

Figure 427 - Hypertrophic vestibular papillae.

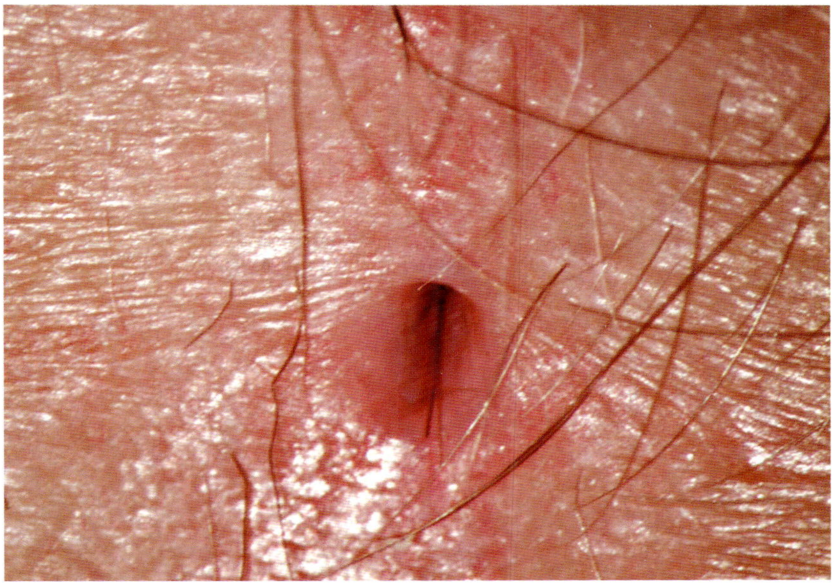

Figure 428 - A tuft of hair comes from the congenital sacral dimple.

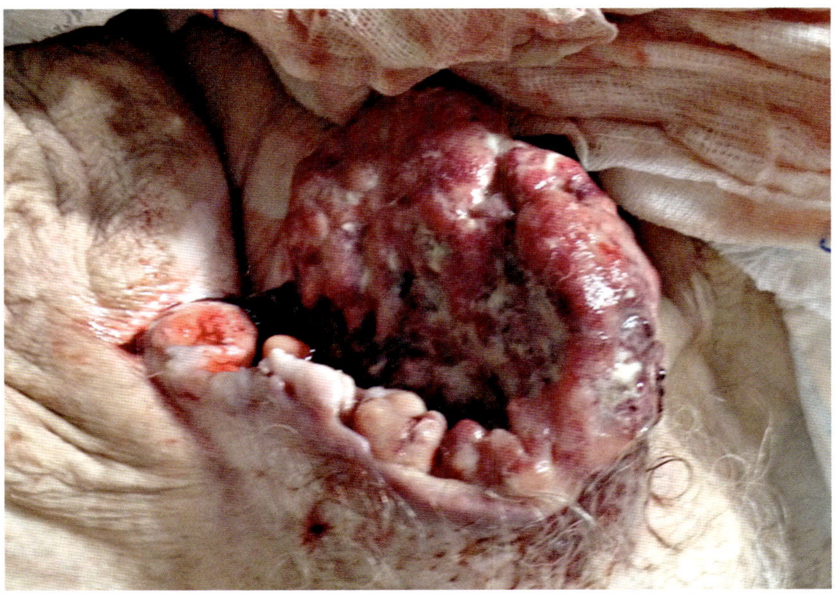

Figure 429 - Ulcerated, invasive carcinoma of the vulva.

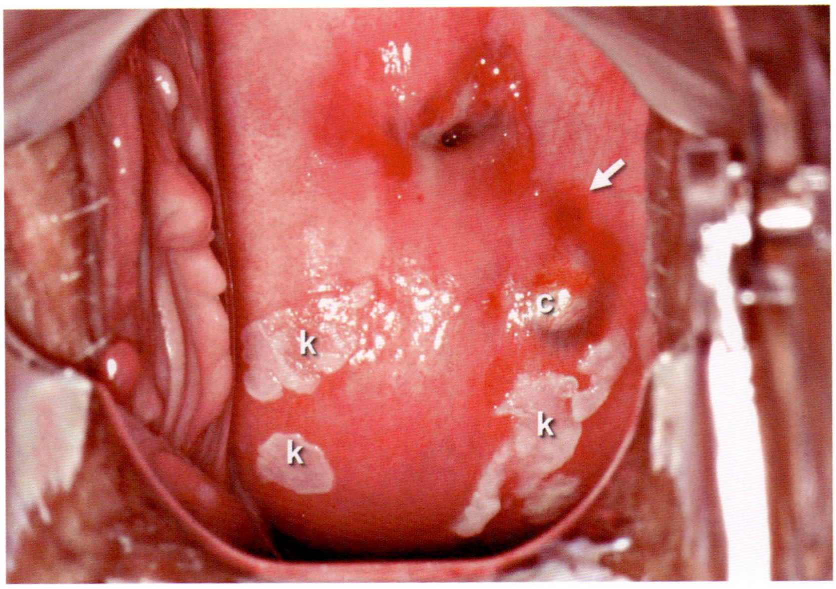

Figure 430 - Patches of keratosis (k), nabothian cyst (c) and hemorrhagic effusions (arrow) following diathermy.

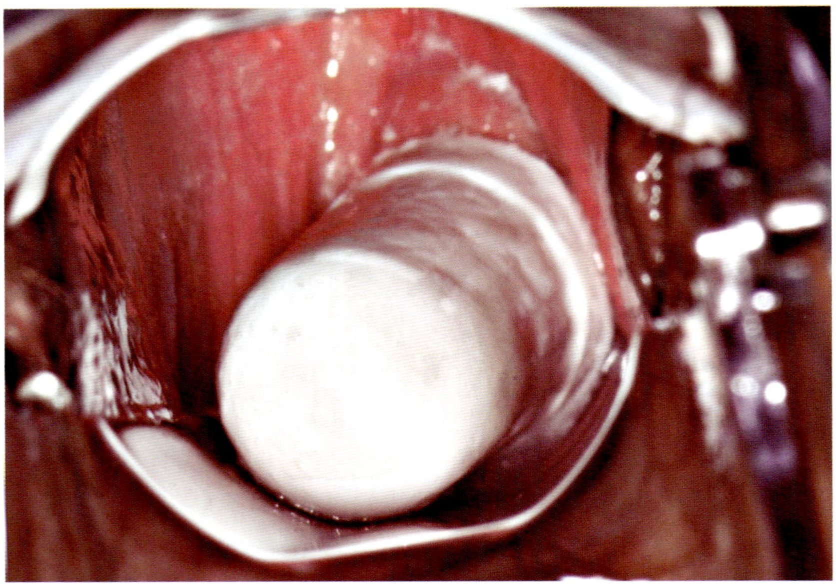

Figure 431 - Retention of the cap of a vaginal douche in the vagina, full of white, malodorous discharge.

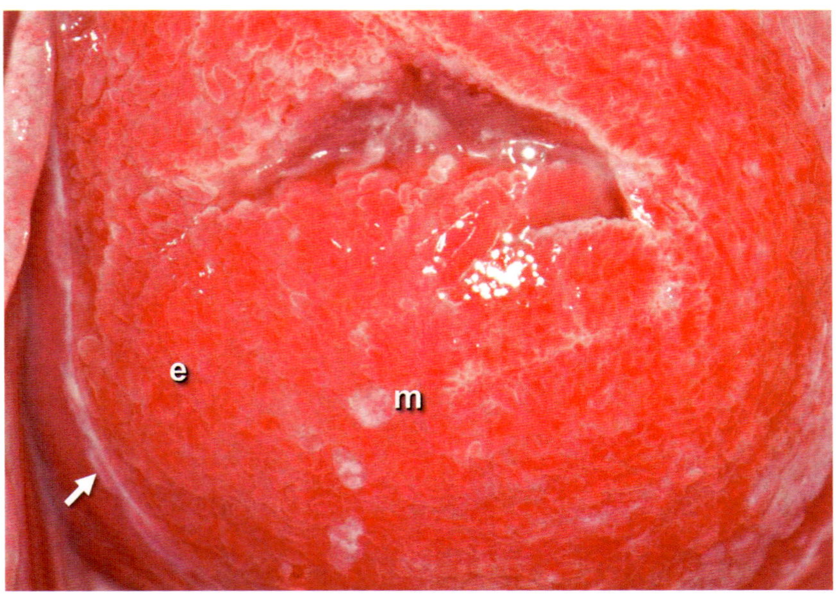

Figure 432 - Extensive exposed columnar epithelium (e). The white opacity corresponds to islands of immature metaplastic epithelium (m).
The arrow indicated the original squamocolumnar junction.

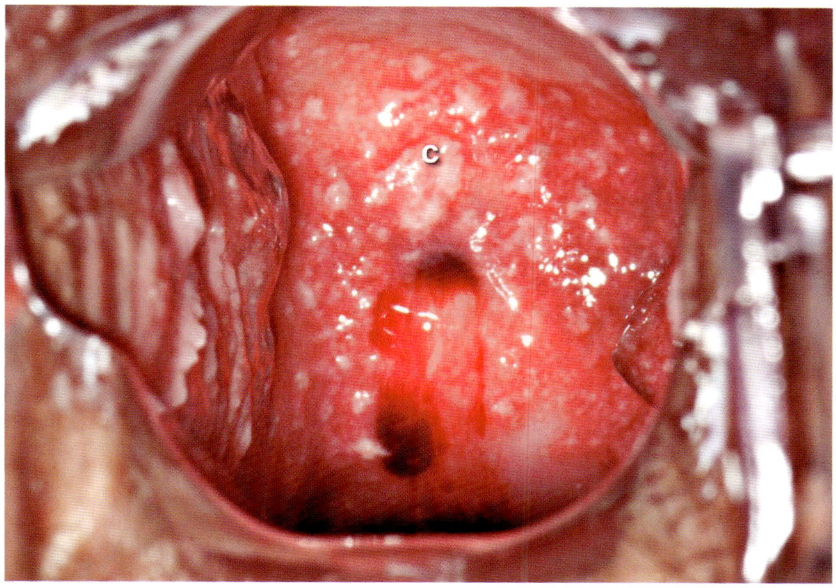

Figure 433 - Diffuse cervical HPV flat condylomas (c).

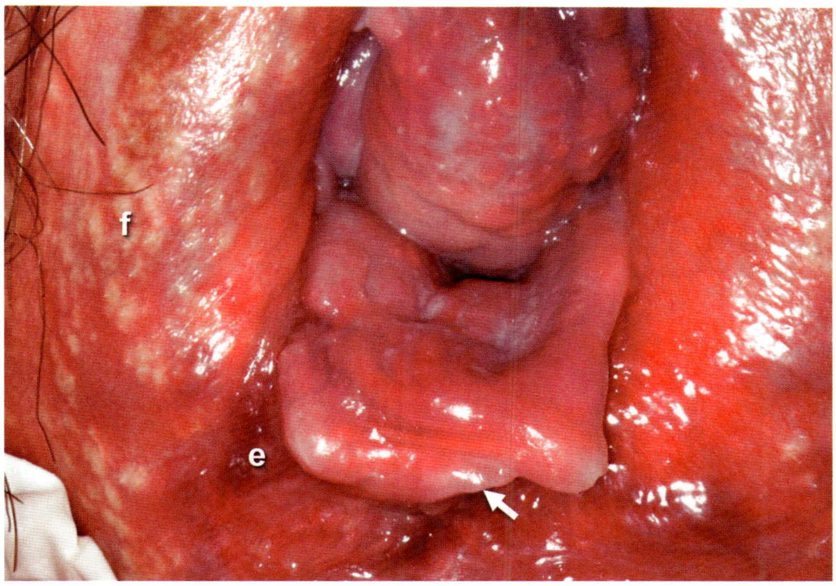

Figure 434 - Babe bib-like hypertrophic hymenal caruncle (arrow), hemorrhagic effusions (e), and Fordyce spots (f).

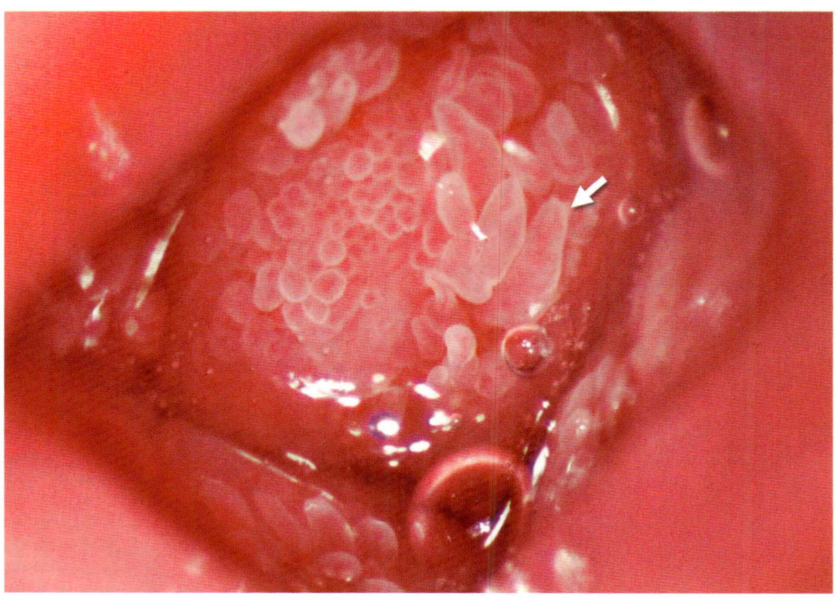

Figure 435 - Hypertrophic villi (arrow) overlap the stem of arbor vitae.

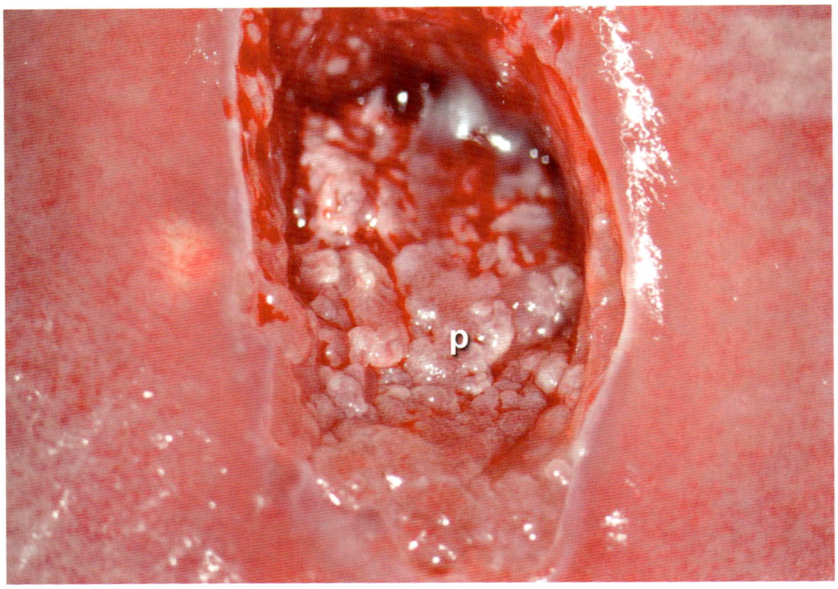

Figure 436 - After application of acetic acid, enlarged and fused papillae (p) turn whitish. Histology disclosed adenocarcinoma.

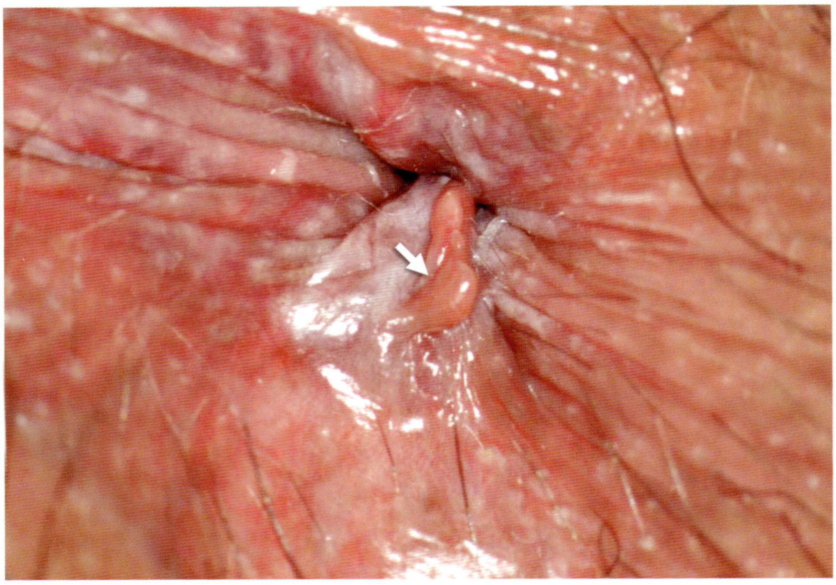

Figure 437 - Anal fibroids (arrow) over an acetowhite area.

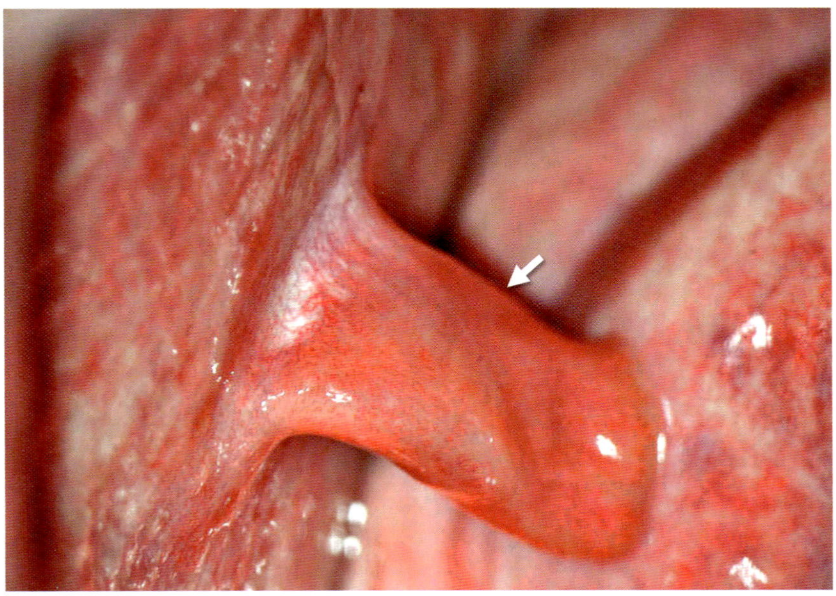

Figure 438 - A bridge of tissue (arrow) connects the right lateral wall to the cervix.

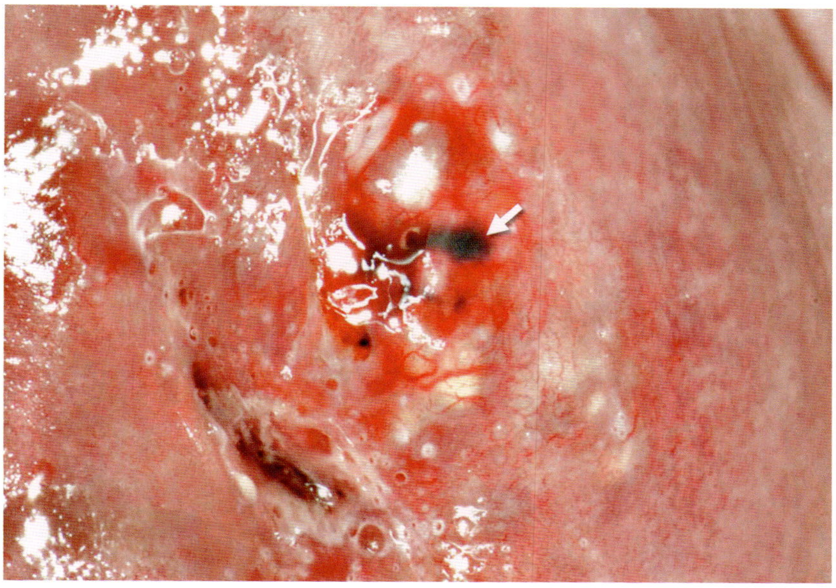

Figure 439 - Endometrial focus (arrow).

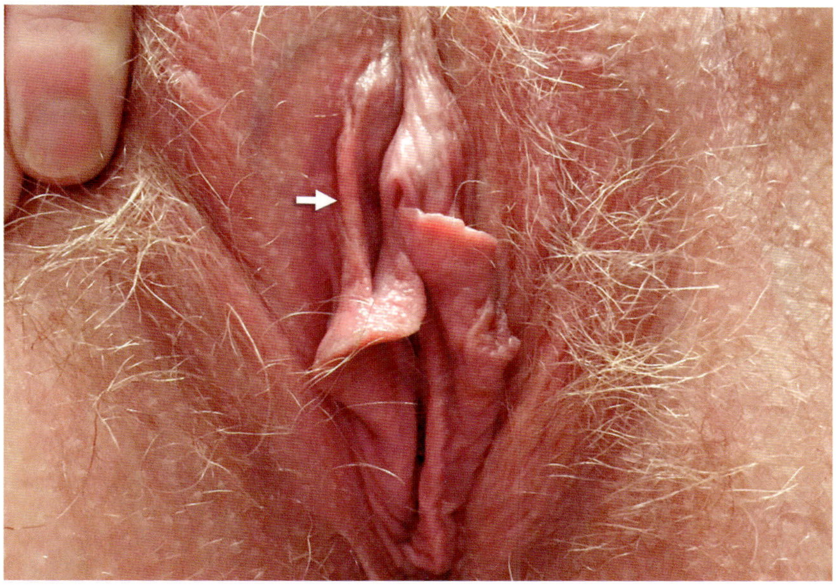

Figure 440 - Duplicated right labium minus (arrow).

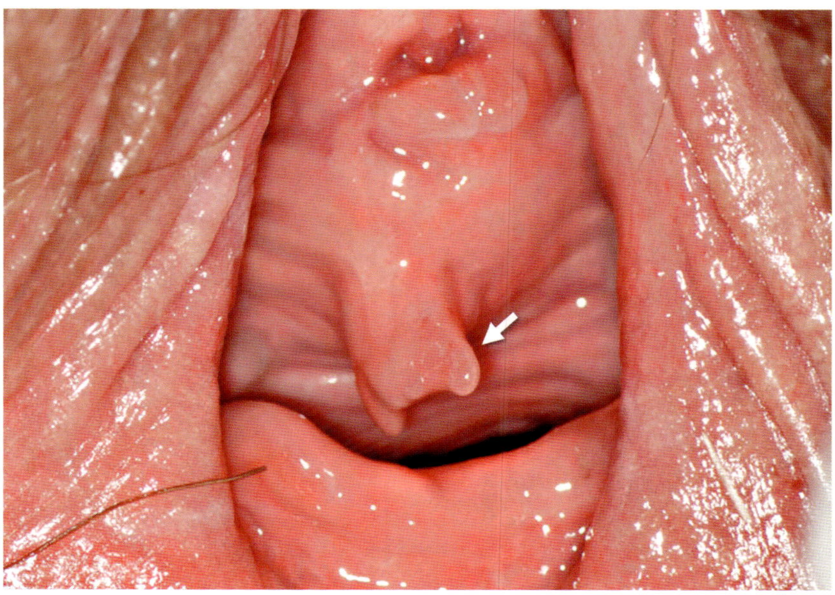

Figure 441 - Hypertrophic structure (arrow) from the anterior vaginal wall.

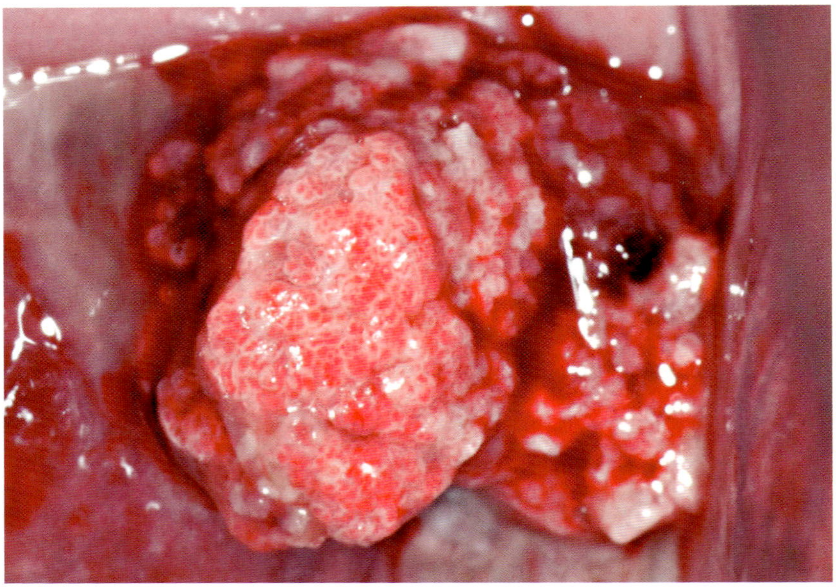

Figure 442 - The polypoid friable and fragile lesion shows fused and enlarged papillae of columnar epithelium, and dilated atypical vessels. Histology disclosed an HPV related adenocarcinoma, usual type.

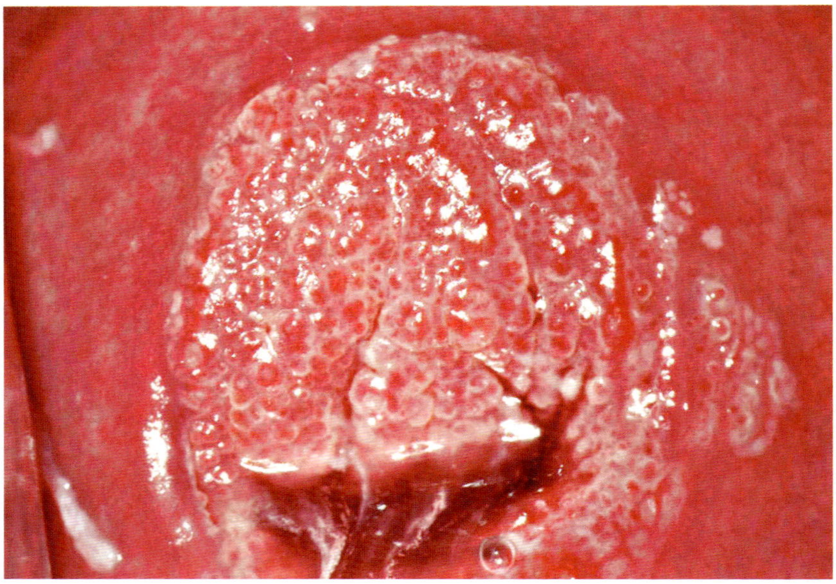

Figure 443 - The coarse punctation displays large and widely separated petechiae over a faint acetowhite epithelium. Despite the coarse punctation, histology showed a low-grade HPV-CIN lesion.

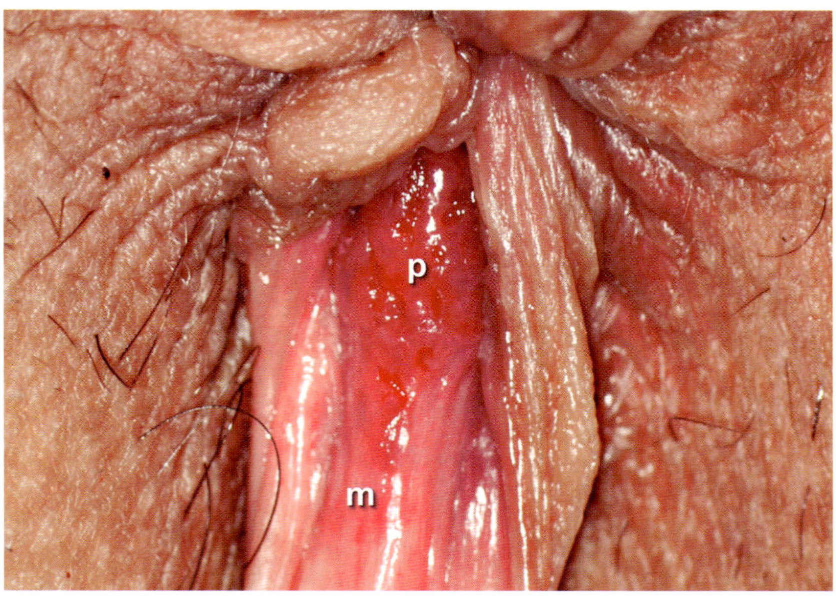

Figure 444 - Pushing aside the anal marisca (m), a prolapsed anal mucosa (p) reveals multiple erosions.

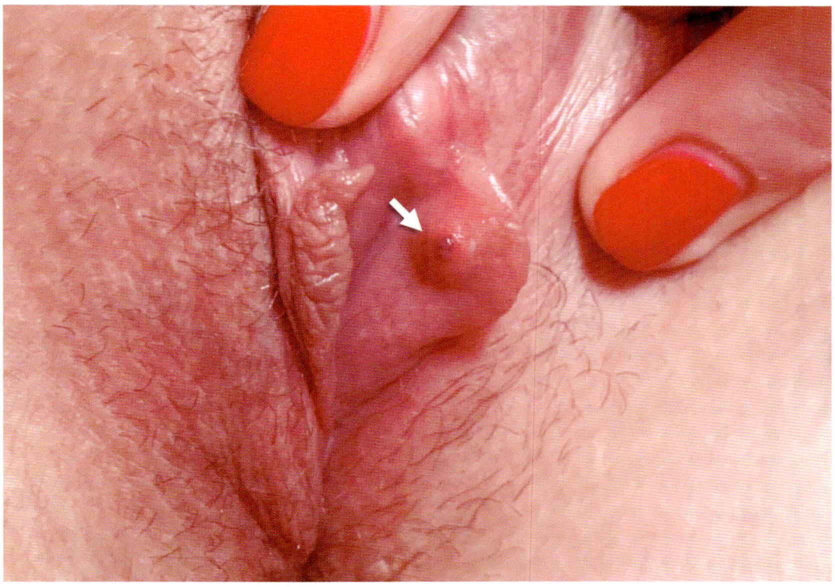

Figure 445 - Gland abscess (arrow) of the left labium minus.

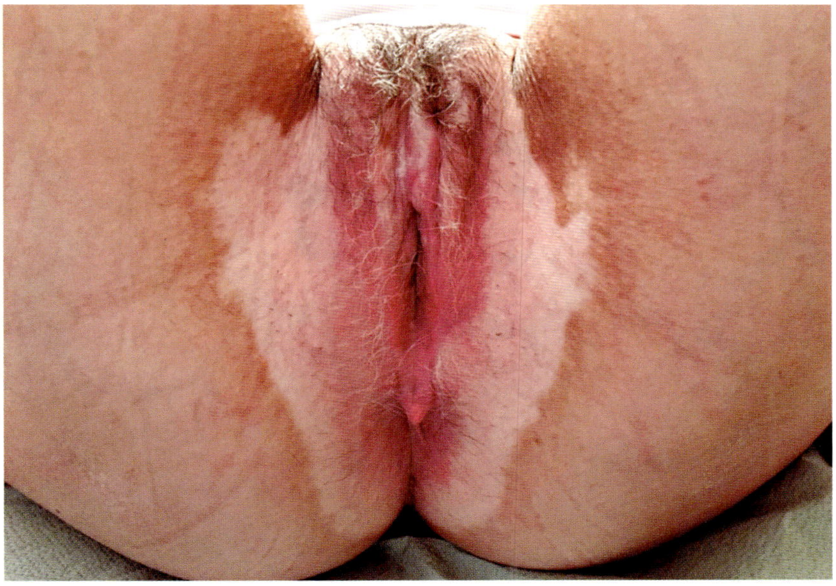

Figure 446 - Vulvar and crural vitiligo.

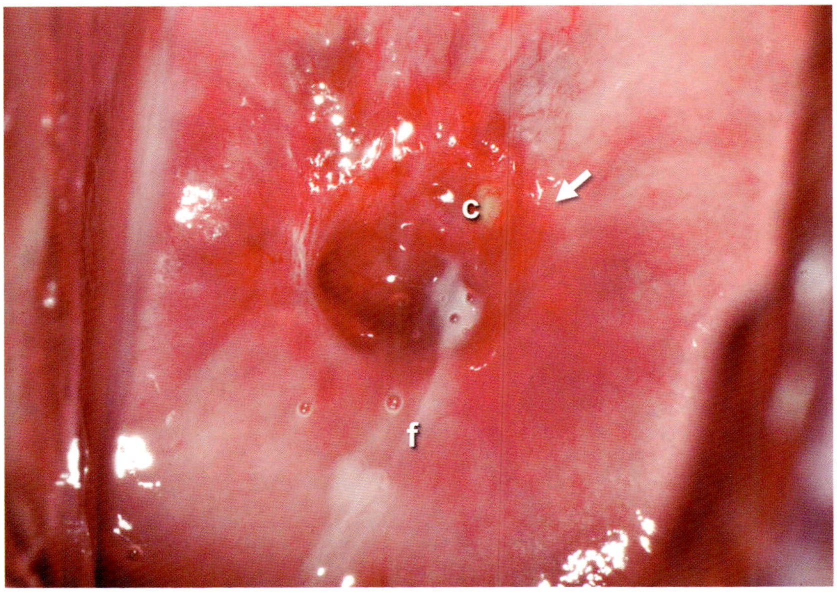

Figure 447 - A visible squamocolumnar junction (arrow) in menopause must make the observer suspect an estrogen stimulation and requires further investigation. Cyto-hormonal evaluation by direct microscopy confirmed an estrogen smear. Endocervical cyst (c) and vaginal fluid (f).

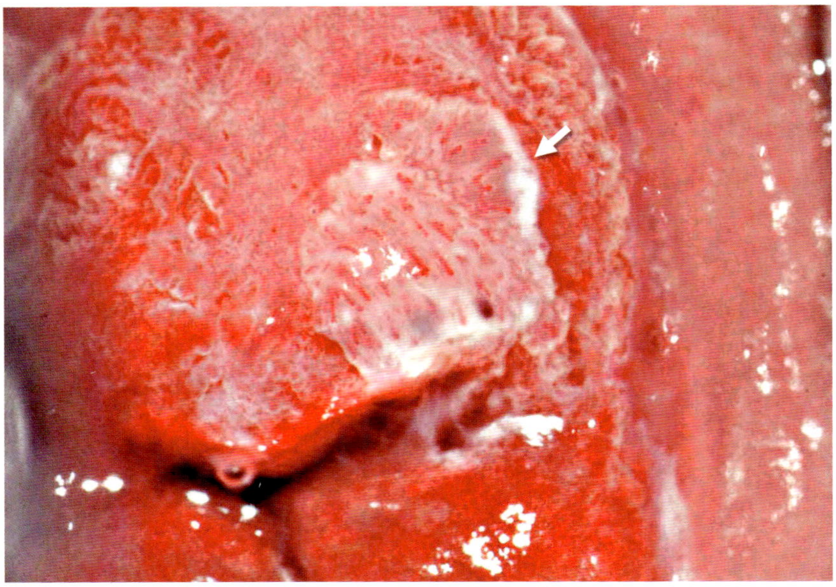

Figure 448 - The arrowed well-defined acetowhite area shows dilated hairpin capillaries. Histology disclosed a low-grade CIN lesion.

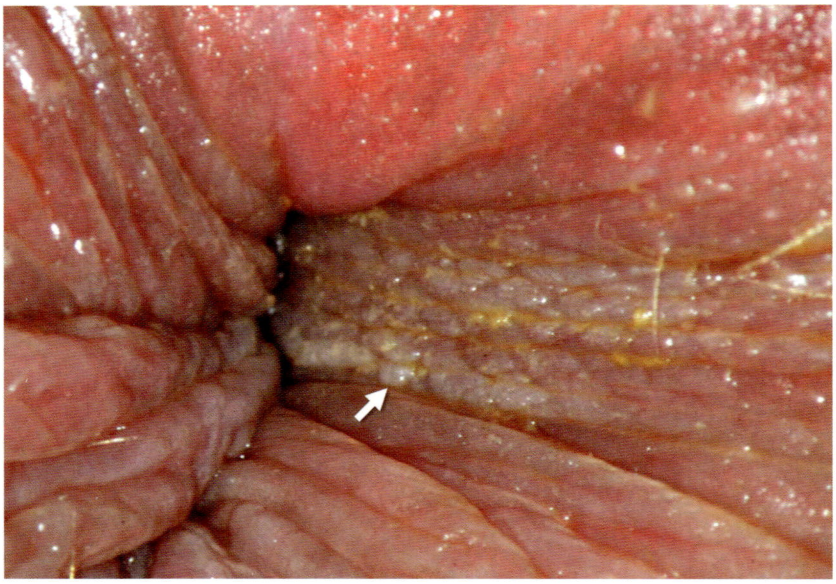

Figure 449 - Anal HPV micropapillary lesions (arrow).

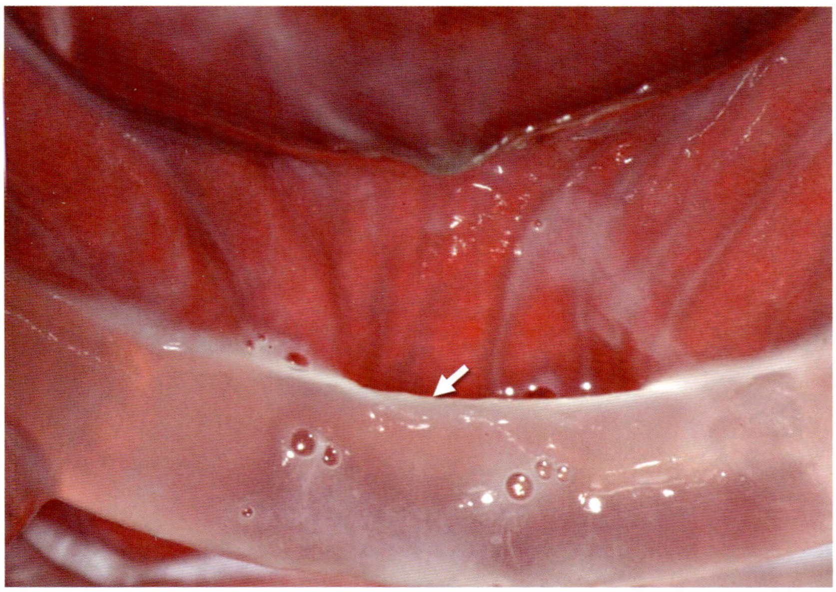

Figure 450 - The contraceptive ring (arrow) harbors a white and frothy discharge in bacterial vaginosis.

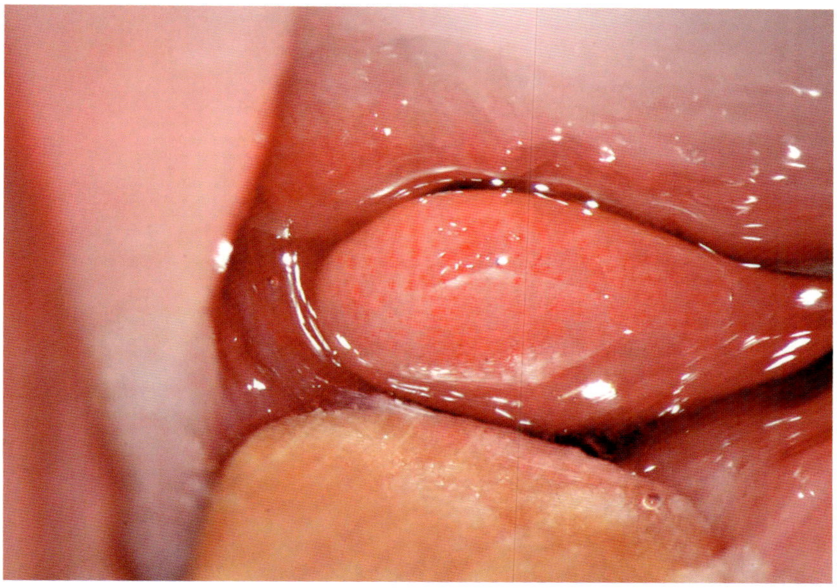

Figure 451 - Cervical polyp showing fine punctation.

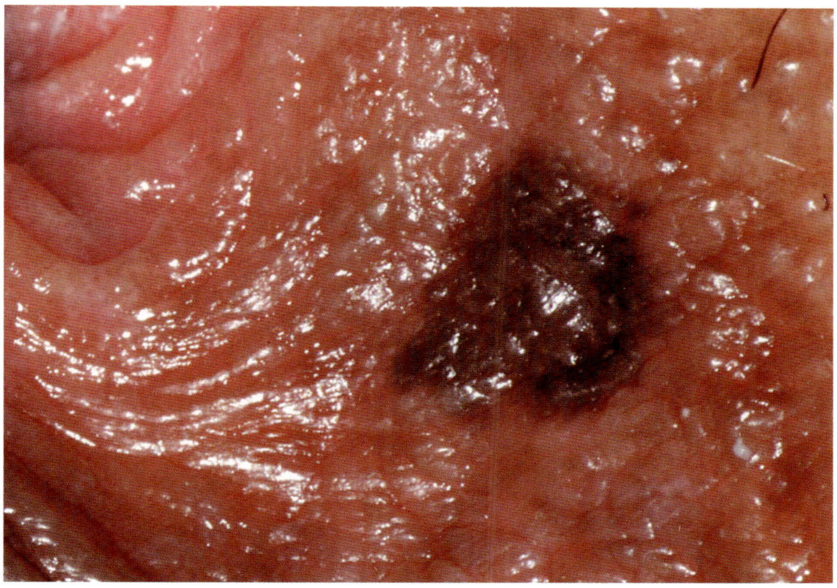

Figure 452 - Melanocytic nevus.

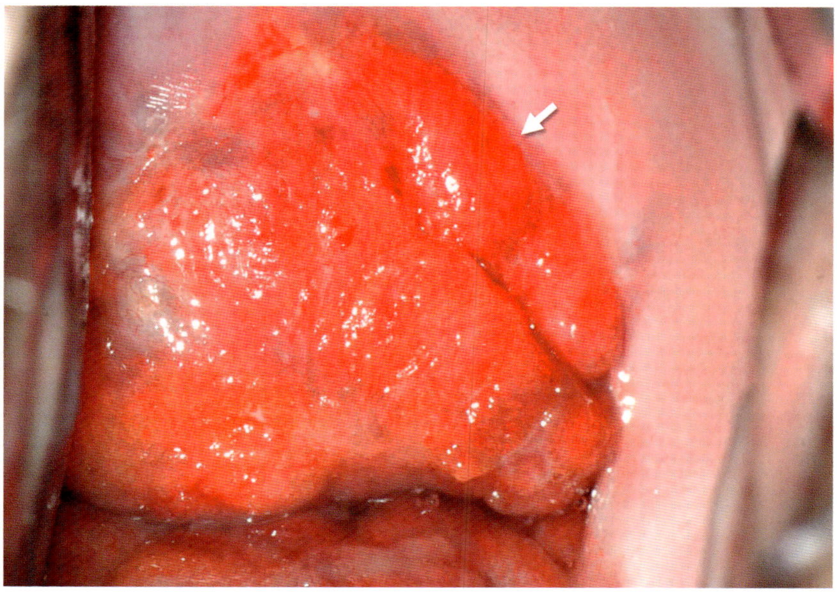

Figure 453 - Ectropion appears as a marked eversion of the endocervical mucosa, strikingly reddish and with raised margins (arrow).

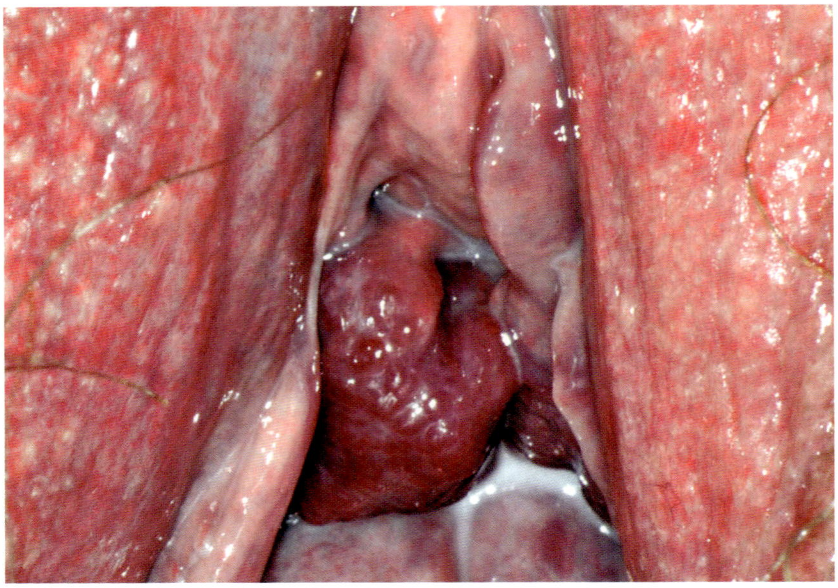

Figure 454 - Periurethral hemangioma.

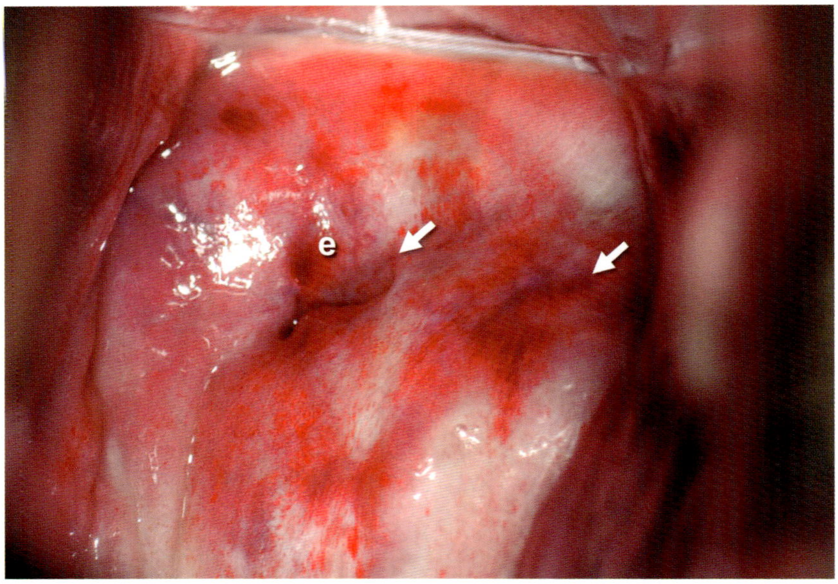

Figure 455 - Severe atrophy of the vaginal vault following hysterectomy, with hemorrhagic effusions (e). The arrows indicate the dog ears.

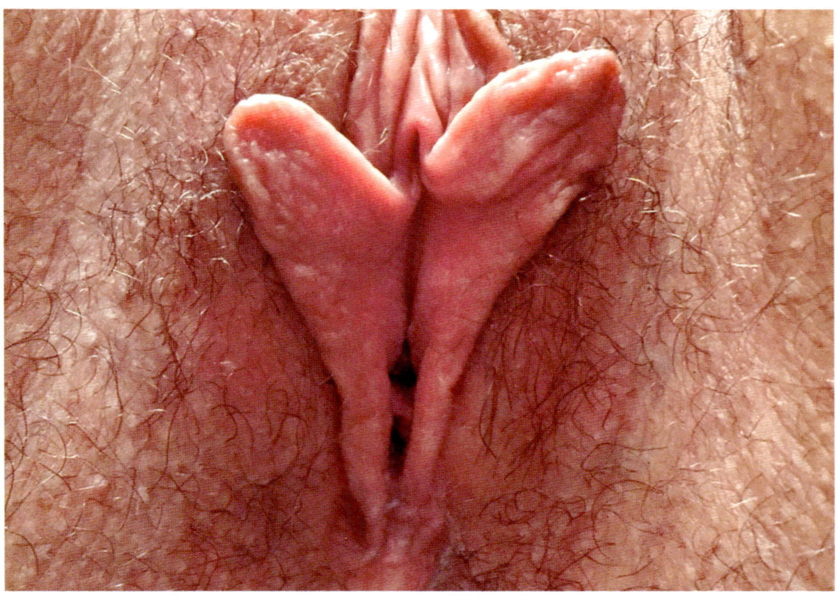

Figure 456 - Butterfly-like labia minora.

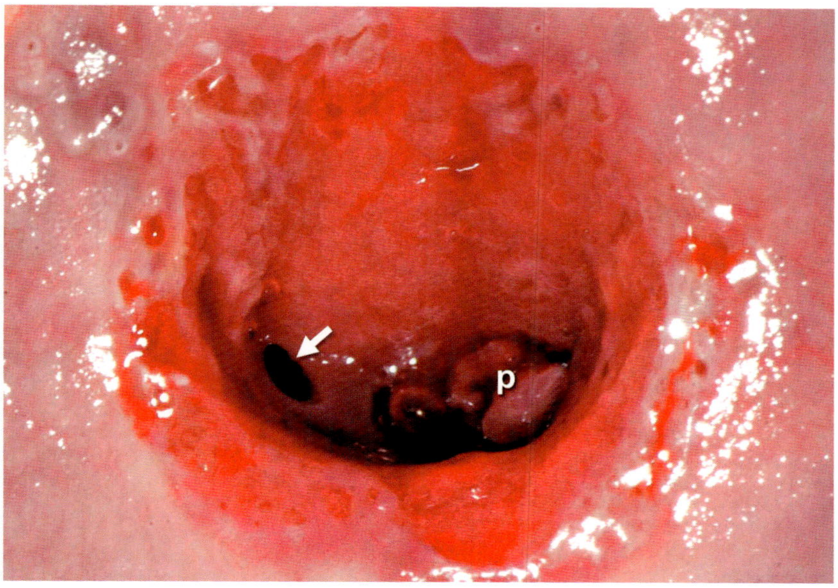

Figure 457 - The cervical canal shows polyps (p) and a spontaneously opened endocervical cyst (arrow).

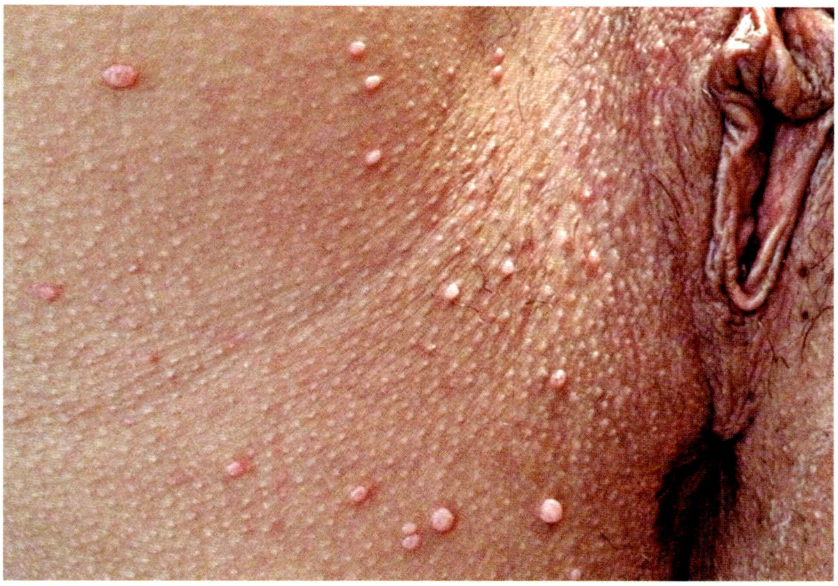

Figure 458 - Overspread molluscum contagiosum.

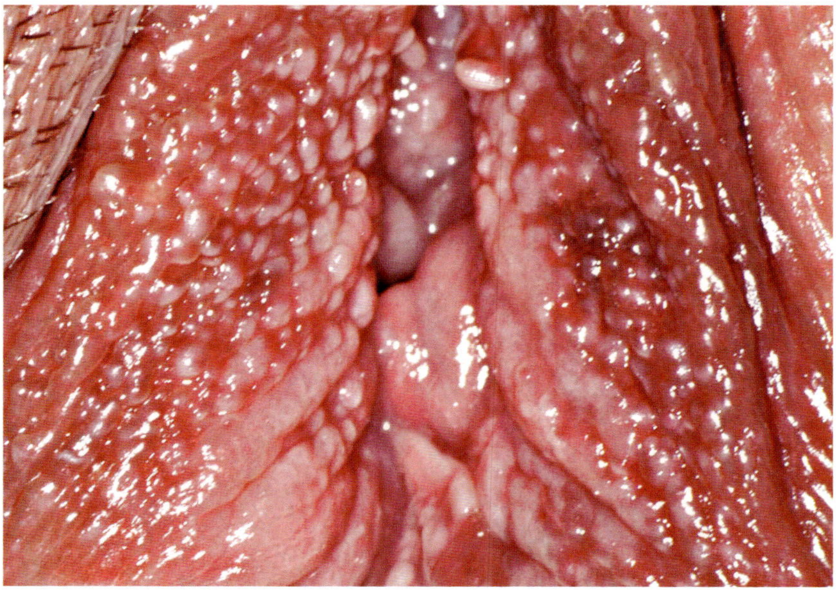

Figure 459 - Diffuse acetowhite areas due to poorly glycogenated epithelium.

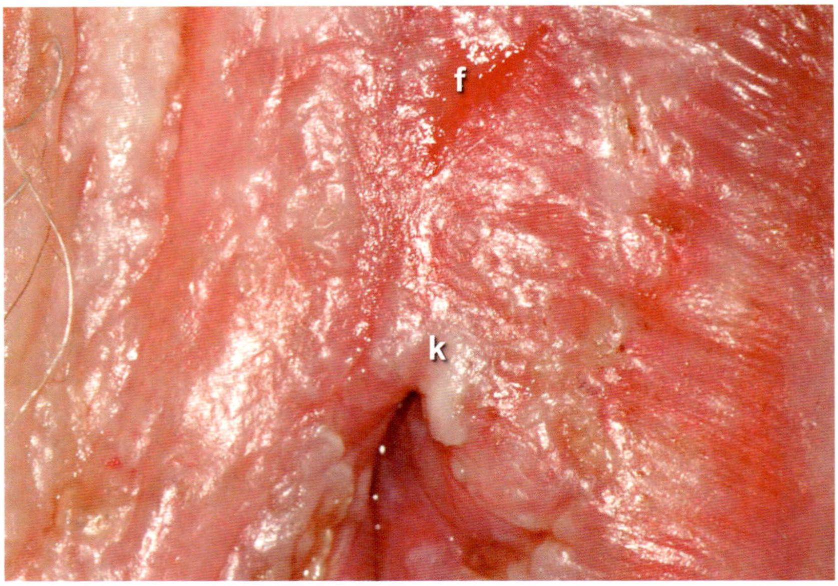

Figure 460 - Cellophane paper-type appearance of the skin in lichen sclerosus. The colpophotograph shows a skin fissure (f) and a plaque of keratosis (k) above the clitoris, completely buried.

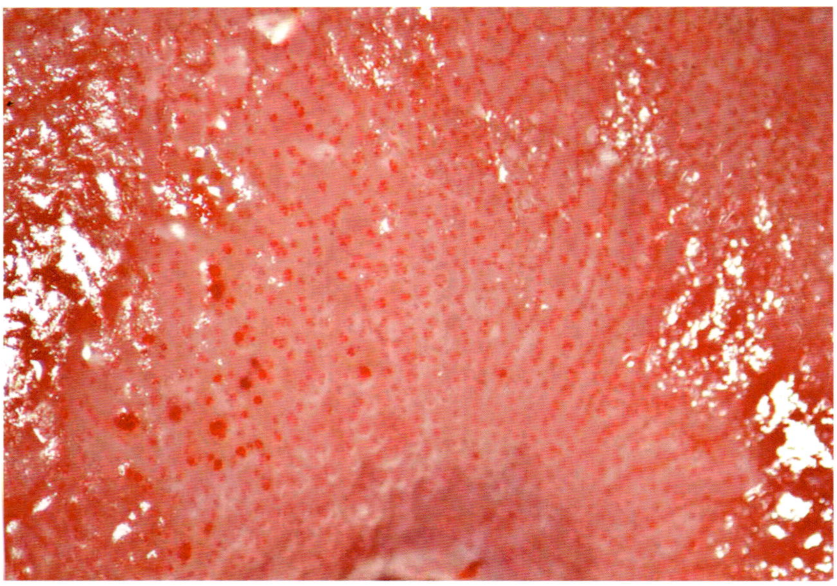

Figure 461 - Healing lines following ablative procedure show irregular in size dots.

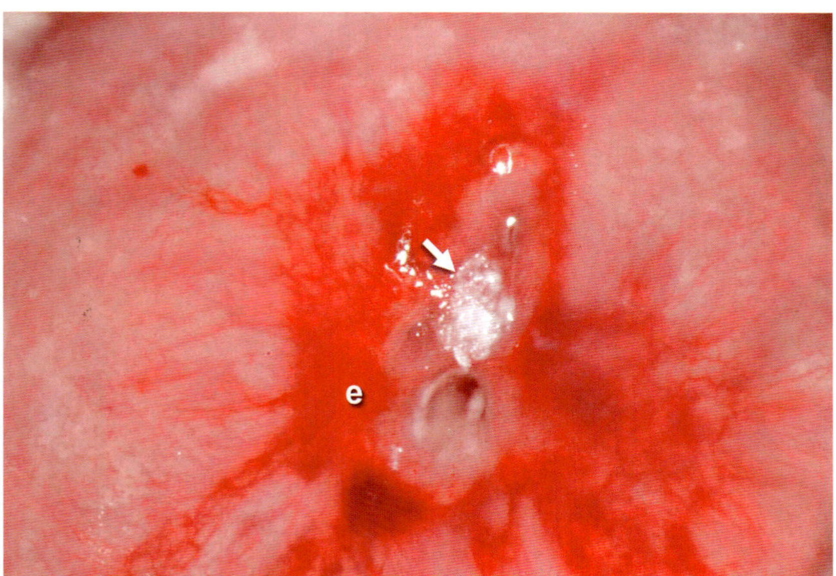

Figure 462 - Hemorrhagic effusions (e) following diathermy surround a thick keratosis (arrow). Histology disclosed carcinoma in situ underlying keratin.

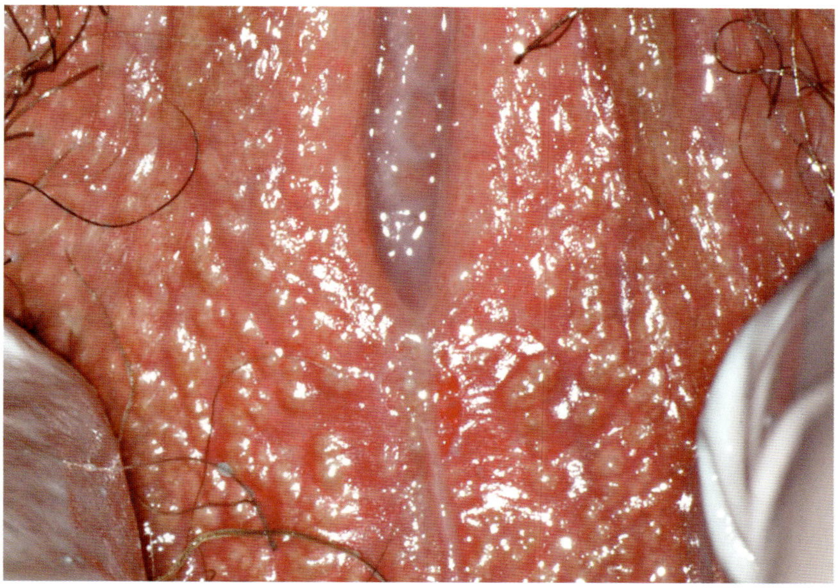

Figure 463 - Vulvar Fordyce dots.

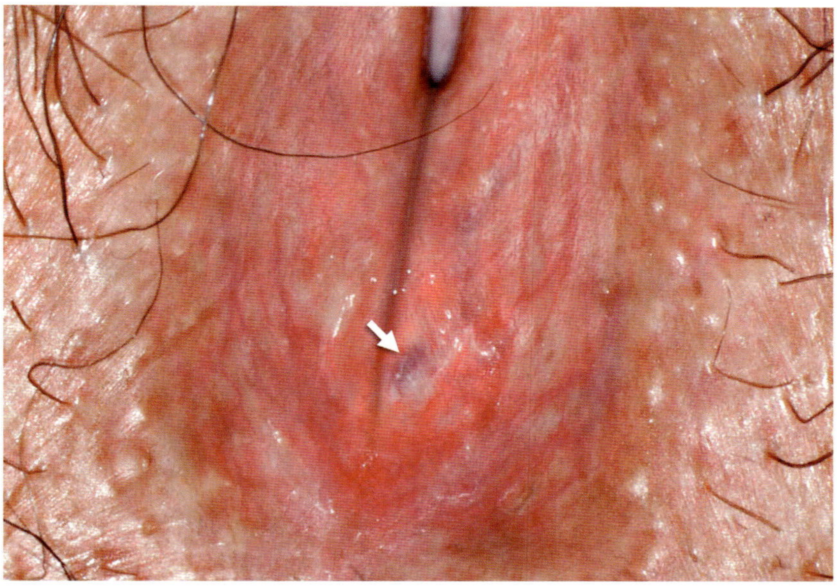

Figure 464 - The arrow indicates the characteristic atrophic dimple in the presence of vulvar vestibulitis.

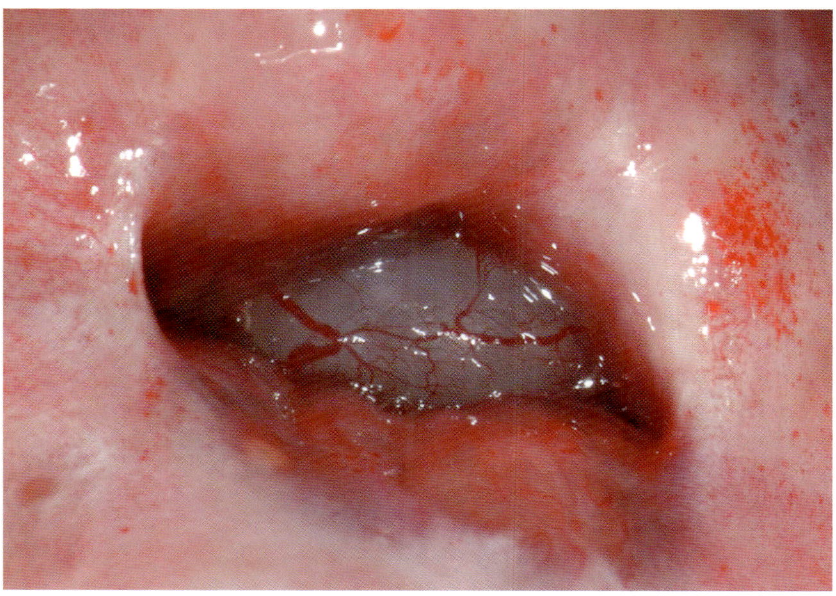

Figure 465 - Endocervical cyst.

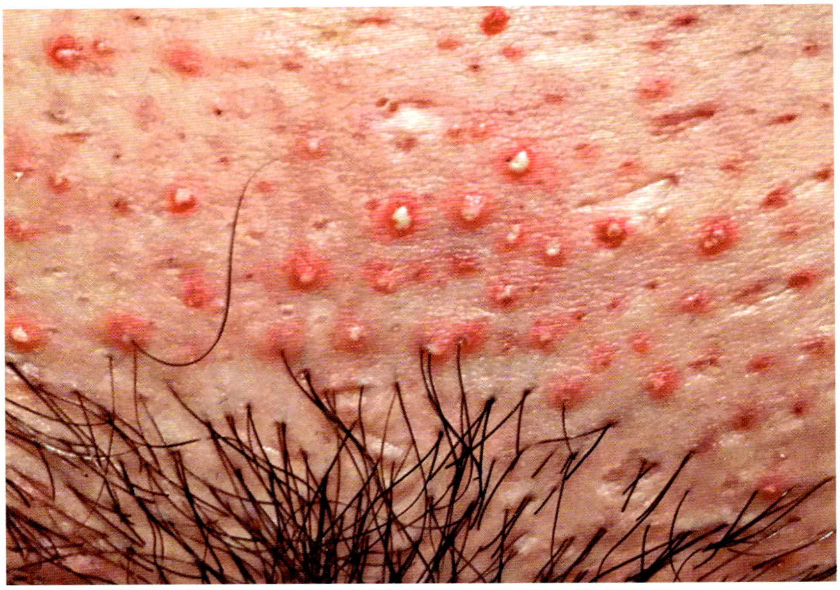

Figure 466 - Folliculitis of the pubic area is characterized by diffuse red bumps or white-headed pimples around hair follicles.

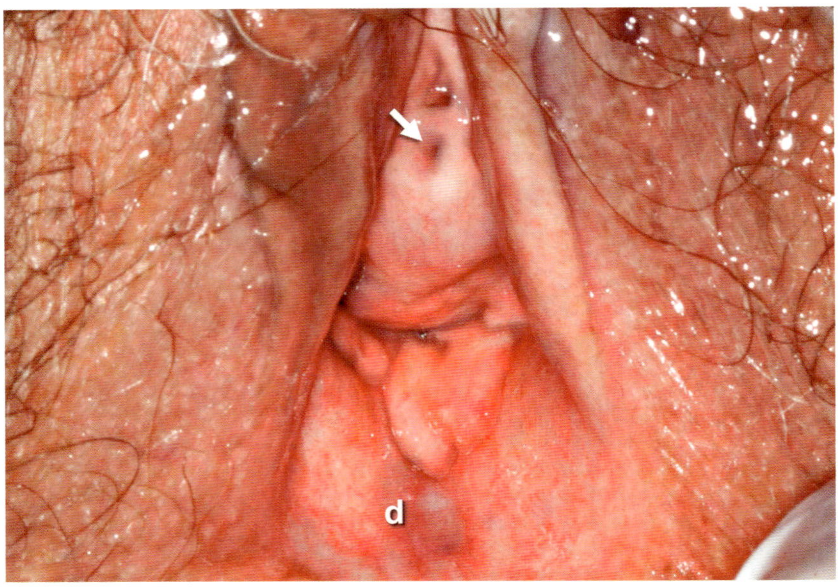

Figure 467 - Rare urethral duplication. The arrow indicates the urethral meatus of the accessory urethra, posterior to the normal channel. Characteristic atrophic dimple (d) in patient affected by vulvar vestibulitis.

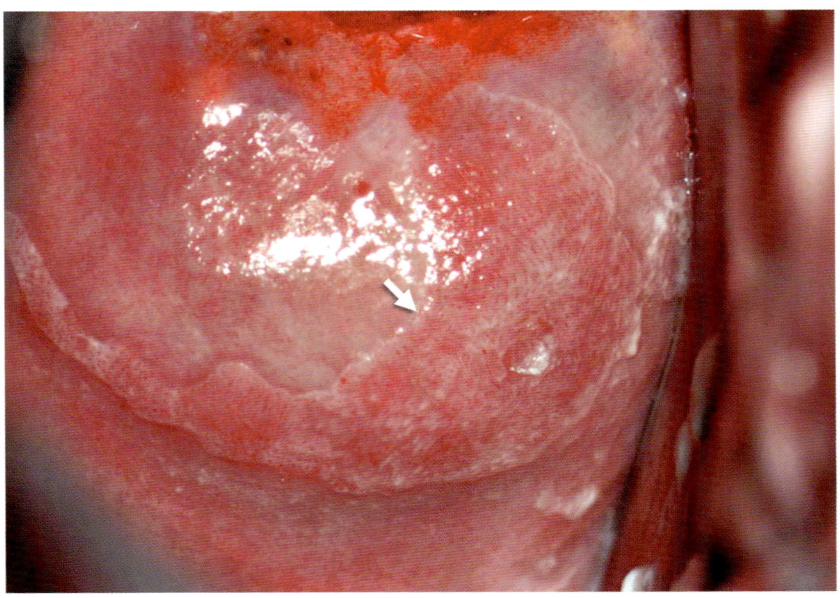

Figure 468 - Semicircular, faint acetowhite and raised lesion (arrow). Excision biopsy and resultant histology revealed HPV flat condyloma.

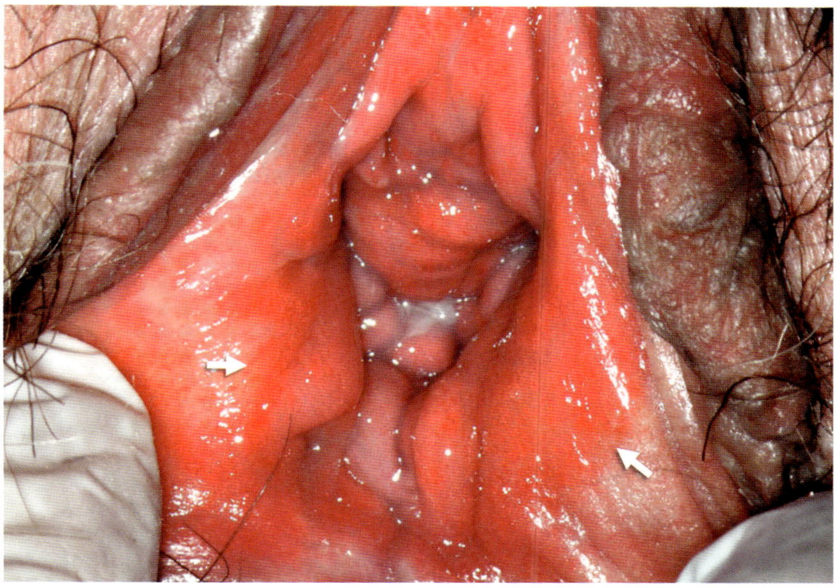

Figure 469 - Vulvar erythema induced by Candida infection. The sharp border (arrows) between the inner reddish area and the outer pale surface is due to the tight contact between the erythematous zones (kissing lesions).

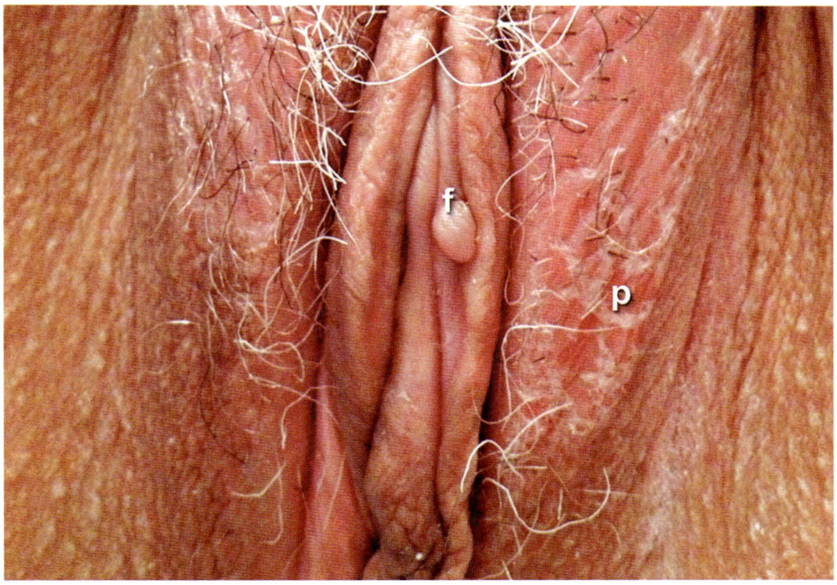

Figure 470 - Vulvar fibroid (f) and psoriasis (p).

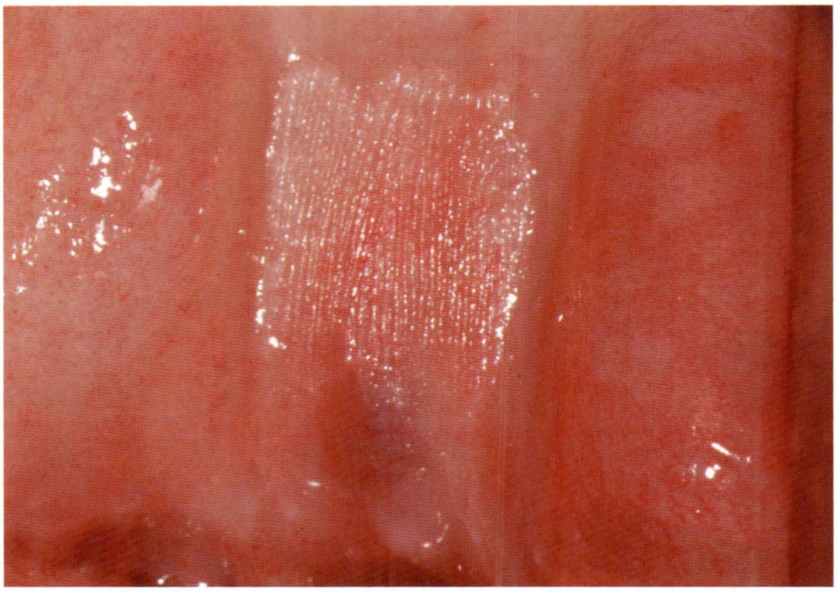

Figure 471 - Keratotic lines.

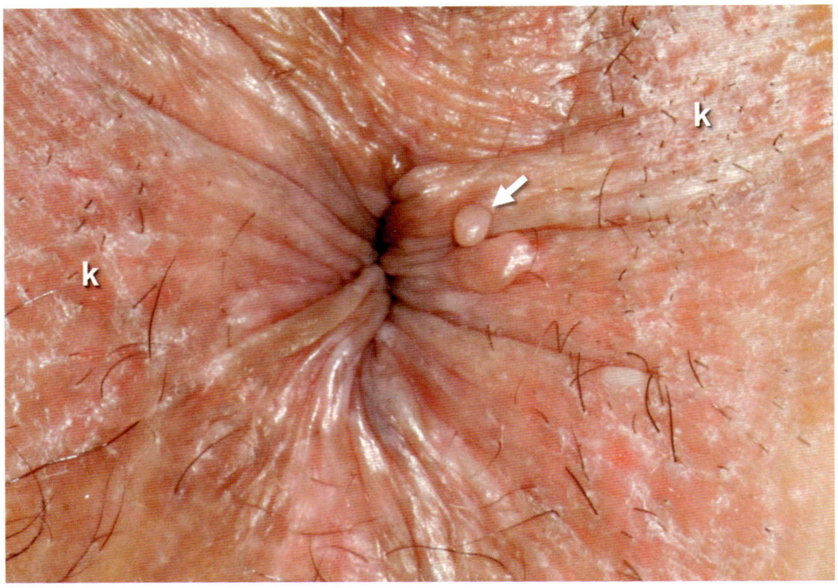

Figure 472 - Perianal keratosis (k) and anal fibroid (arrow).

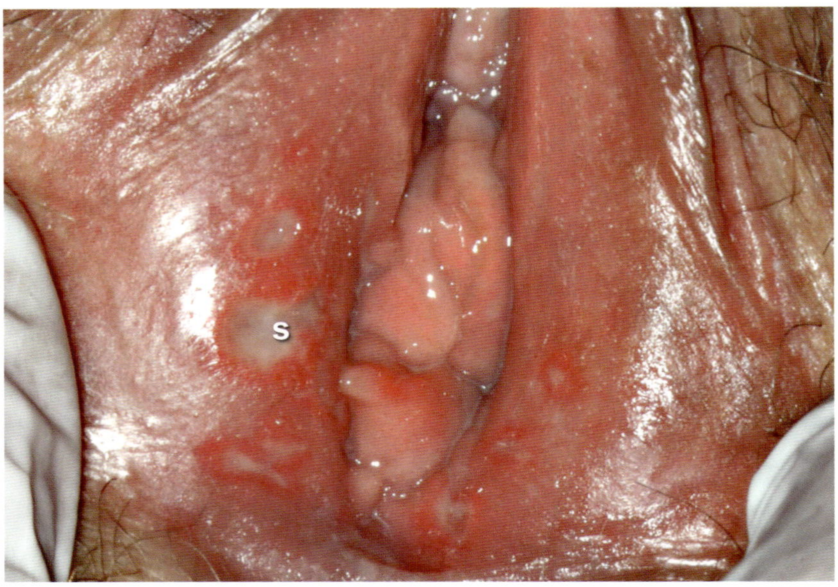

Figure 473 - Vulvar herpetic sores (s).

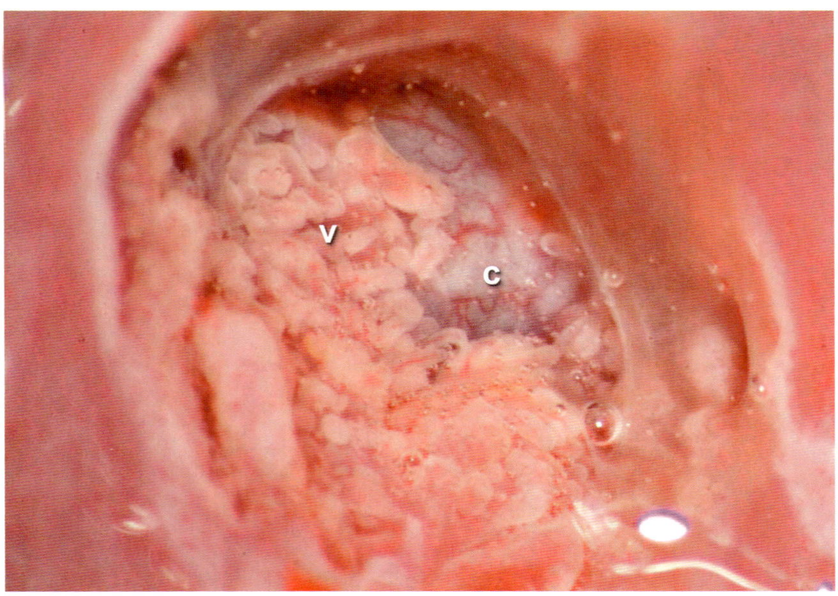

Figure 474 - Endocervical cyst (c) and hypertrophic villi (v).

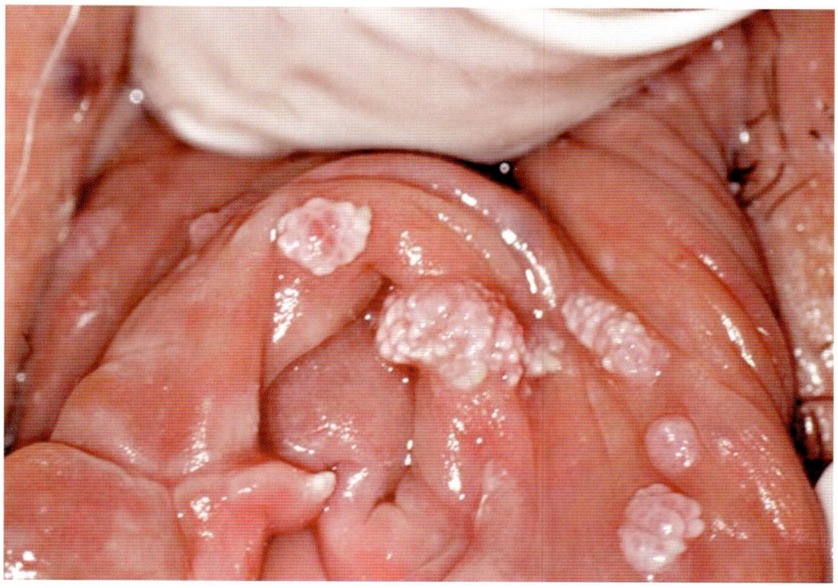

Figure 475 - Paraclitoral exophytic condylomas.

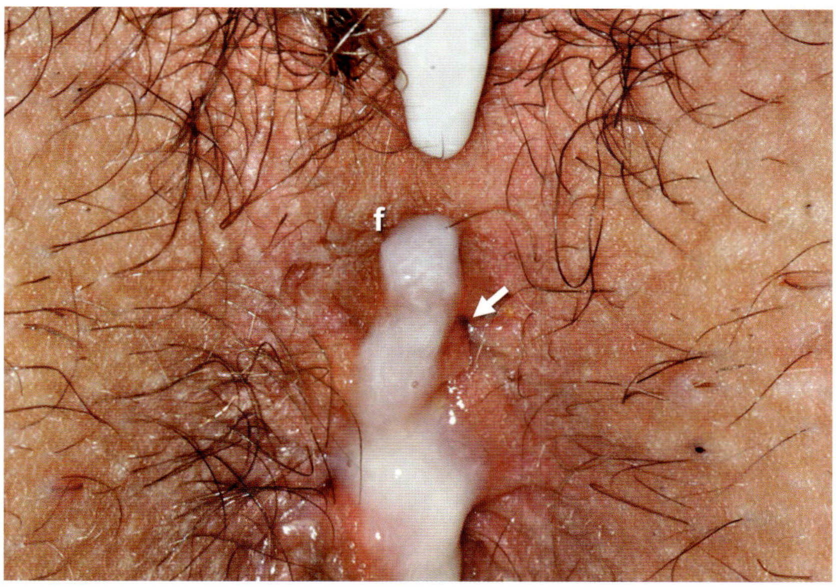

Figure 476 - Vaginal discharge comes out from a perineovaginal fistula (f), following perianal fistulectomy. The arrow indicates another external opening in the skin, near the larger one.

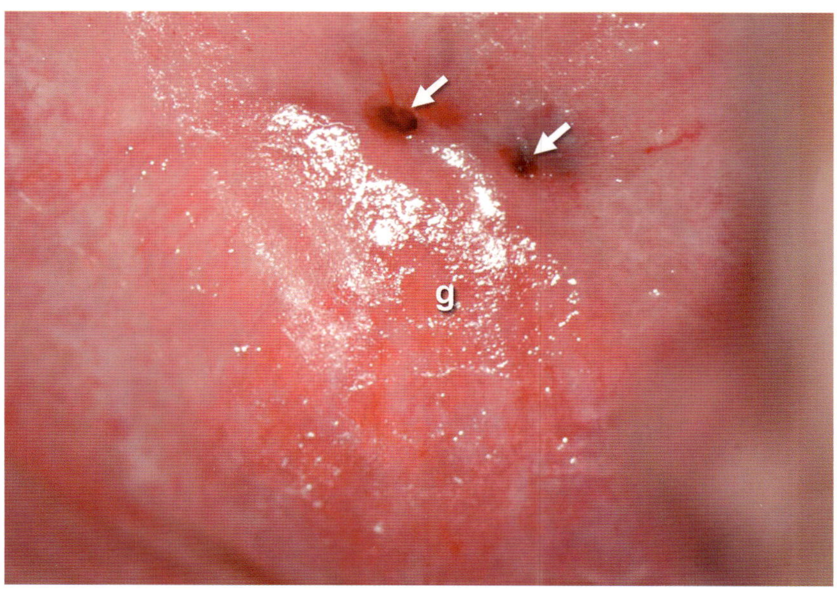

Figure 477 - The colpophotograph shows a double external os (arrows) (septum of the cervical canal). Keratotic granules (g).

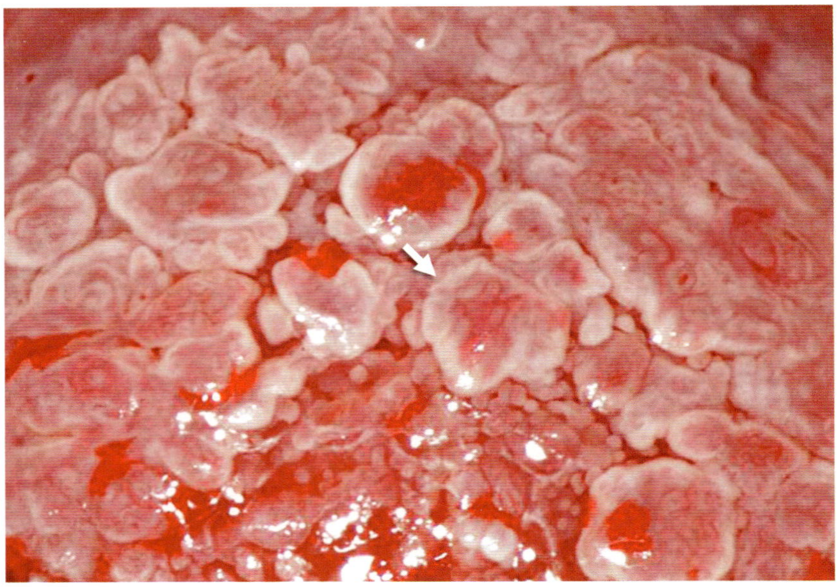

Figure 478 - Hyperplastic, mushroom-shaped columnar villi (arrow). Histology demonstrated a CIN 1 lesion.

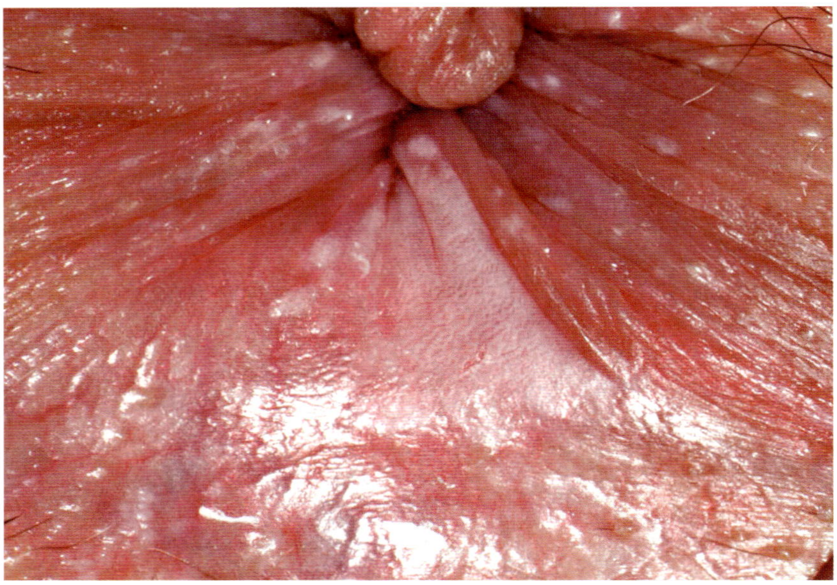

Figure 479 - Perianal acetowhite area with fine punctation. Punch biopsy and histology disclosed a low-grade HPV/AIN.

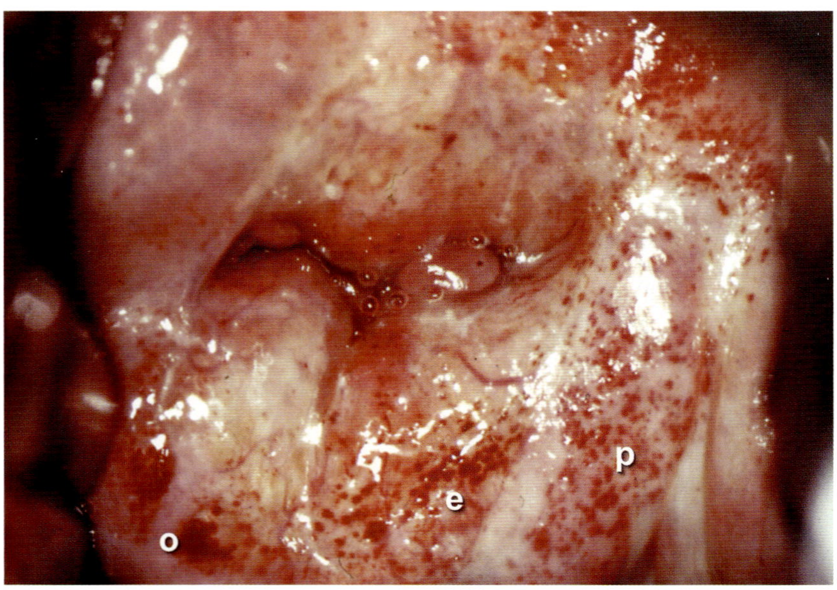

Figure 480 - The thick and dense acetowhite epithelium on the posterior lip of the cervix exhibits capillary oozing (o), hemorrhagic effusions (e) and coarse punctation (p). On histology invasive carcinoma was reported.

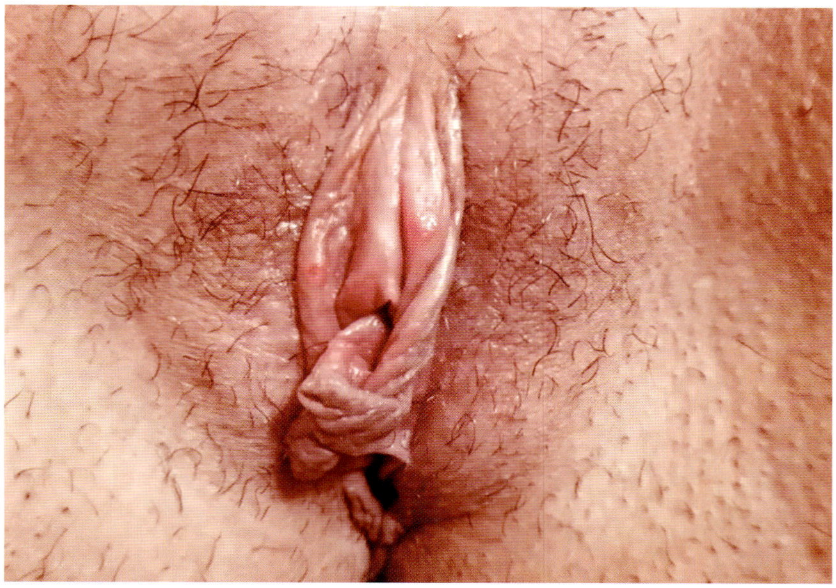

Figure 481 - Hypertrophic inner lips ("with folded arms").

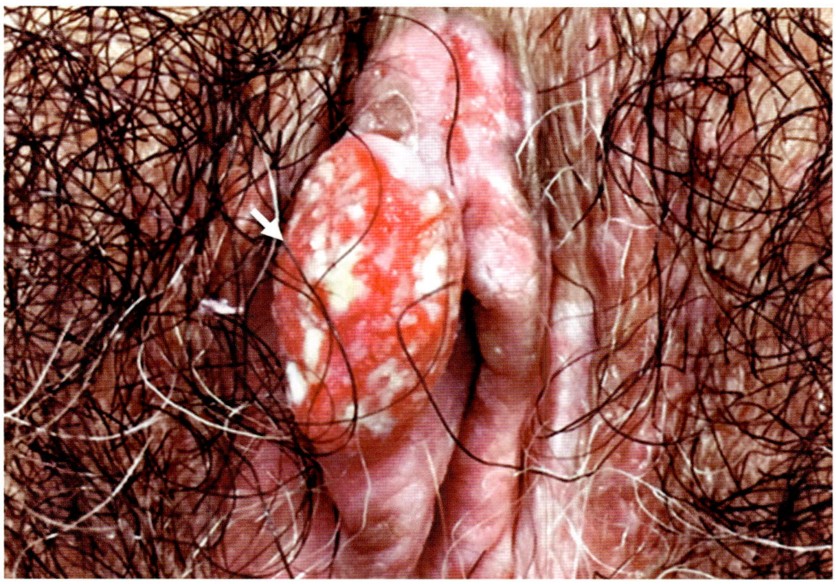

Figure 482 - Vulvar invasive carcinoma (arrow).

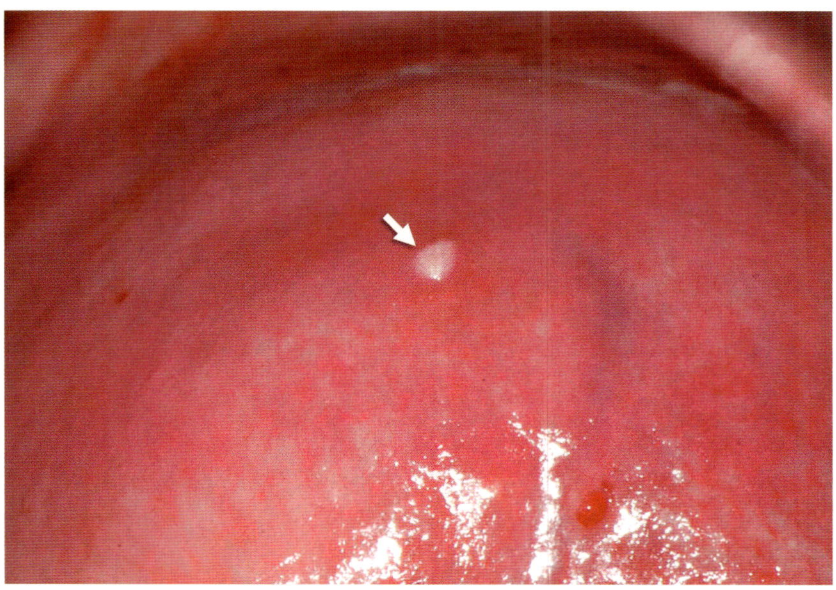

Figure 483 - Discrete cervical flat condyloma (arrow).

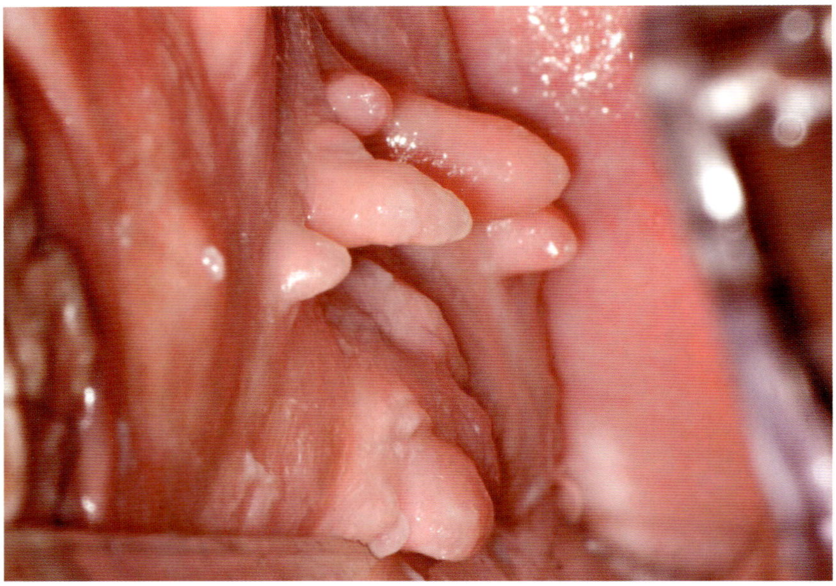

Figure 484 - Multiple fibroids arise from the right vaginal wall.

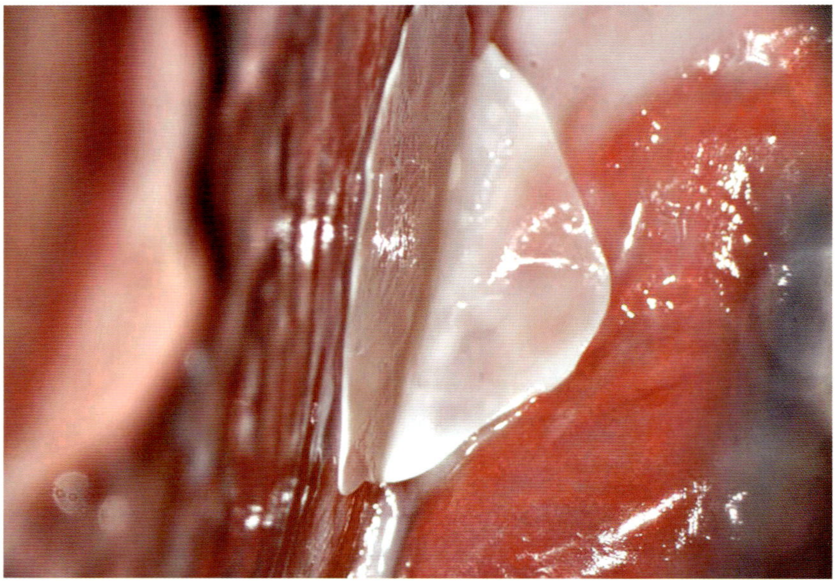

Figure 485 - A fragment of condom is held back in vagina.

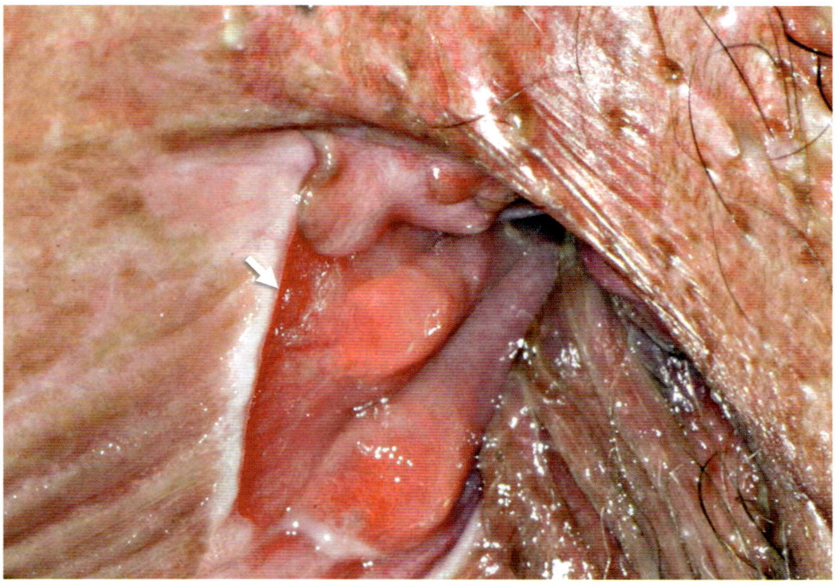

Figure 486 - The arrow indicates an area of bare stroma, following anal fistulectomy.

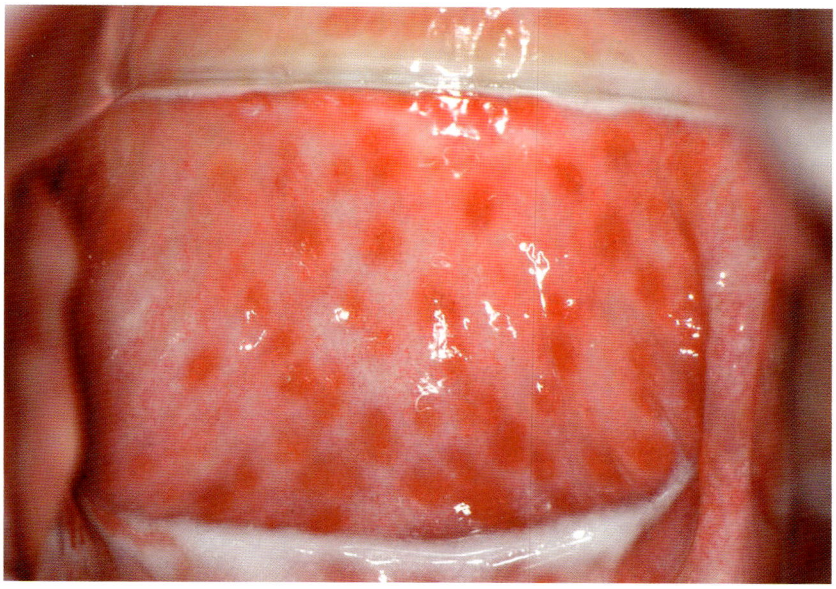

Figure 487 - Erythematous macules, induced by candidiasis.

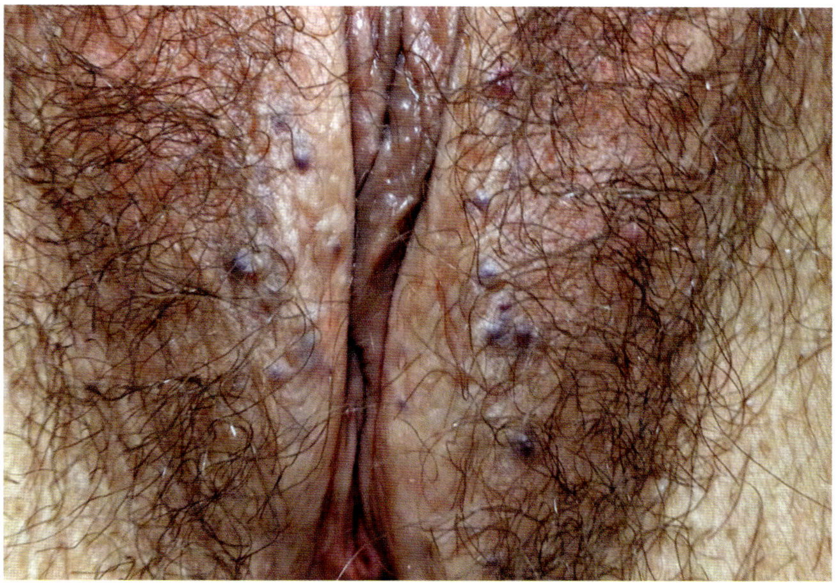

Figure 488 - Scattered angiokeratomas.

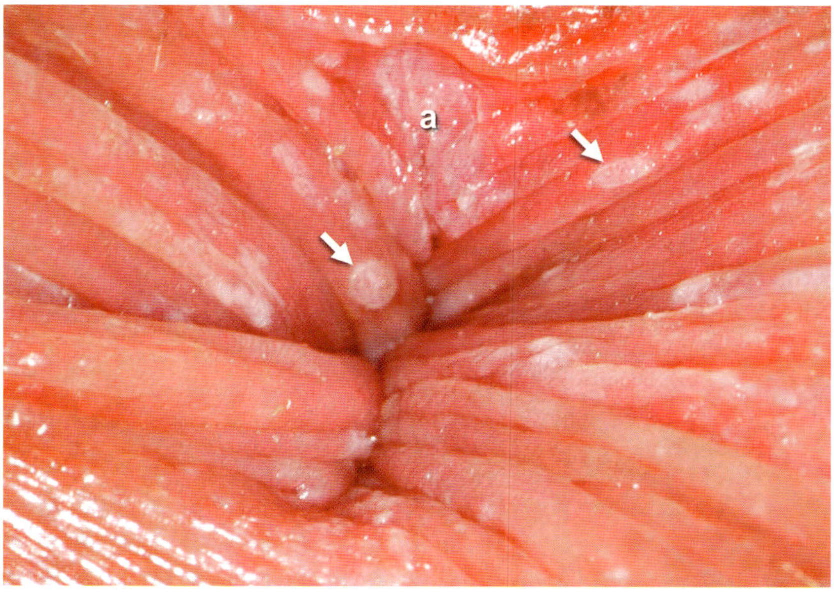

Figure 489 - Perianal acetowhite area (a) and HPV flat condylomas (arrows).

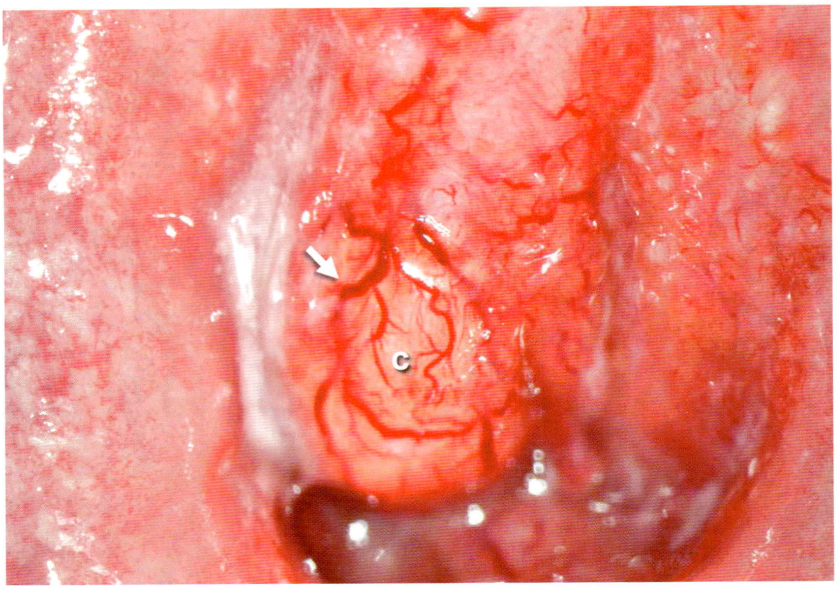

Figure 490 - The arrowed capillary over the nabothian cyst (c) shows an irregular caliber and an abrupt appearance. Despite the abnormal vascular pattern, no atypia is present.

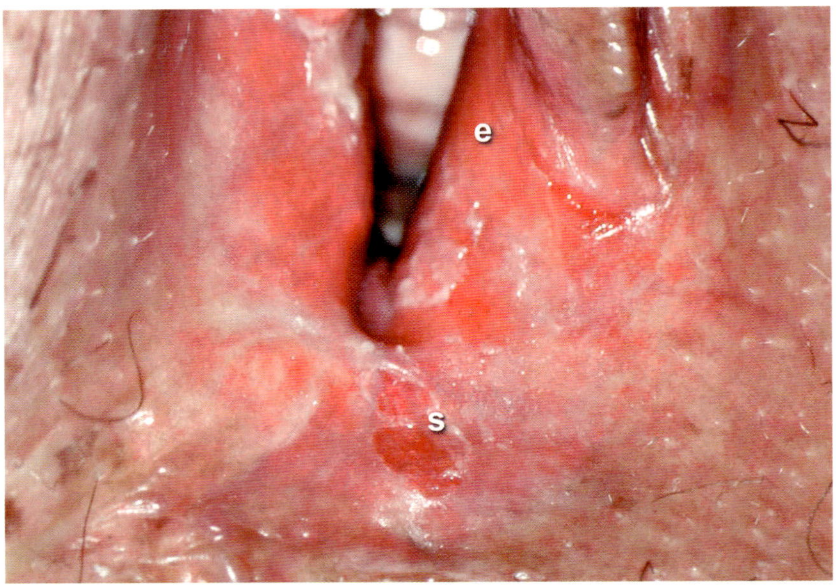

Figure 491 - Lichen planus is characterized by erythema (e) and erosions (s).

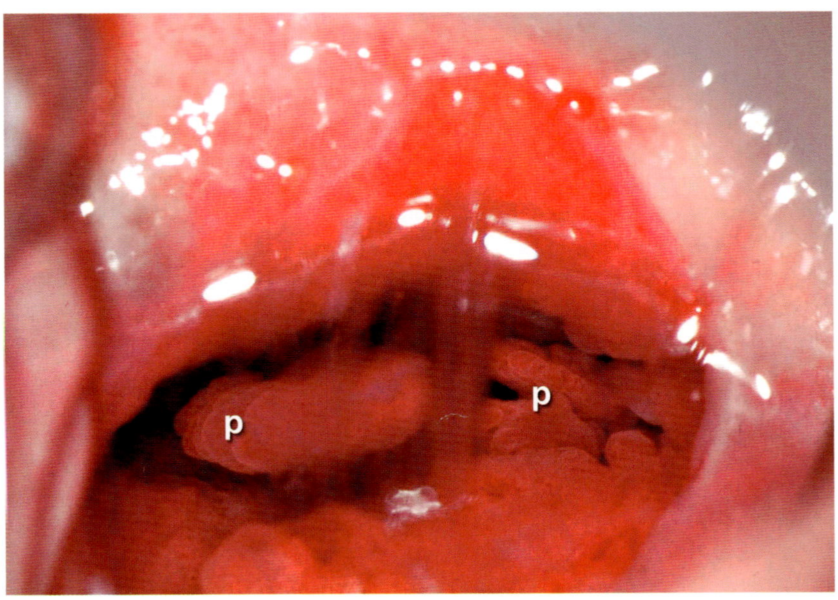

Figure 492 - Multiple endocervical polyps (p).

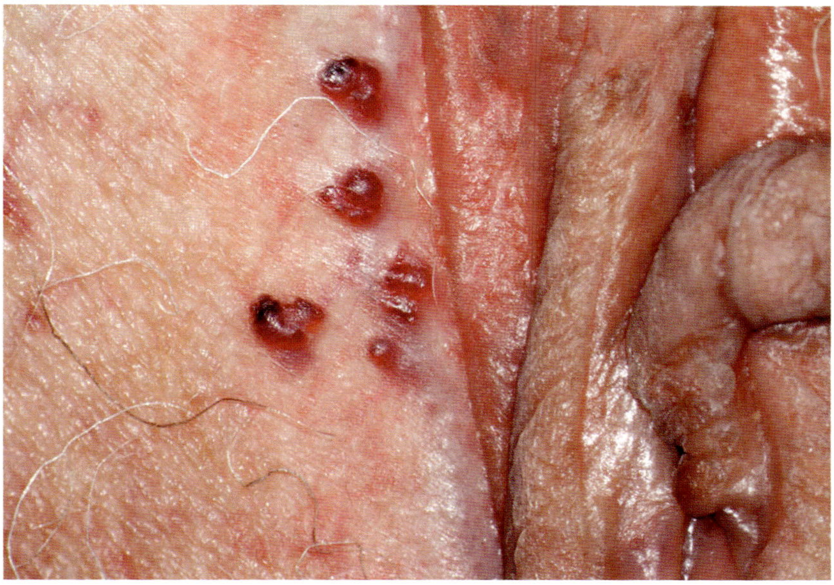

Figure 493 - Vulvar angiokeratomas.

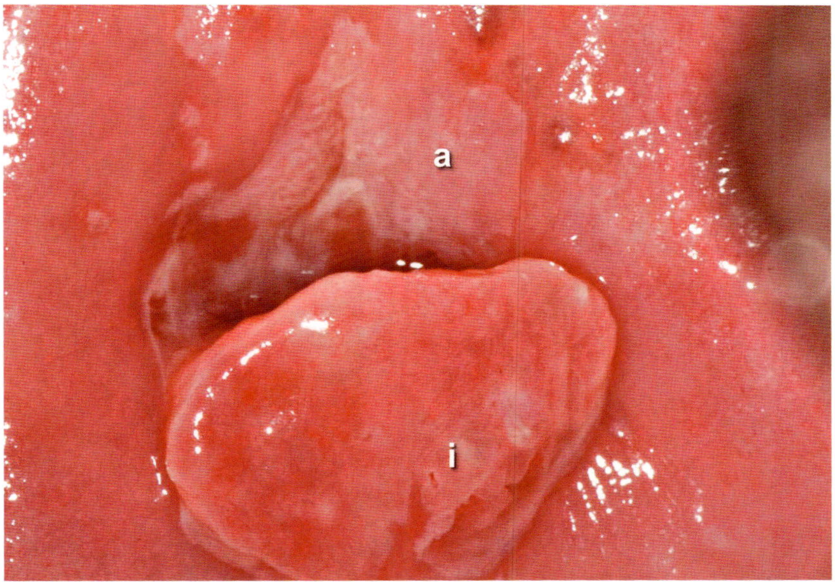

Figure 494 - Pushing down the localized hypertrophy of the posterior cervical lip, lined with an immature metaplastic epithelium (i), a well defined acetowhite area (a) may be observed.

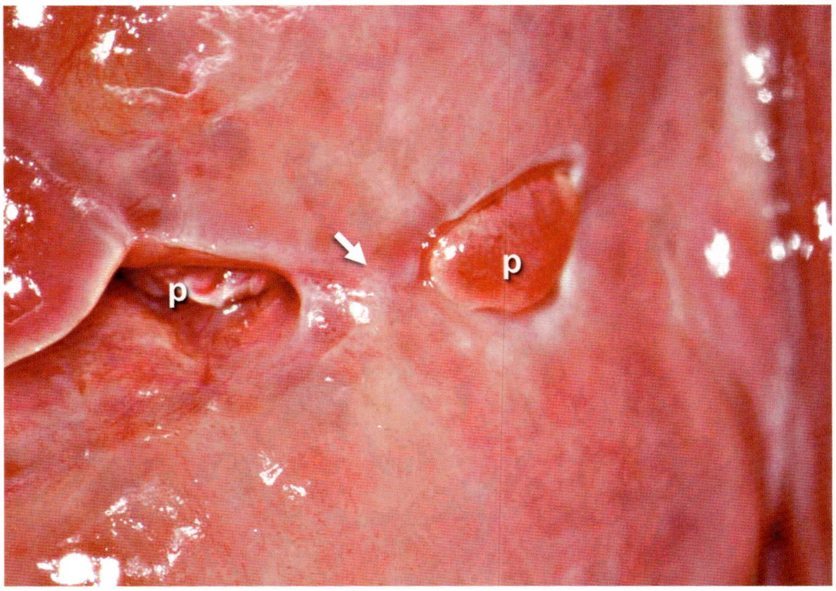

Figure 495 - A bridge of scar tissue (arrow), following trachelorrhaphy, divides the original external os into two segments. Polyps (p) protrude from each partial orifice.

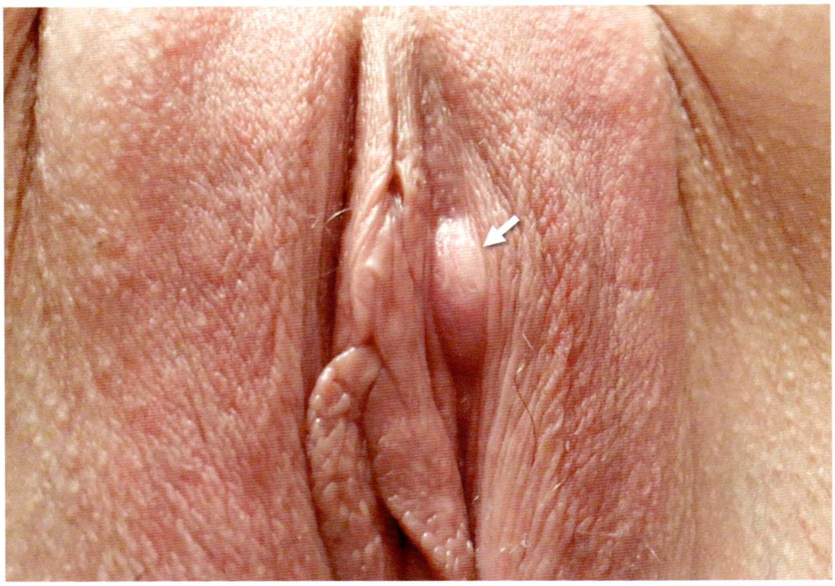

Figure 496 - The arrow indicates an epidermal cyst resulting from obstruction of sebaceous gland duct.

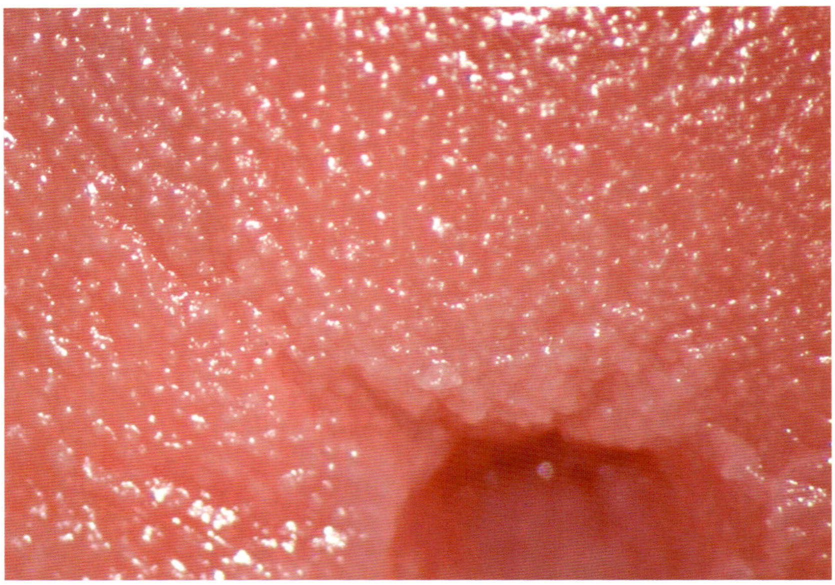

Figure 497 - When the metaplastic replacement is almost completed, the tip of the villi may exceed the height of the smooth surface, developing scattered small humps.

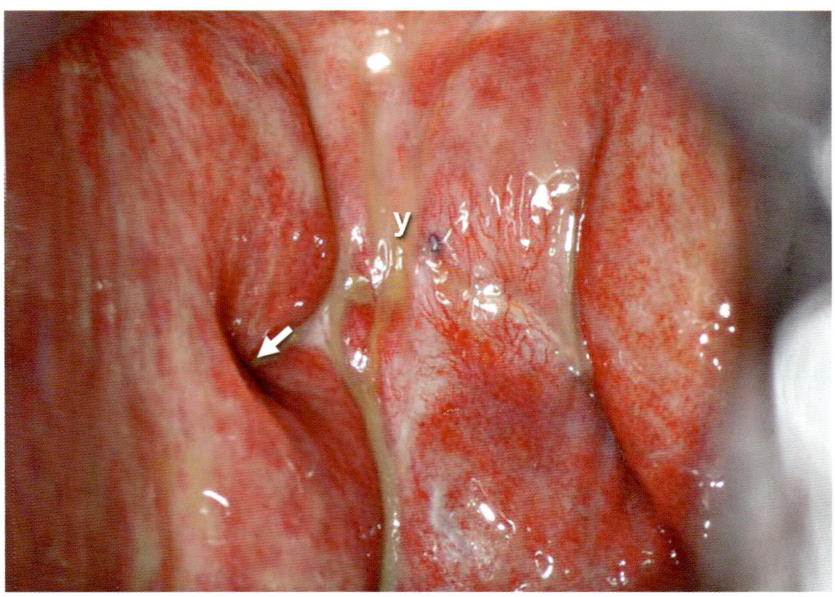

Figure 498 - Yellowish discharge (y) caused by aerobic vaginitis in a congested vaginal vault following hysterectomy. The arrow indicates the right vaginal recess (dog ear).

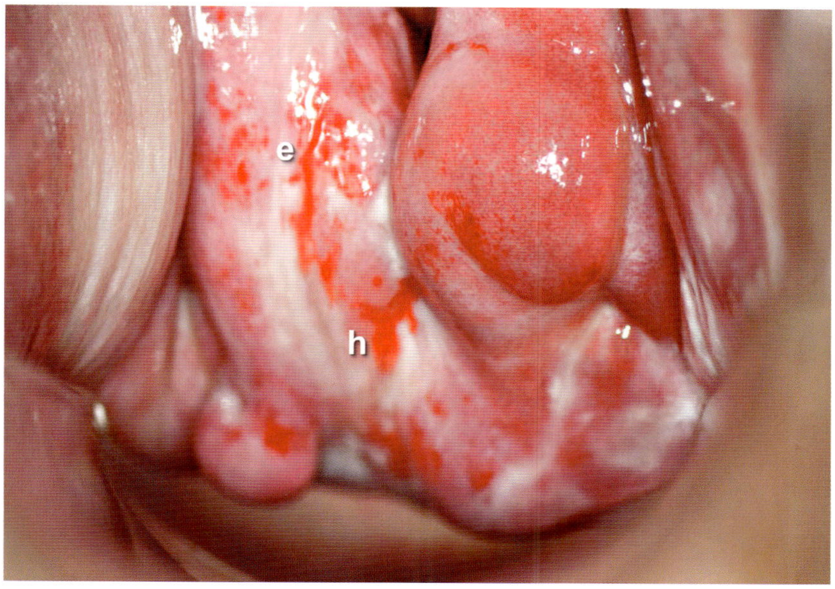

Figure 499 - Sturmdorf suture for hemostasis, after cold-knife conization, is responsible for the dysmorphic cervix which appears inflamed, with hemorrhagic oozing (h) and effusions (e).

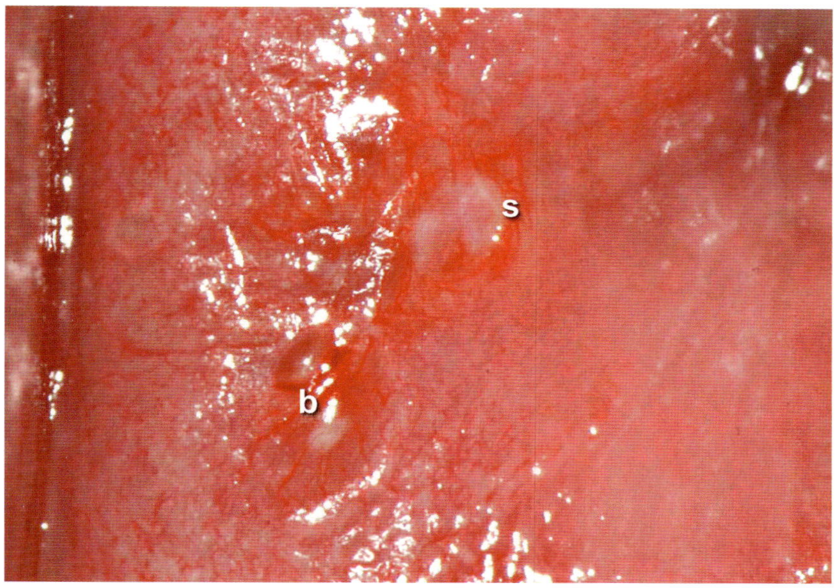

Figure 500 - Genital herpes. Blisters (b) and sore (s).

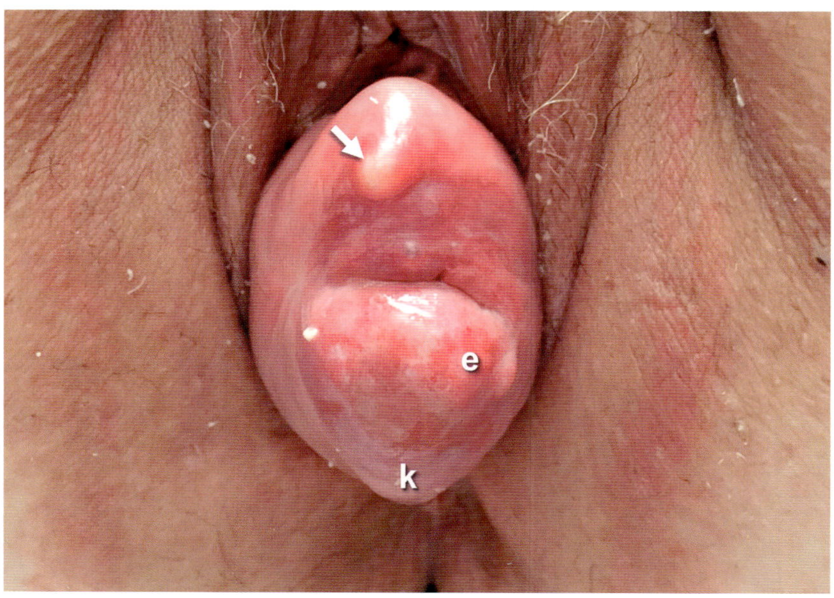

Figure 501 - The cervix, descended outside the introitus, shows an exposed columnar epithelium (e) and a glandular cyst (arrow). Thin keratosis (k).

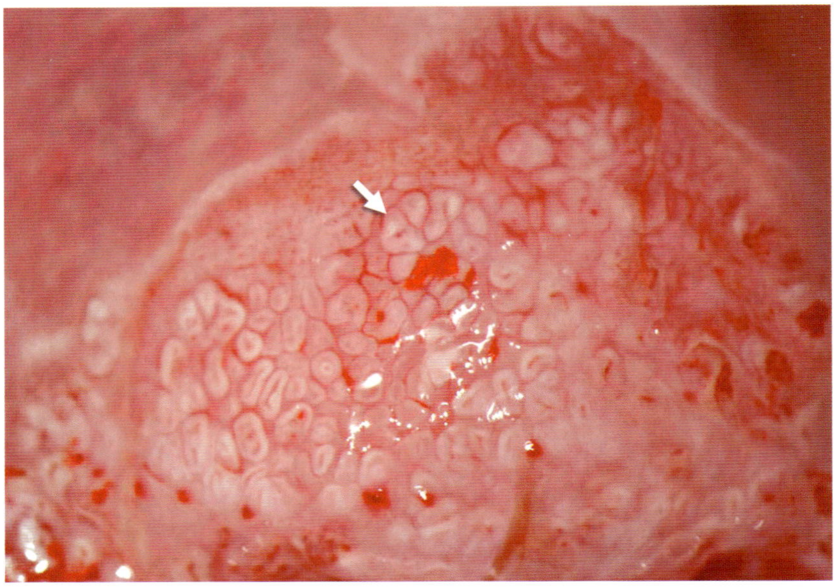

Figure 502 - Coarse mosaic showing umbilication (arrow). Histology disclosed a high-grade HPV-CIN lesion.

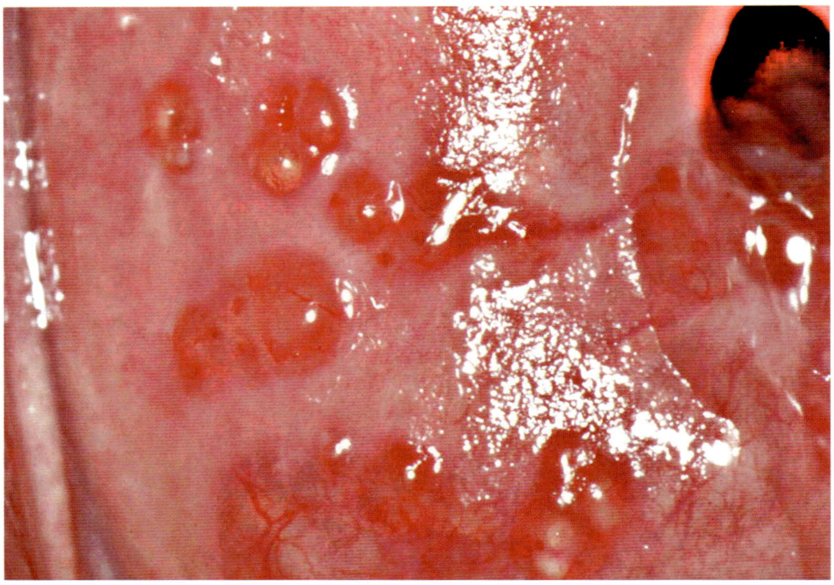

Figure 503 - The cervix appears involved by scattered herpetic blisters surmounting a hyperemic base.

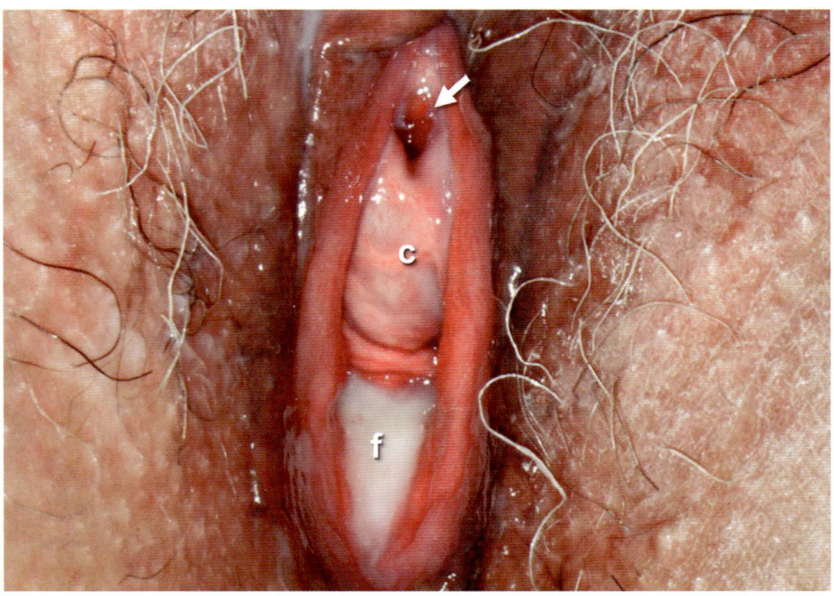

Figure 504 - Despite the thinning of the urethral lining (arrow) in this post-menopausal woman, abundant vaginal fluid (f) may be observed at the introitus. Direct microscopy revealed estrogen stimulation. Cystocele (c).

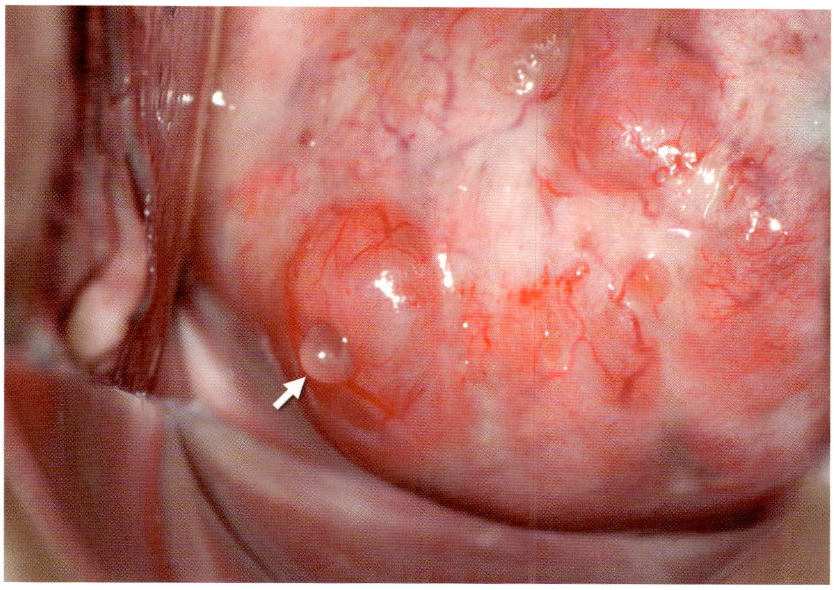

Figure 505 - The arrowed glandular cyst opened spontaneously, letting out a stringy mucus.

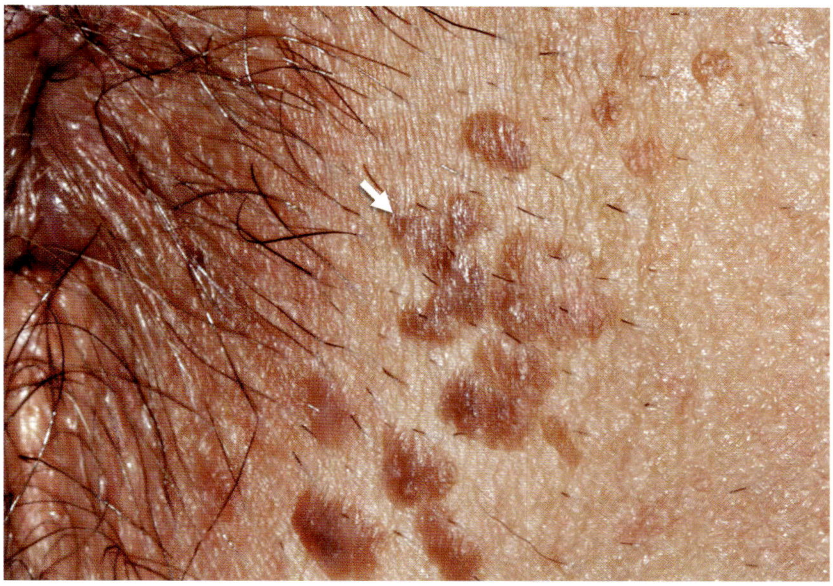

Figure 506 - Perianal bowenoid papulosis (arrow) can mimic perianal warts.

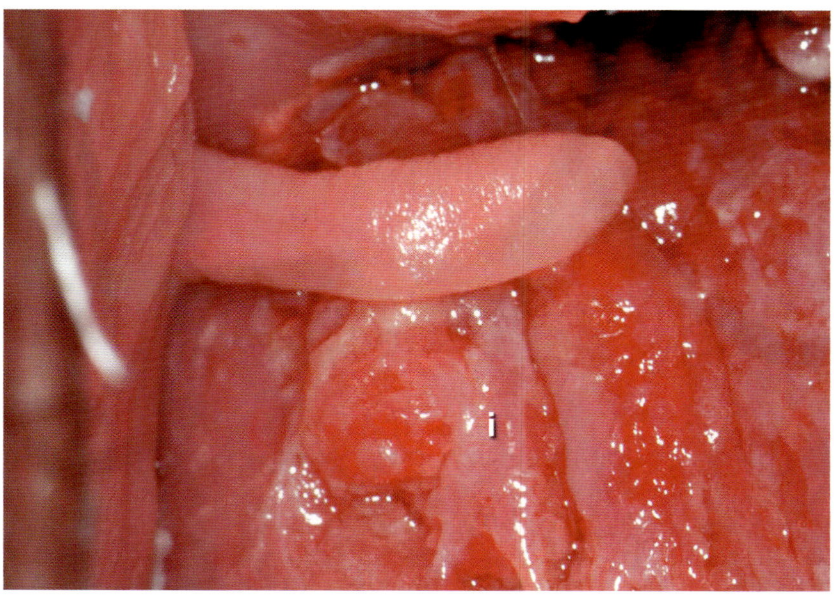

Figure 507 - An elongated fibroid arises from the right vaginal wall. Faint acetowhite immature metaplastic epithelium (i).

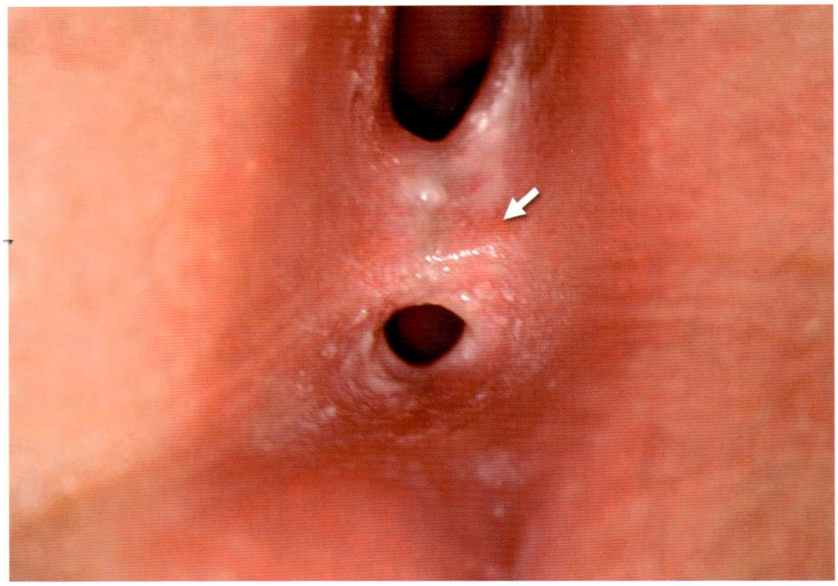

Figure 508 - Partial labial agglutination (arrow) in a five-year-old girl.

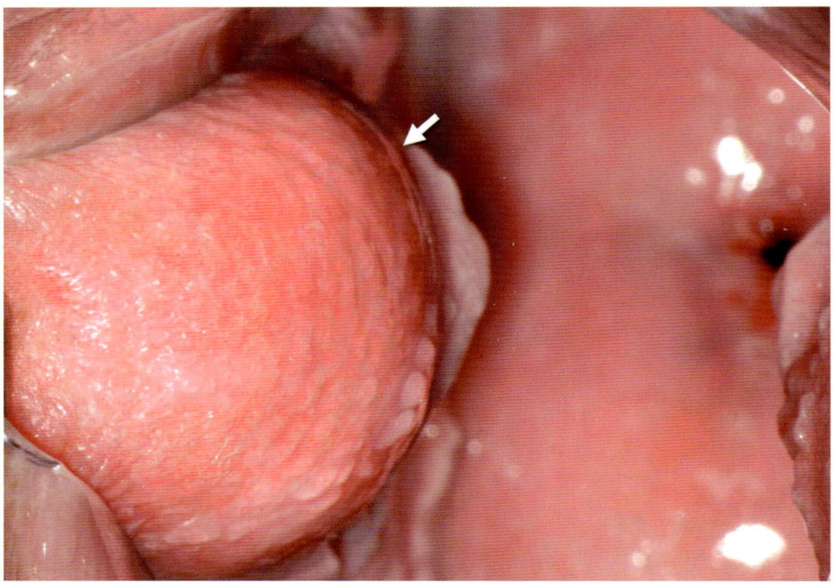

Figure 509 - The arrow indicates a Gartner's duct cyst, deriving from embryonic epithelial remnants at the branching lower ends of the primitive mesonephric tubules.

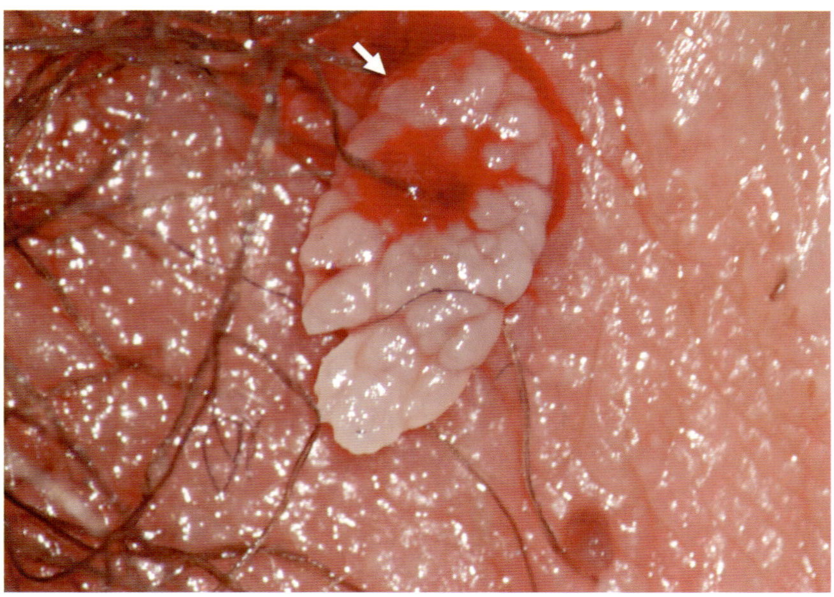

Figure 510 - The base of the vulvar wart is partially detached (arrow) and bleeding due to rubbing with clothing.

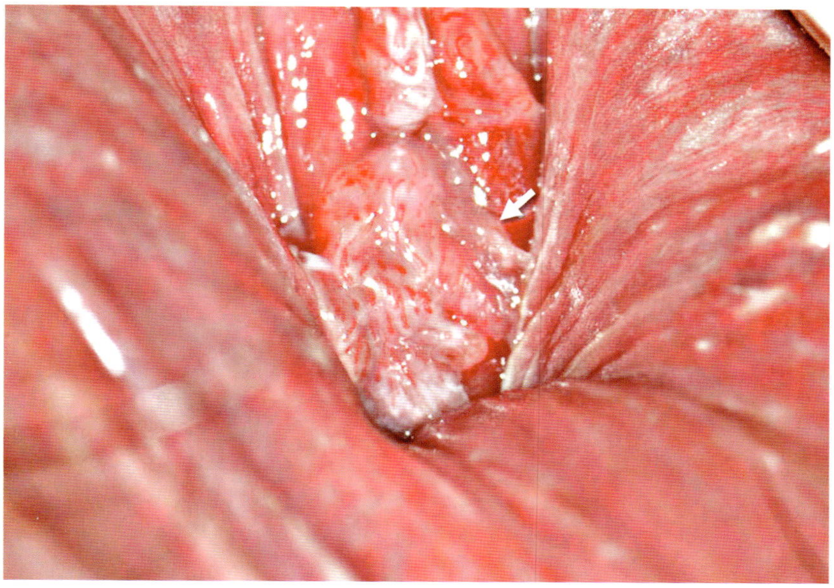

Figure 511 - The deep endocervical acetowhite and raised area (arrow) exhibits abnormal vessels. Histology revealed CIN III.

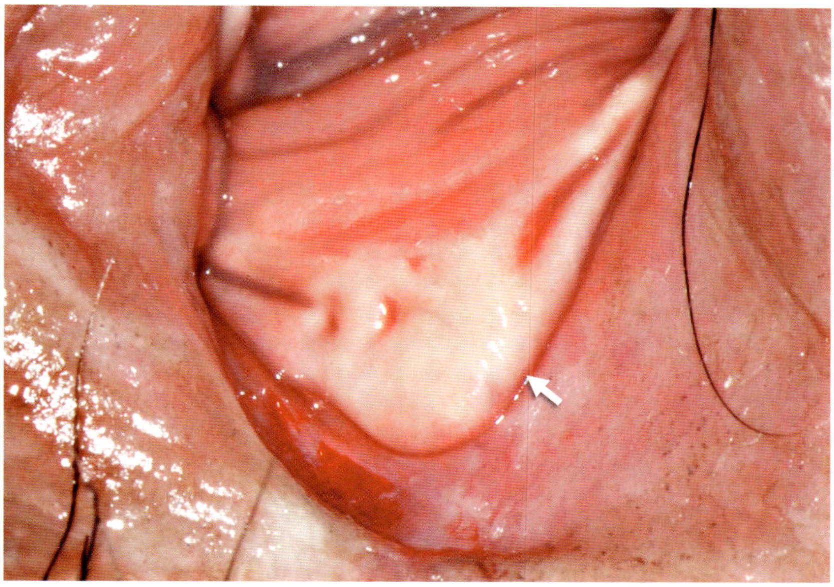

Figure 512 - Thickened, white-ivory epithelium on the posterior vaginal wall (arrow), next to the vulvar introitus. A punch biopsy is recommended.

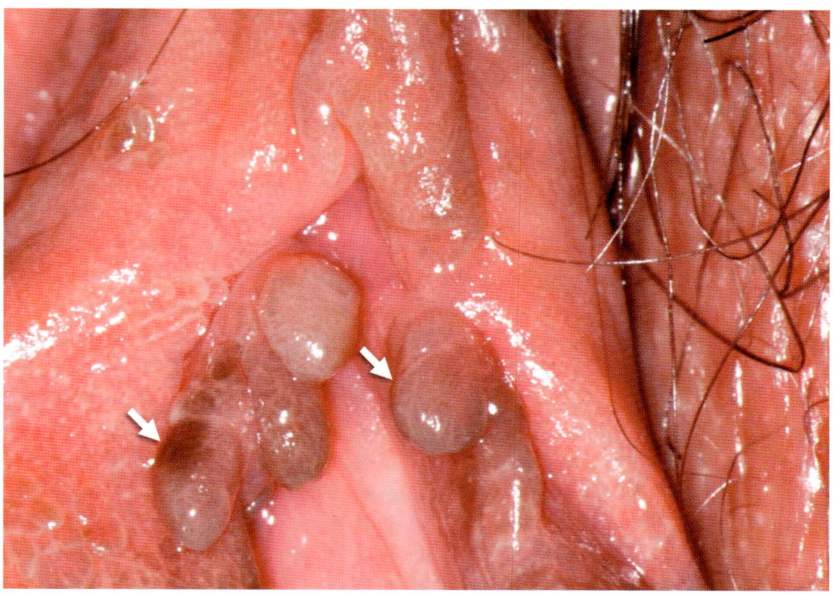

Figure 513 - Hypertrophic fimbriae (arrows) of inner labia.

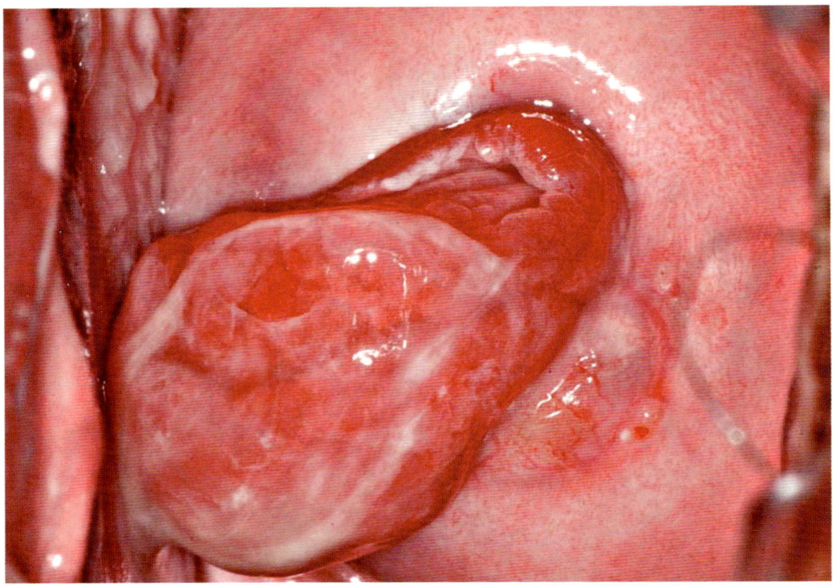

Figure 514 - Elongated uterine submucosal fibroid bulging into the vagina.

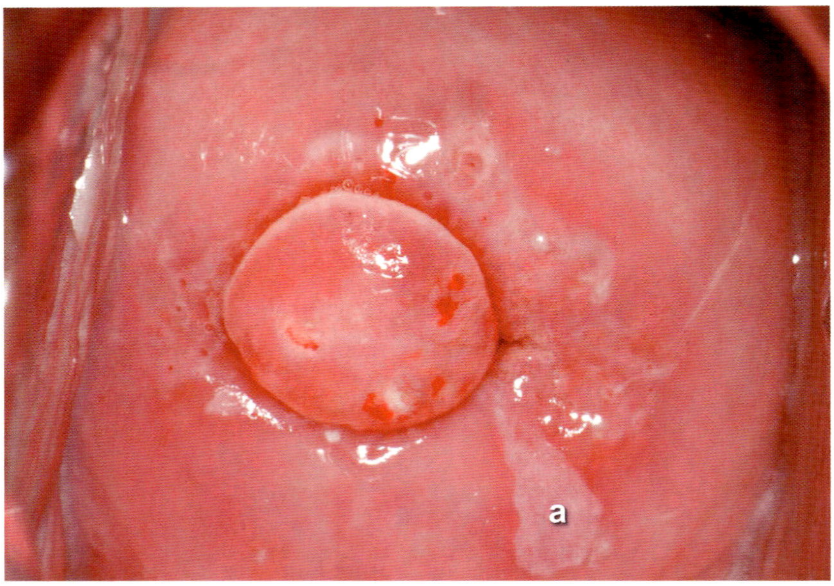

Figure 515 - The cervical polyp, lined with an immature metaplastic epithelium, covers like a cap of the external os, in a young woman eager for offspring. Well-defined faint acetowhite area (a).

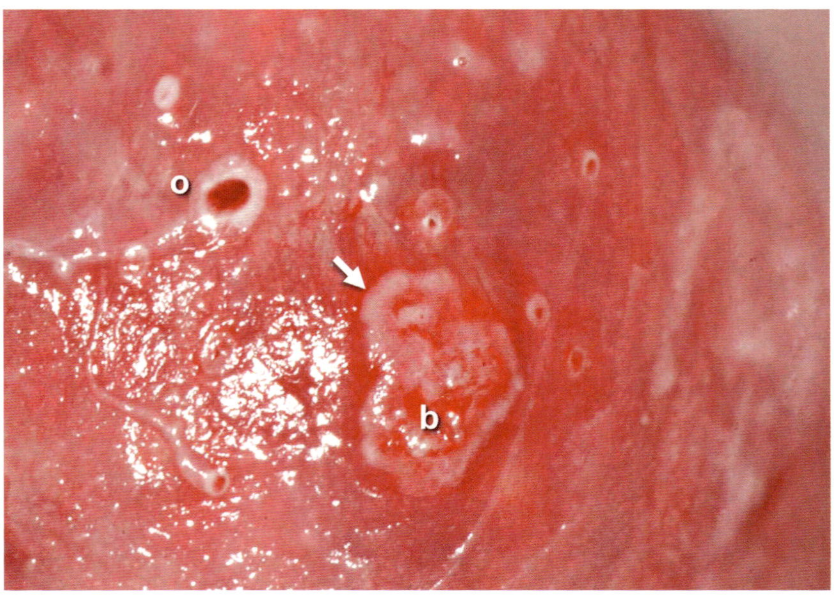

Figure 516 - The arrowed area appears raised, eroded, partially acetowhite, and surmounted by small blisters (b). Excision biopsy disclosed a herpetic lesion. Grade IV gland opening (o).

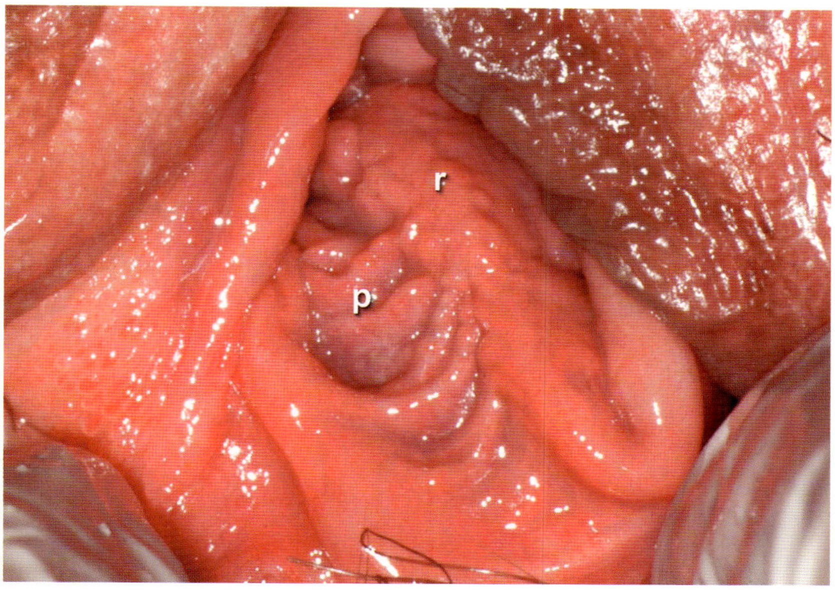

Figure 517 - The vaginal posterior wall shows congenital palmate folds (p), proceeding from a longitudinal ridge (r).

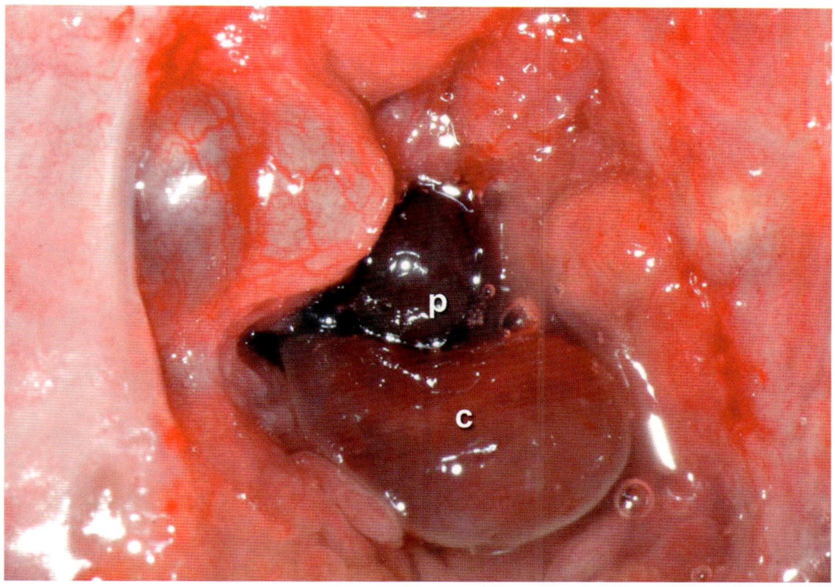

Figure 518 - This colpophotograph shows an endocervical serous cyst (c) and a cystic polyp (p) with hemorrhagic infarction.

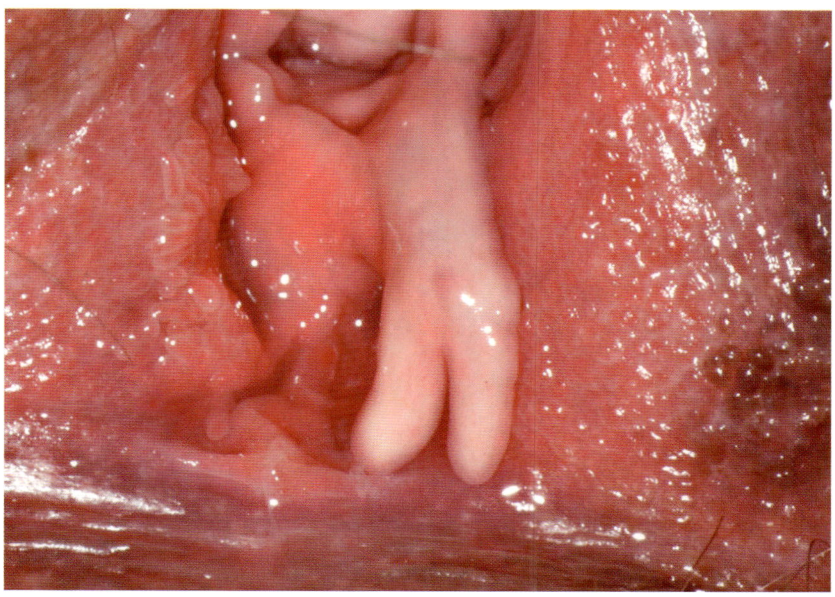

Figure 519 - Hymenal bifid hypertrophic caruncle.

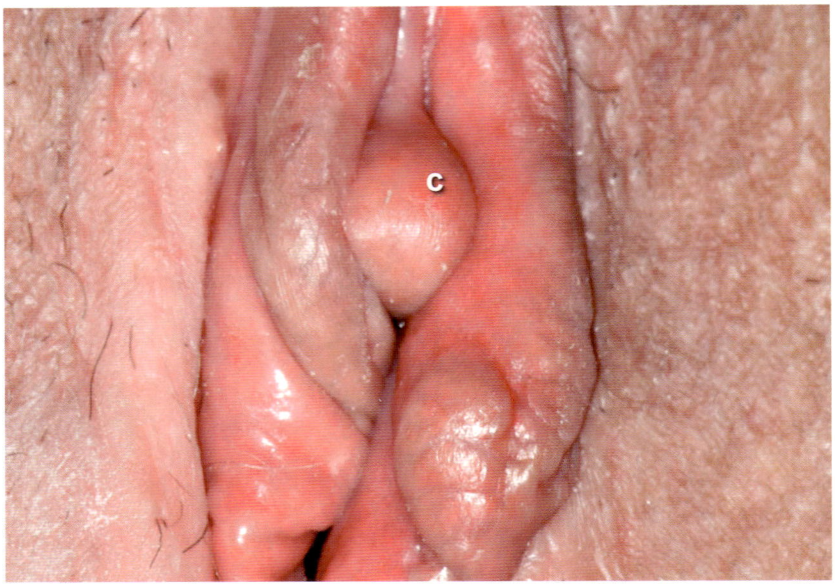

Figure 520 - Paraurethral cyst (c).
The external urethral orifice may be seen under the cyst.

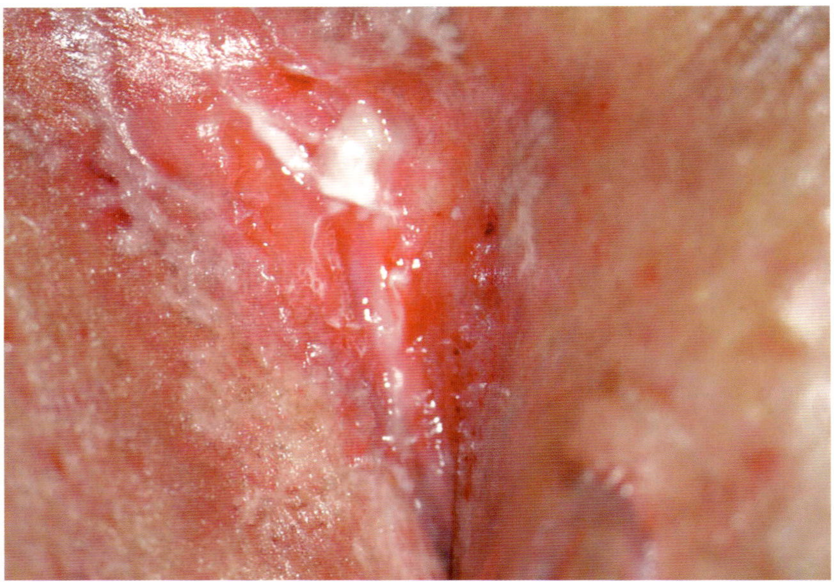

Figure 521 - The eroded psoriatic area involves the intergluteal cleft.

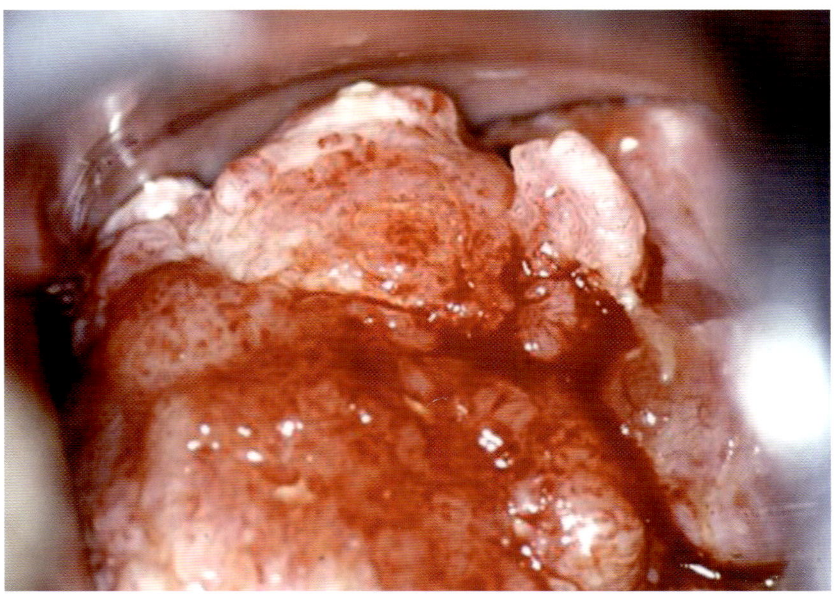

Figure 522 - Advanced invasive carcinoma with exophytic growth pattern.

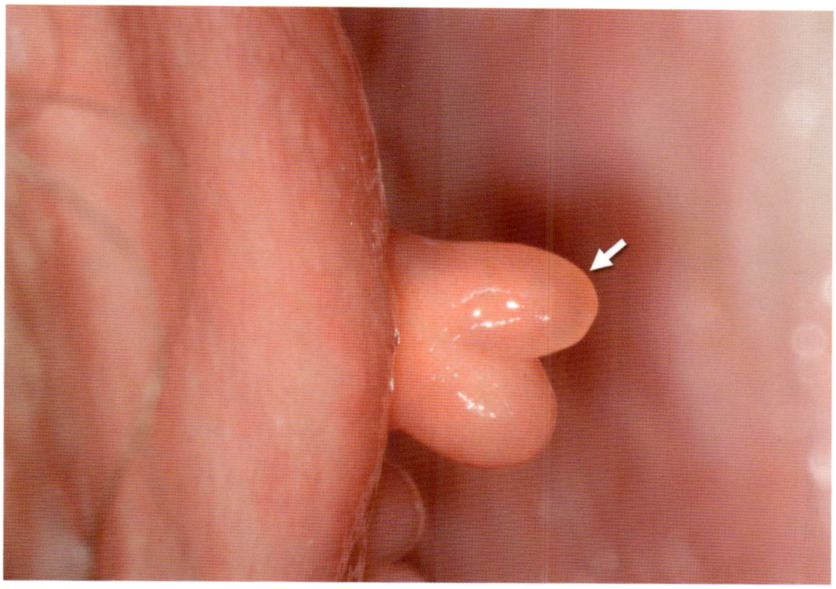

Figure 523 - Bifid vaginal fibroid (arrow).

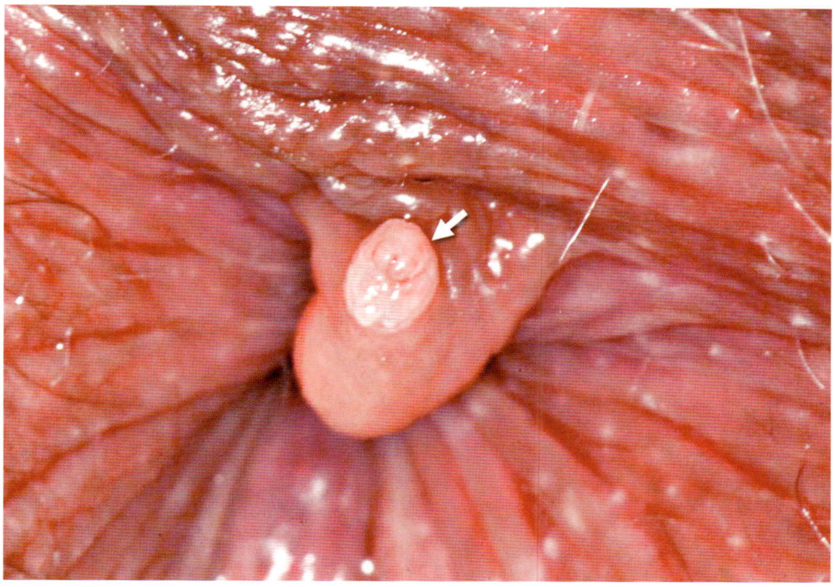

Figure 524 - An exophytic condyloma surmounts an anal skin tag (arrow).

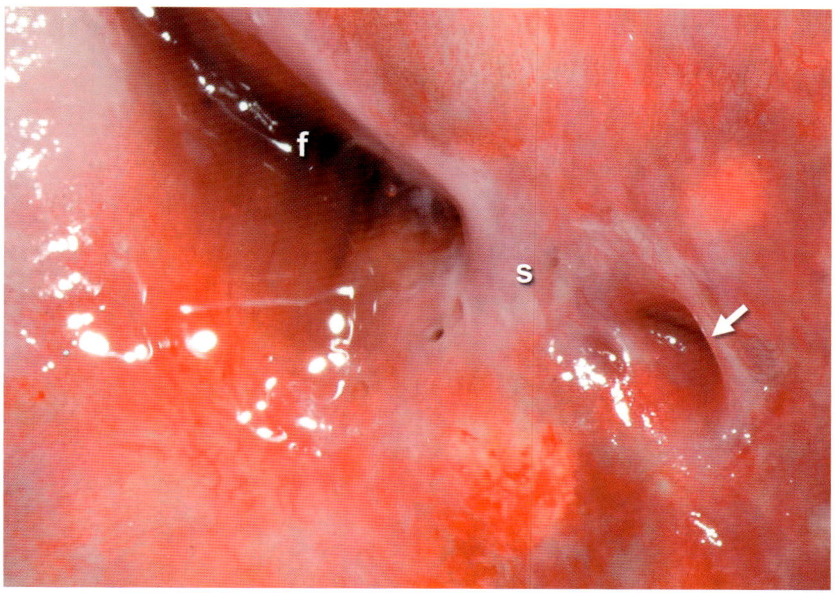

Figure 525 - A bridge of scar tissue (s), following trachelorrhaphy, divides the original external os into a main segment in form of fissure (f), and a peripheral narrow orifice (arrow) that must be checked by cytobrush during PAP test sampling, not to escape cytologic detection.

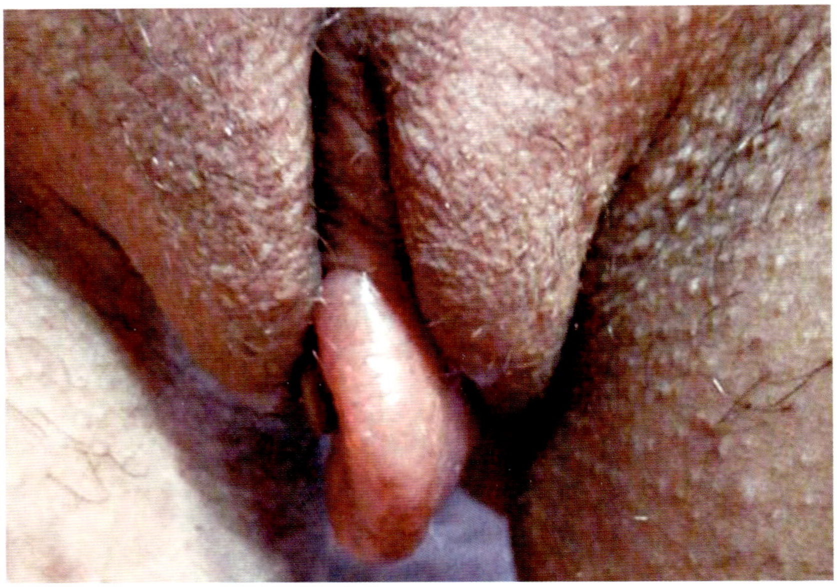

Figure 526 - Phlegmon of the left labium minus. It is distinct from an abscess which is walled-off by peripheral granulation tissue.

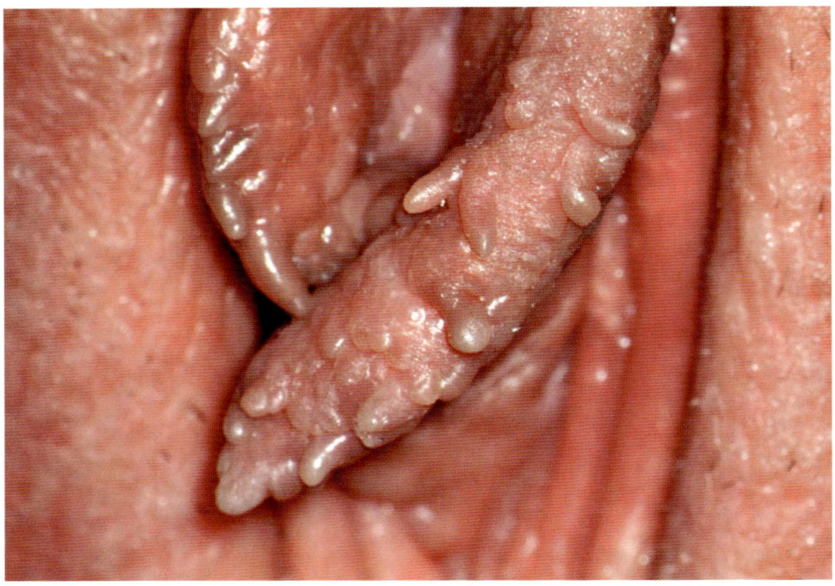

Figure 527 - Longitudinal hypertrophy of the left labium minus, provided with cutaneous papillae.

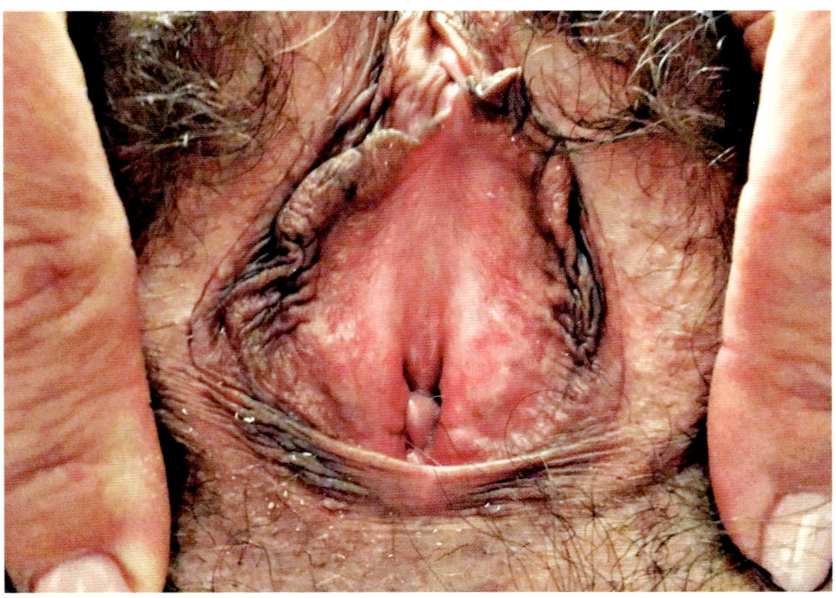

Figure 528 - Female hypospadias is a condition in which the external urethral meatus opens high up in the anterior vaginal wall.

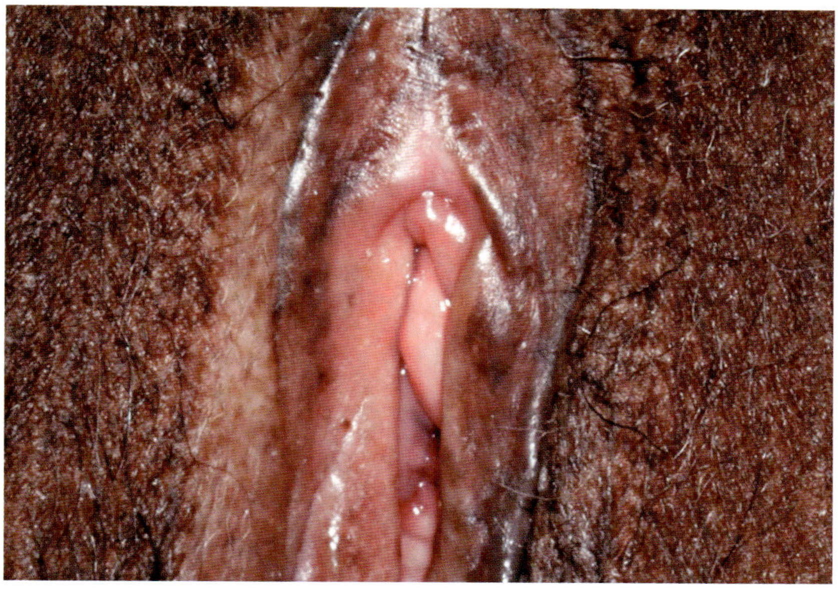

Figure 529 - The darkening of the skin in Addison's disease is sometimes referred to as "bronzing" and is caused by the stimulant effect of excess ACTH on the melanocytes to produce melanin.

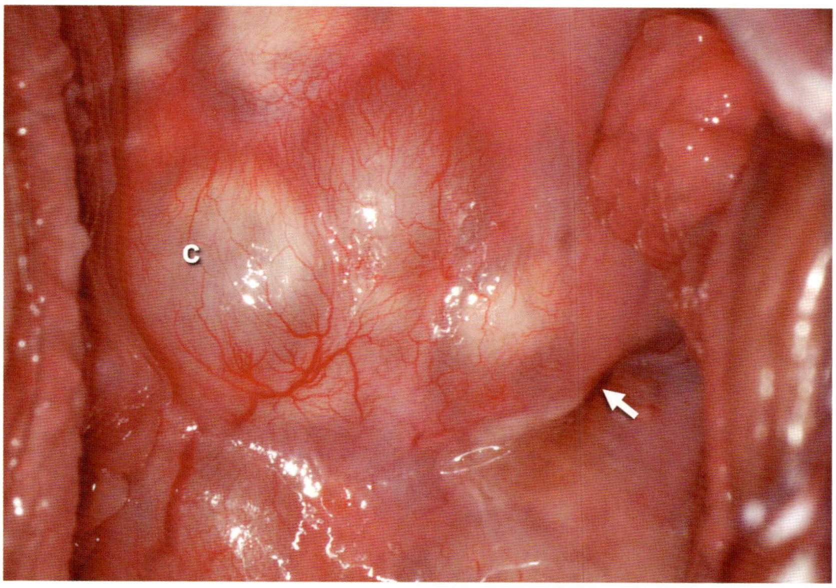

Figure 530 - Multiple nabothian cysts (c). The external os (arrow) is dislocated by the presence of a voluminous uterine fibroid.

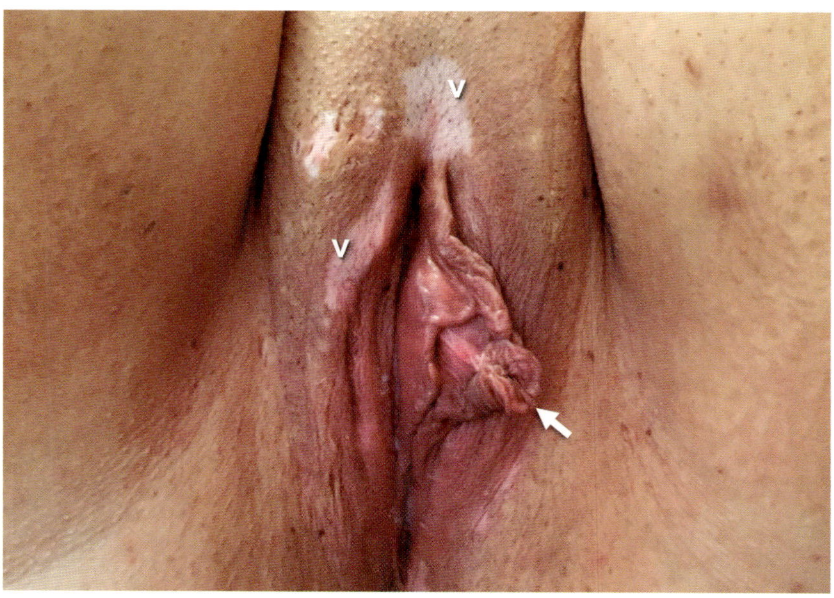

Figure 531 - Areas of vitiligo (v) are associated with hypertrophy of the left inner labium (arrow).

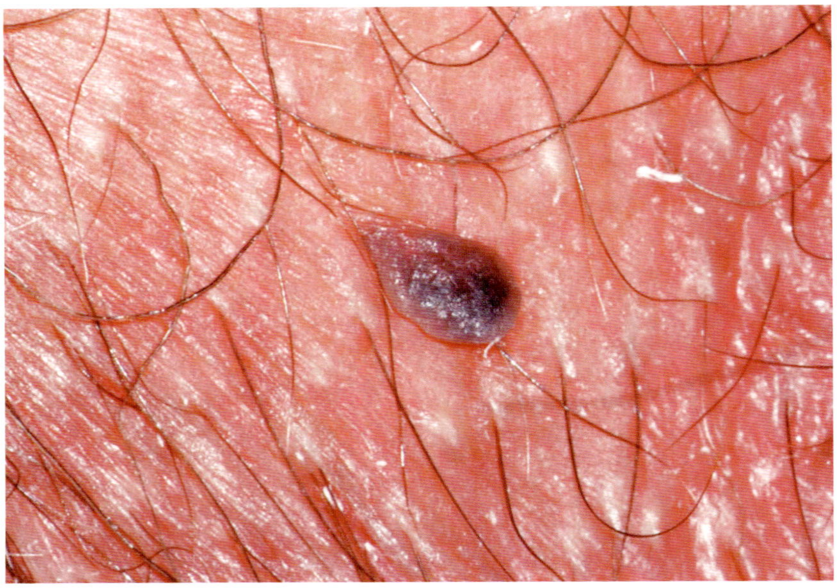

Figure 532 - Vulvar pigmented pedunculated fibroid.

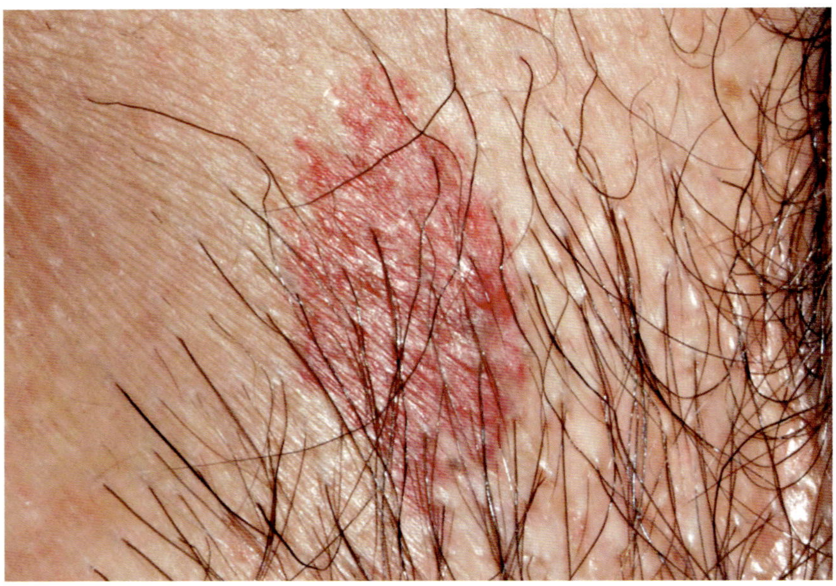

Figure 533 - Extensive flat angiokeratoma.

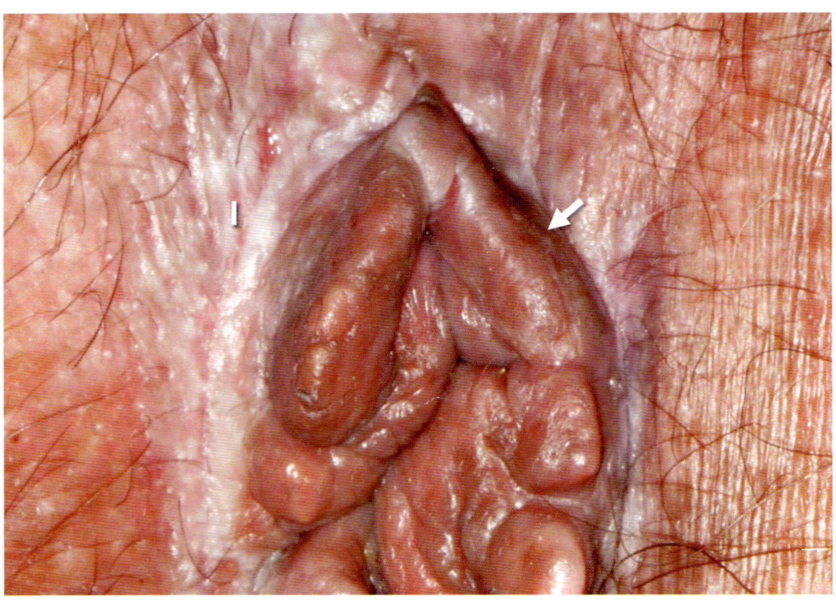

Figure 534 - Perianal lichen sclerosus (I). The arrow indicates anal skin tags (anal marisca). Anal skin tags are small bumps that appear around the anus, but they are not to be confused with warts or hemorrhoids.

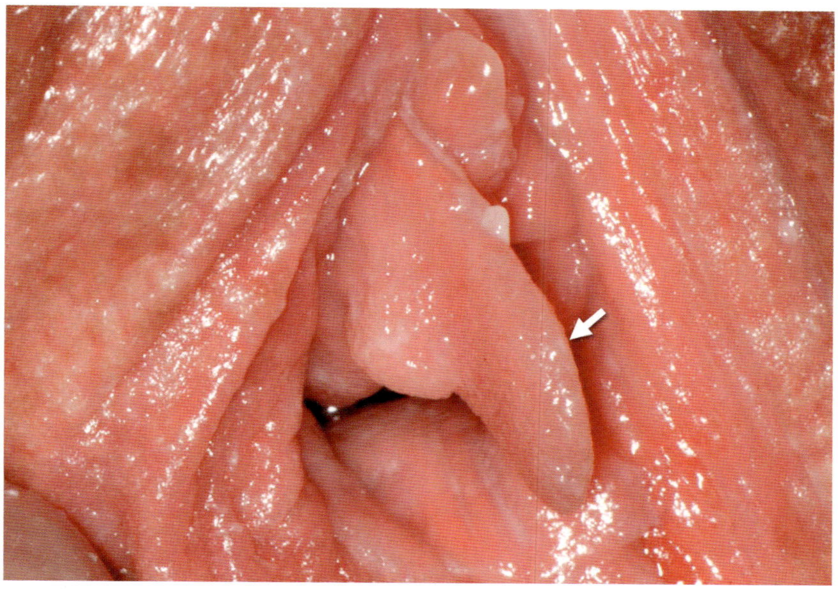

Figure 535 - Hypertrophic tissue (arrow) arises from periurethral area.

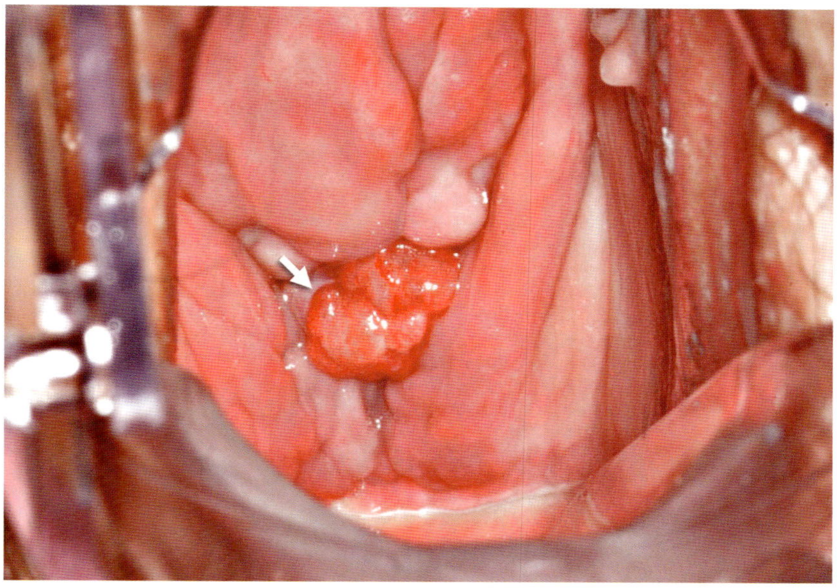

Figure 536 - Polypoid granulation tissue on the vaginal vault (arrow), following hysterectomy.

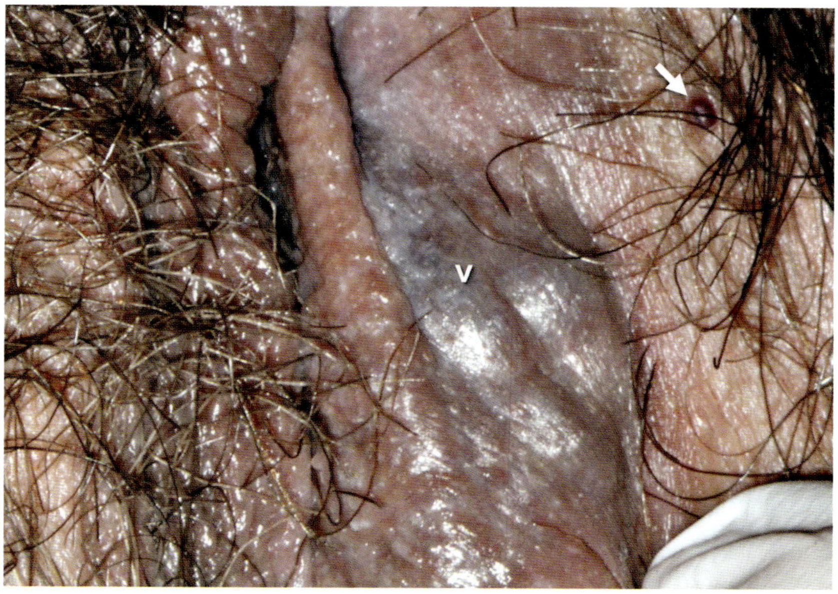

Figure 537 - Vulvar varices (v). The arrow indicates an angiokeratoma.

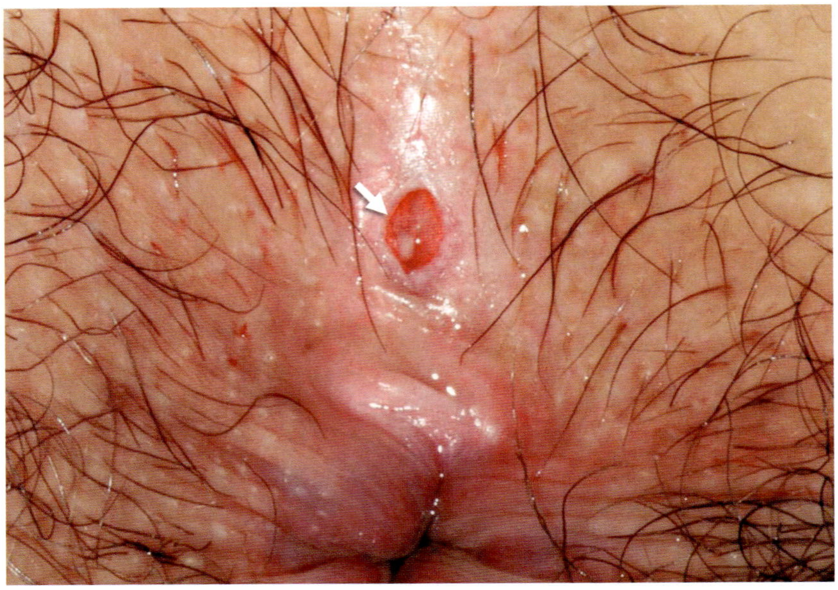

Figure 538 - Perineal fistula (arrow) in Crohn's disease.

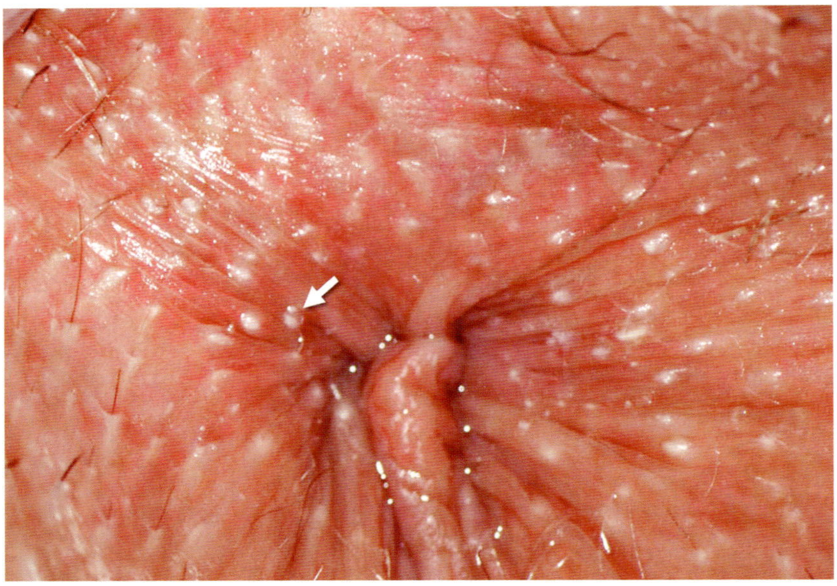

Figure 539 - Sebaceous cysts (arrow) may mimic HPV micropapillary lesions.

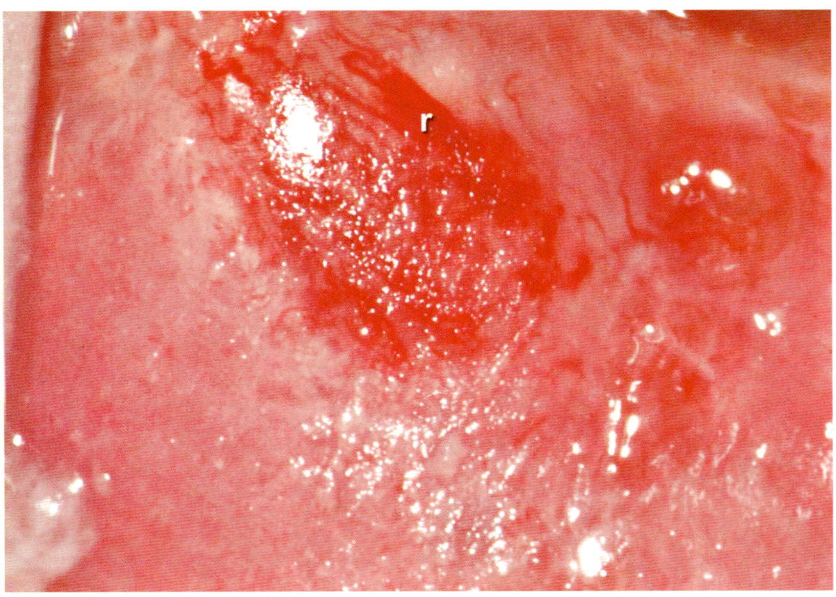

Figure 540 - Keratotic granules are scattered over an inflammatory red area (r).

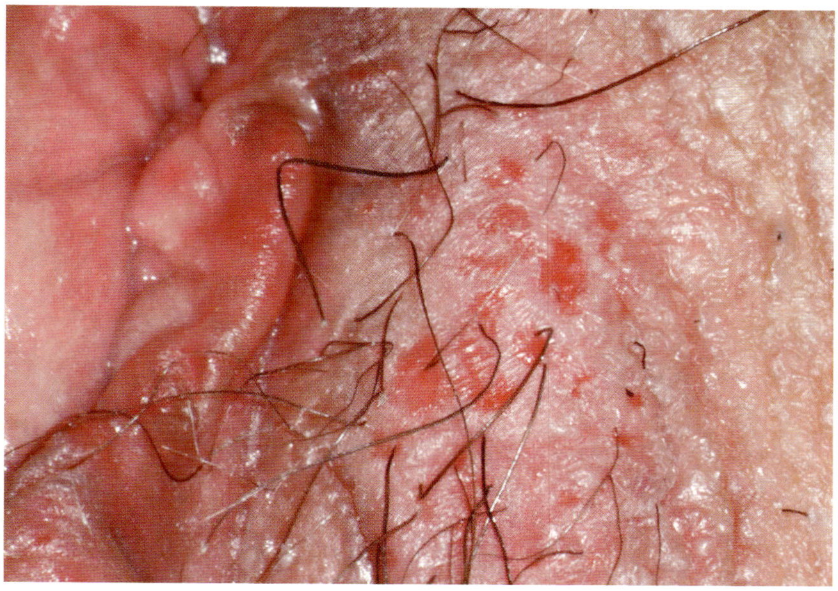

Figure 541 - Vulvar psoriasis.

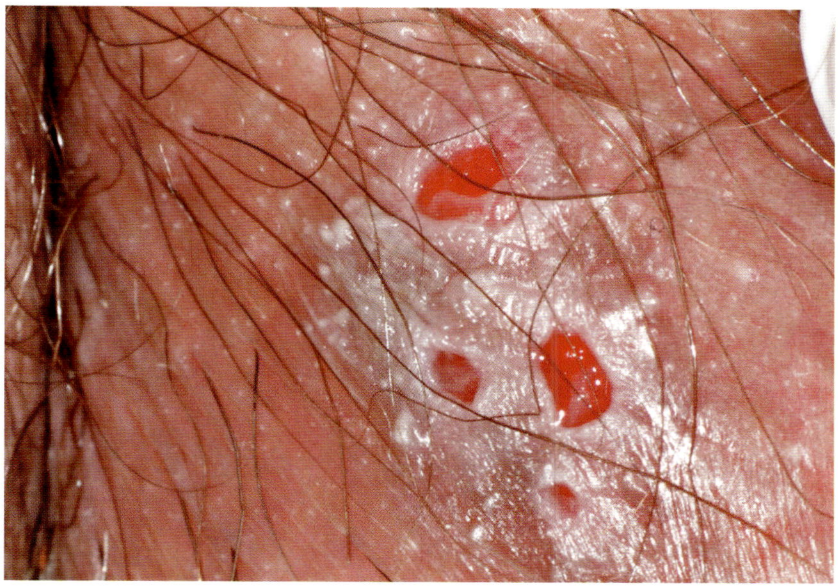

Figure 542 - Lichen sclerosus exhibits scattered erosions in a plaque of sclerosis and hyperkeratosis.

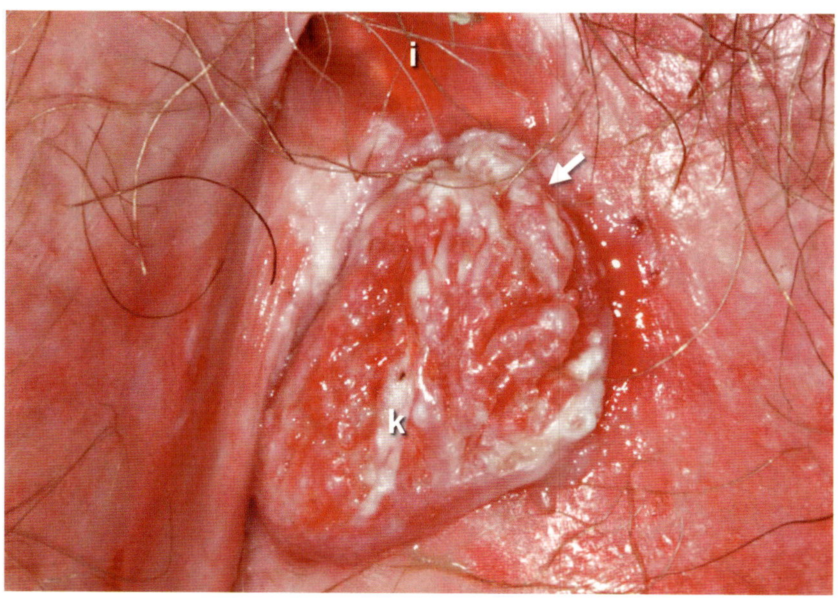

Figure 543 - An elevated red lump (arrow), covered with keratosis (k) involves the lower portion of vulva. Excision biopsy and resultant pathology demonstrated squamous cell carcinoma. Severe vulvar atrophy is responsible for intraoital constriction (i).

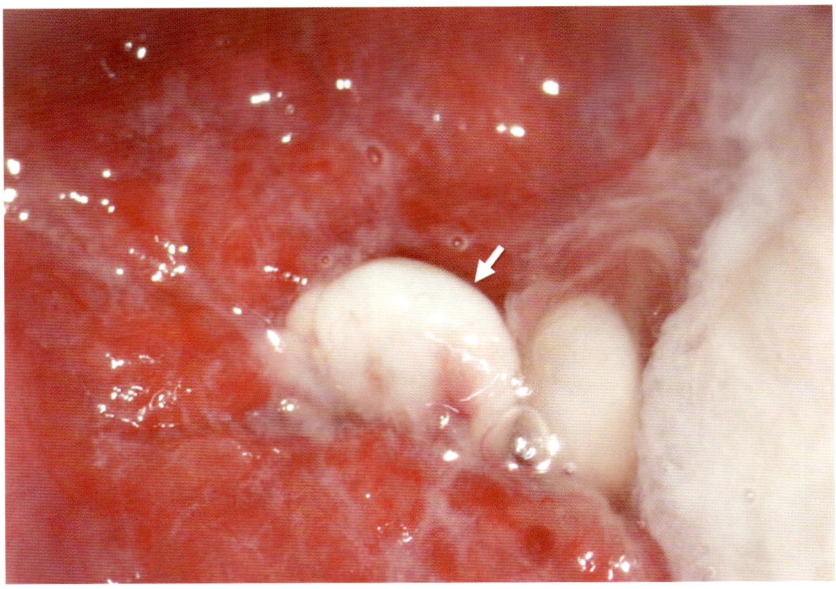

Figure 544 - Endocervical dense acetowhite lesion with snow-white appearance (arrow). Histology disclosed adenocarcinoma.

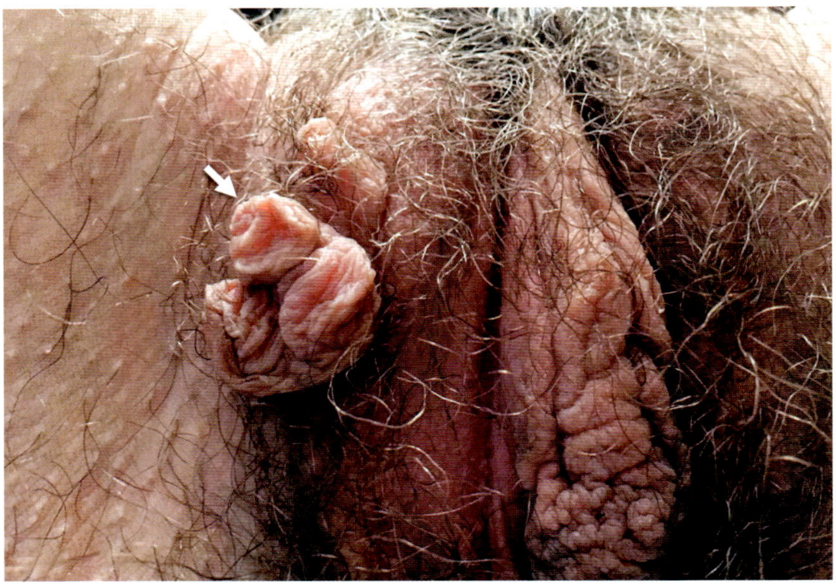

Figure 545 - Nevus lipomatosus cutaneous superficialis (arrow) is a rare idiopathic abnormality characterized by ectopic adipose tissue in the dermis.

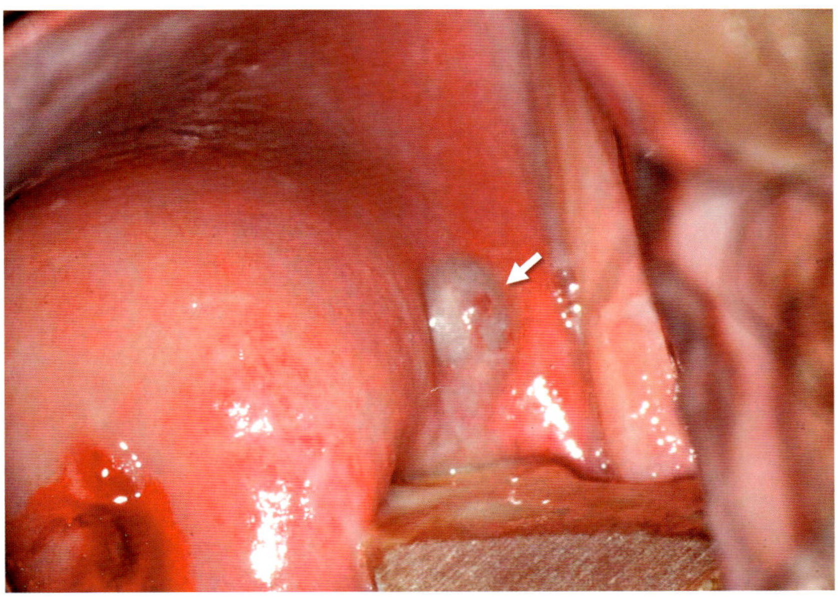

Figure 546 - The position of the arrowed glandular cyst in the vaginal lateral fornix suggests the outcome of a congenital metaplasia.

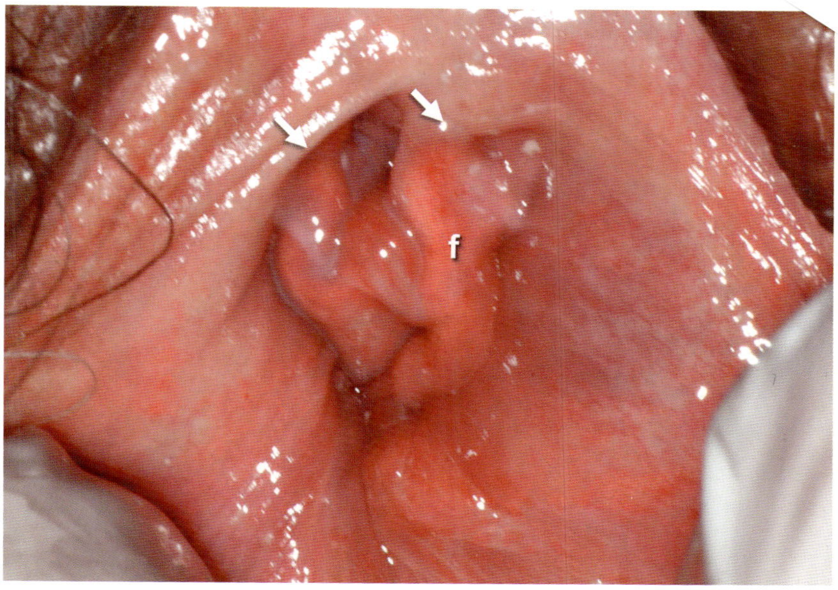

Figure 547 - Hypertrophic hymenal folds (f) are anchored to the upper contour of the vaginal introitus (arrows).

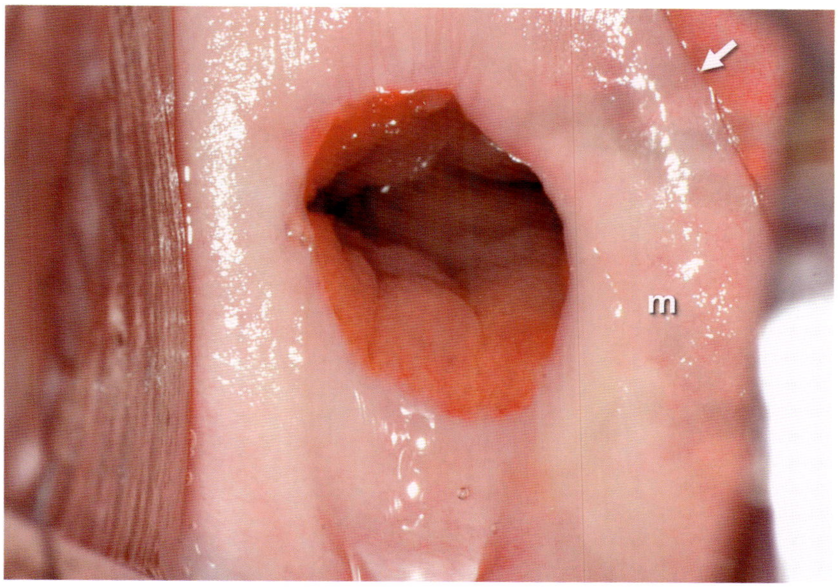

Figure 548 - Mature metaplastic epithelium (m), following diathermy, appears pale and raised (arrow).

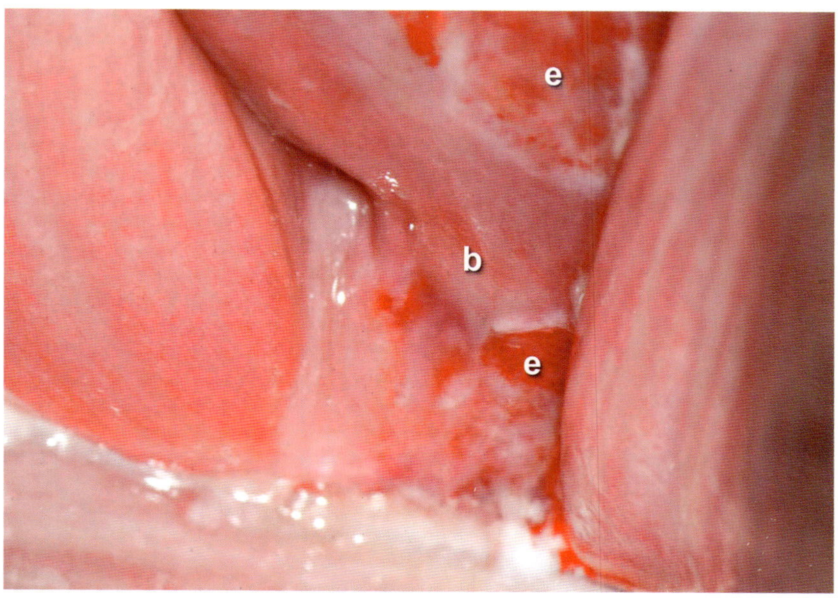

Figure 549 - A bridge of scar tissue (b) fixes the cervix to the posterior vaginal wall. The application of the speculum causes epithelial erosions (e).